New Advances in Insulin—100 Years Since Its Discovery

New Advances in Insulin—100 Years Since Its Discovery

Guest Editor

Tomislav Bulum

MDPI

Basel • Beijing • Wuhan • Barcelona • Belgrade • Novi Sad • Cluj • Manchester

Guest Editor
Tomislav Bulum
Medical Faculty
University of Zagreb
Zagreb
Croatia

Editorial Office
MDPI AG
Grosspeteranlage 5
4052 Basel, Switzerland

This is a reprint of the Special Issue, published open access by the journal *Biomedicines* (ISSN 2227-9059), freely accessible at: https://www.mdpi.com/journal/biomedicines/special_issues/E600W6QG3M.

For citation purposes, cite each article independently as indicated on the article page online and as indicated below:

Lastname, A.A.; Lastname, B.B. Article Title. *Journal Name* **Year**, *Volume Number*, Page Range.

ISBN 978-3-7258-7308-1 (Hbk)
ISBN 978-3-7258-7309-8 (PDF)
https://doi.org/10.3390/books978-3-7258-7309-8

Contents

About the Editor

Tomislav Bulum

Tomislav Bulum is employed at the Vuk Vrhovac University Clinic for Diabetes, Endocrinology, and Metabolic Diseases, University Hospital Merkur, Croatia's Referral Center for Diabetes, where he currently serves as a Specialist in Internal Medicine and a Subspecialist in Endocrinology and Diabetology. He received his PhD in 2010 from the Faculty of Science, University of Zagreb. Since 2016, he has been employed at the Medical School, University of Zagreb, where he currently holds the positions of Associate Professor and Scientific Adviser. He lectures in undergraduate courses as well as postgraduate specialist and PhD studies in biomedicine and health sciences at the Medical School, University of Zagreb. He has participated in multiple scientific and clinical projects in the field of type 1 and type 2 diabetes, with a particular focus on chronic diabetic complications.

He has authored over 100 scientific papers published in Web of Science, Scopus, and Index Medicus-indexed journals, as well as over 100 scientific and professional abstracts, with his work cited over 1000 times. He has served as a Guest Editor for over 10 Special Issues in first-quartile (Q1) journals, including *Biomedicines*, *Journal of Clinical Medicine*, *International Journal of Molecular Sciences*, *Diagnostics*, *Frontiers in Endocrinology*, and *Biology*. In 2023, he received the annual award from the Croatian Medical Chamber for scientific advancement in medicine and professional excellence. He is a member of the Croatian Academy of Medical Sciences.

biomedicines

MDPI

Editorial

Special Issue "New Advances in Insulin—100 Years Since Its Discovery"

Tomislav Bulum [1,2]

[1] Department of Diabetes and Endocrinology, Vuk Vrhovac University Clinic for Diabetes, Endocrinology and Metabolic Diseases, Merkur University Hospital, Dugi dol 4a, 10000 Zagreb, Croatia; tomobulum@gmail.com; Tel.: +385-12353887; Fax: +385-12331515

[2] School of Medicine, University of Zagreb, Šalata 3, 10000 Zagreb, Croatia

The discovery of insulin in 1921 represented a milestone in the treatment of diabetes. In 1923, the Nobel Prize for Medicine was awarded for its discovery, and it is considered one of the most valuable scientific events of the 20th century, affecting millions of people worldwide [1–3]. Before the discovery of insulin, children diagnosed with type 1 diabetes typically survived for less than a year after diagnosis, and those with type 2 diabetes also faced significantly reduced life expectancy. At that time, treatment options were extremely limited, and patients were often placed on strict diets with minimal carbohydrate intake in an attempt to control their symptoms. While this approach could slightly prolong patients' lives, it was not a cure and, in some cases, it led to death by starvation due to severe caloric restriction.

Since insulin discovery, thousands of lives have been saved, and the life expectancy of people with diabetes has been significantly extended. Since its discovery, insulin has been continuously improved through pharmacological development and optimized for therapeutic purposes, including the development of intermediate- and long-acting insulins, the production of human insulin, and finally, the development of insulin analogs with improved properties using recombinant-DNA technology [4].

Despite over a century of using insulin as a standard treatment for type 1 diabetes—with continuing advances in diabetes research and technology, continuous glucose monitoring and insulin administration via insulin pumps—we are far from being able to achieve a real cure for type 1 diabetes. Moreover, in the last 15 years, the number of people diagnosed with type 1 diabetes has increased by 45% [5,6]. Despite the rapid development of a wide range of new drugs for the treatment of diabetes, particularly in the context of protection from cardiorenovascular diseases, insulin remains one of the most potent therapeutic options for patients with type 2 diabetes, and the only treatment for those with type 1 diabetes [7]. In addition, despite increasing awareness of diabetes and its devastating complications, it is one of the leading causes of death and disability worldwide, irrespective of gender, age, and country, and health expenditures associated with diabetes and its chronic complications will reach more than USD 1054 billion by 2045 [8].

Although recent trends show a decline in complications among patients with type 1 diabetes—largely due to improved management practices and advancements in care technologies such as continuous glucose monitoring and modern insulin delivery systems—the risk of microvascular and macrovascular complications remains high [9,10]. In this context, this Special Issue aims to highlight the latest research and advances related to insulin and its actions in a broad sense, featuring six original research articles, four review articles, and one systematic review.

The first research article investigated potential factors associated with post-bariatric hypoglycemia. It is well known that post-bariatric hypoglycemia is a challenging condition affecting the quality of life of patients after bariatric surgery [11]. In this study, risk of post-bariatric postprandial hypoglycemia was observed over 12 months in a cohort of 24 patients with type 2 diabetes mellitus and a body mass index of $\geq$40 kg/m^2 who had undergone laparoscopic Roux-en-Y gastric bypass. All patients filled in a questionnaire based on the Edinburgh hypoglycemia scale. The results of the study suggest that pre-existing β-cell hyperfunction, which persists postoperatively after weight loss, and consequent postprandial insulin values at 30 min and 6 months seem to be strong predictors for post-bariatric hypoglycemia, while GLP-1 and glucagon values were not significantly associated with post-bariatric hypoglycemia.

The second research article was a real-world, retrospective study of patients with type 1 diabetes using multiple daily insulin injections. The study aimed to assess overnight glucose levels based on insulin type and timing. Nocturnal hypoglycemia is frequent, and episodes are often prolonged for several hours, particularly in those who undertake physical activity during the day [12]. In this study, continuous glucose monitoring and insulin injection data were collected for ten hours after dinner using the Insulclock® connected cap. Higher glucose was observed in subjects with delayed injections, while those using ultrarapid insulin had fewer hypoglycemic events. Those on glargine U300 had a higher time in range than those on degludec, while use of a correction injection was associated with a higher number of hypoglycemic events. The results of the study suggest that the time of rapid insulin injection before dinner, insulin type, and use of correction injections affect nocturnal glucose profiles in patients with type 1 diabetes.

The third research article was a pilot study that investigated the relationship between the proteomics profiles of serum exosomes from normal individuals and those with obesity and insulin resistance. The researchers identified 23 upregulated and 46 downregulated proteins between normal individuals and those with obesity and insulin resistance. Those affecting insulin resistance, β-cell activation, and inflammation were upregulated in subjects with obesity and insulin resistance compared to lean/overweight insulin-sensitive subjects. The researchers concluded that in subjects with obesity and insulin resistance, serum exosomal proteins can be used as biomarkers to identify the future risk of diabetes and as a therapeutic target to prevent or slow down the progression of diabetes.

The fourth research article explores the effect of insulin and metformin on the mortality of patients with type 2 diabetes with symptomatic COVID-19 infection. Previous observational analyses have shown that prevalent metformin use is associated with favorable outcomes after COVID-19 infection in adults with type 2 diabetes [13]. On the other hand, insulin treatment is associated with increased mortality in patients with COVID-19 and type 2 diabetes [14]. In this study, the association of death with insulin and metformin therapy was weak and could not be included in the multivariate model. However, the interaction of both drugs with other factors, including remdesivir and low-molecular-weight heparin (metformin), age, and C-reactive protein (insulin), modulated the odds of death. The role of metformin and insulin in the mortality of patients with type 2 diabetes and symptomatic COVID-19 may vary depending on a more personalized risk assessment model that includes and explores their interactions with various patient characteristics. In contrast, most other studies examining metformin and insulin in the context of COVID-19-related mortality lack such an exploration of interaction effects.

The fifth research article investigated the risk factors for lower transcutaneous oxygen pressure as a measure of microvascular circulation in the feet of patients with type 2 diabetes. Transcutaneous oxygen pressure is an excellent prognostic tool for wound healing in the population of diabetic patients with foot problems [15]. This study included 119 patients with type 2 diabetes. Those with lower transcutaneous oxygen pressure (<40 mmHg), indicating lower tissue oxygenation and a risk of delayed wound healing, were younger; had higher systolic blood pressure, glycated hemoglobin, fasting plasma glucose, and total and LDL cholesterol; and smoked more frequently than those with normal transcutaneous oxygen pressure. However, in association with other risk factors, smoking was the main predictor for lower transcutaneous oxygen pressure in patients with type 2 diabetes. Additional efforts are needed in everyday clinical practice to actively encourage patients with type 2 diabetes and peripheral arterial disease to quit smoking.

The sixth research article examined the relationship between hyperglycemia and prognostic value in patients with COVID-19 infection admitted to a hospital in Lithuania. Admission hyperglycemia is a predictor of mortality in patients hospitalized with COVID-19, even in patients without a previous history of diabetes, and hyperglycemia is also associated with increased mortality in critically ill patients with COVID-19 [16,17]. This study aimed to evaluate the association between hyperglycemia at admission with the need for invasive mechanical ventilation and in-hospital mortality in patients without diabetes who were hospitalized for COVID-19 infection. Over 10% of hospitalized patients had intermittent hyperglycemia at admission (blood glucose levels $\geq$ 7.8 mmol/L and <11.1 mmol/L), and those patients had a hazard ratio of 3 for 30-day in-hospital mortality compared to those with normoglycemia at admission.

The first narrative review comprises data from preclinical animal studies, longitudinal cohort studies, cross-sectional studies, machine learning analyses, and randomized controlled trials. It examines the role of insulin in maintaining health and preventing disease. This review proposes an expanded view of insulin as a metabolic–socio-psychological substance within the mitochondrial information processing framework, suggesting its roles beyond metabolism, particularly in cooperating with mitochondria to process psychosocial factors into the biological fabric, and providing new insights into the interplay between socio-psychological factors and biological systems in chronic diseases, such as type 2 diabetes.

The second review examines the potential impact of insulin, metformin, and glucagon-like peptide-1-based therapies on the progression of osteoarthritis in patients with diabetes. Evidence suggests that diabetes and osteoarthritis coexist within the same population, and that diabetes is associated with a greater degree of osteoarthritic pain [18]. The results of this review indicate that insulin, beyond its role in glycemic control, may potentially influence joint health by modulating inflammatory pathways relevant to osteoarthritis. Metformin also shows promise in mitigating osteoarthritis via its anti-inflammatory properties and reducing inflammatory markers. Glucagon-like peptide-1-based therapies also exhibit anti-inflammatory effects that may suppress cytokine-mediated joint inflammation and support cartilage repair mechanisms, with beneficial effects on osteoarthritis. Targeting common underlying mechanisms, insulin, metformin, and glucagon-like peptide-1-based therapies have therapeutic potential in osteoarthritis.

The third review focuses on the role of basal weekly insulin in clinical practice, and its use in patients with type 1 and 2 diabetes, by examining its safety, efficacy, and manageability, and therapeutic compliance. Several new weekly insulins have been developed, and they have demonstrated a significant decrease in blood glucose in pre-clinical studies. Therapy with basal weekly long-acting insulin in patients with type 1 and type 2 diabetes shows similar and better glycemic efficacy than daily basal insulin due to its association with reduced hypoglycemia, a reduction in the number of injections, and its proven effectiveness. Icodec insulin would likely be the most effective primary basal weekly insulin, as supported by the results of the ONWARDS clinical program, due to its tolerability, safety in terms of hypoglycemia, and increased patient compliance [19].

The fourth review summarized the last 100 years of insulin research, from its discovery to the insulins of the future. The discovery of insulin had a profound impact not only within the field of diabetes but also across medicine as a whole, emphasizing the importance of collaboration between clinicians, researchers, and pharmaceutical companies committed to improving the lives of people with diabetes. Notably, decision of the original discover not to commercialize or profit from their discovery enabled rapid and widespread progress in the early years. This stands in contrast with more recent developers who have patented new insulin formulations, potentially limiting their broader accessibility. Although a century has passed since the discovery of insulin and significant progress has been made in diabetes research, a true cure for type 1 diabetes—one that prevents the autoimmune destruction of pancreatic beta cells—remains elusive. Nevertheless, ongoing advancements continue to improve the quality of life for individuals living with the disease year after year.

The final review is a systematic review that explores the efficacy and safety of Icodec compared to once-daily insulin analogs (Degludec U100, Glargine U100, Glargine U300, and Detemir) in type 1 and type 2 diabetes. The review included 4347 patients with type 1 and type 2 diabetes with glycated hemoglobin over 7%. Those treated with Icodec had a greater probability of achieving glycated hemoglobin A1c < 7% without severe hypoglycemic events, but with slight and statistically significant weight gain. No difference in fasting glucose levels, time in range, and time above range was observed. Icodec demonstrated slightly greater efficacy compared to its competitors when used in a basal-only regimen rather than in a basal-bolus approach. While weight gain and the risk of hypoglycemia were relatively low, they remain clinically relevant and should not be overlooked.

In conclusion, this Special Issue offers a comprehensive overview of insulin secretion and action, as well as the development and action of insulin analogs and their impact on glycemic control and the chronic complications of diabetes. Advances in diabetes treatment have been numerous in the 100 years since the discovery of insulin, resulting in extraordinary progress in the development of novel molecules to improve glucose control, simplify insulin regimens, and enhance quality of life. However, insulin remains the only replacement therapy for type 1 diabetes, and the data presented here may encourage and support further research in this important field.

Conflicts of Interest: The author declares no conflicts of interest.

List of Contributions:

1. Kehagias, D.; Lampropoulos, C.; Vamvakas, S.-S.; Kehagia, E.; Georgopoulos, N.; Kehagias, I. Post-Bariatric Hypoglycemia in Individuals with Obesity and Type 2 Diabetes after Laparoscopic Roux-en-Y Gastric Bypass: A Prospective Cohort Study. *Biomedicines* **2024**, *12*, 1671. https://doi.org/10.3390/biomedicines12081671.
2. Gómez-Peralta, F.; Valledor, X.; Abreu, C.; Fernández-Rubio, E.; Cotovad, L.; Pujante, P.; Azriel, S.; Pérez-González, J.; Vallejo, A.; Ruiz-Valdepeñas, L.; et al. Nocturnal Glucose Profile According to Timing of Dinner Rapid Insulin and Basal and Rapid Insulin Type: An Insulclock® Connected Insulin Cap-Based Real-World Study. *Biomedicines* **2024**, *12*, 1600. https://doi.org/10.3390/biomedicines12071600.
3. Saraswathi, V.; Ai, W.; Kumar, V.; Sharma, K.; Gopal, T.; Kumar, N.; Malhi, H.; Sehrawat, T.; Desouza, C.V. A Pilot Study on the Proteomics Profile of Serum Exosome-Enriched Extracellular Vesicles from Normal versus Individuals with Obesity-Related Insulin Resistance. *Biomedicines* **2024**, *12*, 799. https://doi.org/10.3390/biomedicines12040799.
4. Lewandowski, Ł.; Bronowicka-Szydełko, A.; Rabczyński, M.; Bednarska-Chabowska, D.; Adamiec-Mroczek, J.; Doroszko, A.; Trocha, M.; Kujawa, K.; Matera-Witkiewicz, A.; Kuźnik, E.; et al. Insulin and Metformin Administration: Unravelling the Multifaceted Association with Mortality across Various Clinical Settings Considering Type 2 Diabetes Mellitus and COVID-19. *Biomedicines* **2024**, *12*, 605. https://doi.org/10.3390/biomedicines12030605.

5. Bulum, T.; Brkljačić, N.; Tičinović Ivančić, A.; Čavlović, M.; Prkačin, I.; Tomić, M. In Association with Other Risk Factors, Smoking Is the Main Predictor for Lower Transcutaneous Oxygen Pressure in Type 2 Diabetes. *Biomedicines* **2024**, *12*, 381. https://doi.org/10.3390/biomedicines12020381.
6. Zabuliene, L.; Kubiliute, I.; Urbonas, M.; Jancoriene, L.; Urboniene, J.; Ilias, I. Hyperglycaemia and Its Prognostic Value in Patients with COVID-19 Admitted to the Hospital in Lithuania. *Biomedicines* **2024**, *12*, 55. https://doi.org/10.3390/biomedicines12010055.
7. Wevers, A.; San Roman-Mata, S.; Navarro-Ledesma, S.; Pruimboom, L. The Role of Insulin Within the Socio-Psycho-Biological Framework in Type 2 Diabetes—A Perspective from Psychoneuroimmunology. *Biomedicines* **2024**, *12*, 2539. https://doi.org/10.3390/biomedicines12112539.
8. Halabitska, I.; Babinets, L.; Oksenych, V.; Kamyshnyi, O. Diabetes and Osteoarthritis: Exploring the Interactions and Therapeutic Implications of Insulin, Metformin, and GLP-1-Based Interventions. *Biomedicines* **2024**, *12*, 1630. https://doi.org/10.3390/biomedicines12081630.
9. Argano, C.; Priola, L.; Manno, F.; Corrao, S. What Is the Role of Basal Weekly Insulin in Clinical Practice? The State of the Art. *Biomedicines* **2024**, *12*, 900. https://doi.org/10.3390/biomedicines12040900.
10. Lisco, G.; De Tullio, A.; De Geronimo, V.; Giagulli, V.A.; Guastamacchia, E.; Piazzolla, G.; Disoteo, O.E.; Triggiani, V. Once-Weekly Insulin Icodec in Diabetes Mellitus: A Systematic Review and Meta-Analysis of Randomized Clinical Trials (ONWARDS Clinical Program). *Biomedicines* **2024**, *12*, 1852. https://doi.org/10.3390/biomedicines12081852.

References

1. Tan, S.Y.; Merchant, J. Frederick Banting (1891–1941): Discoverer of insulin. *Singap. Med. J.* **2017**, *58*, 2–3. [CrossRef]
2. Hegele, R.A.; Maltman, G.M. Insulin's centenary: The birth of an idea. *Lancet Diabetes Endocrinol.* **2020**, *8*, 971–977. [CrossRef] [PubMed]
3. Marshall, S.M. Celebrating 100 years of insulin. *Diabetologia* **2021**, *64*, 944–946. [CrossRef] [PubMed]
4. Lambert, C.; Delgado, E. 100 years since the discovery of insulin, from its discovery to the insulins of the future. *Biomedicines* **2024**, *12*, 533. [CrossRef] [PubMed]
5. Ogrotis, I.; Koufakis, T.; Kotsa, K. Changes in the global epidemiology of type 1 diabetes in an evolving landscape of environmental factors: Causes, challenges, and opportunities. *Medicina* **2023**, *59*, 668. [CrossRef] [PubMed]
6. GBD 2021 Diabetes Collaborators. Global, regional, and national burden of diabetes from 1990 to 2021, with projections of prevalence to 2050: A systematic analysis for the global burden of disease study 2021. *Lancet* **2023**, *402*, 203–234. [CrossRef] [PubMed]
7. Sebastian, S.A.; Padda, I.; Johal, G. Cardiovascular-kidney-metabolic (CKM) syndrome: A state-of-the-art review. *Curr. Probl. Cardiol.* **2024**, *49*, 102344. [CrossRef] [PubMed]
8. Sun, H.; Saeedi, P.; Karuranga, S.; Pinkepank, M.; Ogurtsova, K.; Duncan, B.B.; Stein, C.; Basit, A.; Chan, J.C.N.; Mbanya, J.C.; et al. IDF diabetes atlas: Global, regional and country-level diabetes prevalence estimates for 2021 and projections for 2045. *Diabetes Res. Clin. Pract.* **2022**, *183*, 109119. [CrossRef] [PubMed]
9. Longendyke, R.; Grundman, J.B.; Majidi, S. Acute and chronic adverse outcomes of type 1 diabetes. *Endocrinol. Metab. Clin. N. Am.* **2024**, *53*, 123–133. [CrossRef] [PubMed]
10. Poulsen, C.G.; Jesse, K.; Carstensen, B.; Frimodt-Møller, M.; Hansen, T.W.; Persson, F.; Vistisen, D.; Rossing, P. Prognosis for type 1 diabetes with diabetic nephropathy between 2000 and 2020—Changes in kidney function decline over time and development of cardiovascular disease, kidney failure, and mortality. *Kidney Int. Rep.* **2024**, *9*, 3403–3413. [CrossRef] [PubMed]
11. Lüscher, A.; Vionnet, N.; Pasquier, J.; Chartoumpekis, D.; Mantziari, S.; Wojtsusizyn, A.; Favre, L. Predictors and weight impact of postbariatric hypoglycemia after Roux-en-Y gastric bypass surgery: A prospective observational cohort study. *Surg. Obes. Relat. Dis.* **2024**, *20*, 1187–1195. [CrossRef] [PubMed]
12. Leutheuser, H.; Bartholet, M.; Marx, A.; Pfister, M.; Burckhardt, M.A.; Bachmann, S.; Vogt, J.E. Predicting risk for nocturnal hypoglycemia after physical activity in children with type 1 diabetes. *Front. Med.* **2024**, *11*, 1439218. [CrossRef] [PubMed]
13. Johnson, S.G.; Abedian, S.; Stürmer, T.; Huling, J.D.; Lewis, V.C.; Buse, J.B.; Brosnahan, S.B.; Mudumbi, P.C.; Erlandson, K.M.; McComsey, G.A.; et al. Prevalent metformin use in adults with diabetes and the incidence of long COVID: An EHR-based cohort study from the RECOVER program. *Diabetes Care* **2024**, *47*, 1930–1940. [CrossRef] [PubMed]
14. Yu, B.; Li, C.; Sun, Y.; Wang, D.W. Insulin treatment is associated with increased mortality in patients with COVID-19 and type 2 diabetes. *Cell Metab.* **2020**, *33*, 65–77.e2. [CrossRef] [PubMed]

15. Pinelo, A.; Loureiro, L.; Martins, J.; Sommerset, J.; Carvalho, R.; Machado, R. Correlation between pedal acceleration time and transcutaneous oxygen pressures—A prognostic tool for wound healing in the diabetic foot population. *Ann. Vasc. Surg.* **2024**, *106*, 400–407. [CrossRef] [PubMed]
16. Mazori, A.Y.; Bass, I.R.; Chan, L.; Mathews, K.S.; Altman, D.R.; Saha, A.; Soh, H.; Wen, H.H.; Bose, S.; Leven, E.; et al. Hyperglycemia is associated with increased mortality in critically ill patients with COVID-19. *Endocr. Pract.* **2021**, *27*, 95–100. [CrossRef] [PubMed]
17. Carrasco-Sánchez, F.J.; López-Carmona, M.D.; Martínez-Marcos, F.J.; Pérez-Belmonte, L.M.; Hidalgo-Jiménez, A.; Buonaiuto, V.; Suárez Fernández, C.; Freire Castro, S.J.; Luordo, D.; Pesqueira Fontan, P.M.; et al. Admission hyperglycaemia as a predictor of mortality in patients hospitalized with COVID-19 regardless of diabetes status: Data from the spanish SEMI-COVID-19 registry. *Ann. Med.* **2021**, *53*, 103–116. [CrossRef] [PubMed]
18. Alenazi, A.M.; Alhowimel, A.S.; Alshehri, M.M.; Alqahtani, B.A.; Alhwoaimel, N.A.; Segal, N.A.; Kluding, P.M. Osteoarthritis and diabetes: Where are we and where should we go? *Diagnostics* **2023**, *13*, 1386. [CrossRef] [PubMed]
19. Aktas, G.; Duman, T.T. Current usage of long-acting insulin analogs in patients with type 2 diabetes mellitus. *Expert Rev. Endocrinol. Metab.* **2024**, *19*, 155–161. [CrossRef] [PubMed]

biomedicines

MDPI

Article

Post-Bariatric Hypoglycemia in Individuals with Obesity and Type 2 Diabetes after Laparoscopic Roux-en-Y Gastric Bypass: A Prospective Cohort Study

Dimitrios Kehagias [1], Charalampos Lampropoulos [2], Sotirios-Spyridon Vamvakas [3], Eirini Kehagia [1], Neoklis Georgopoulos [1] and Ioannis Kehagias [1,*]

1 Department of Medicine, University of Patras, 26504 Patras, Greece; dimikech@gmail.com (D.K.); up1084196@ac.upatras.gr (E.K.); neoklisgeorgo@gmail.com (N.G.)
2 Intensive Care Unit, Saint Andrew's General Hospital, 26504 Patras, Greece; x_lamp@hotmail.com
3 Department of Nutritional Science & Dietetics, School of Health Sciences, University of Peloponnese, 24100 Kalamata, Greece; sotvam74@gmail.com
* Correspondence: ikehag@upatras.gr

Abstract: Post-bariatric hypoglycemia (PBH) is an increasingly recognized complication after metabolic bariatric surgery (MBS). The aim of this study is to investigate potential factors associated with PBH. A cohort of 24 patients with type 2 diabetes mellitus (T2DM) and body mass index (BMI) $\geq$40 kg/m^2 who underwent laparoscopic Roux-en-Y gastric bypass (LRYGBP) was retrospectively investigated for PBH at 12 months. PBH was defined as postprandial glucose at 120 min below 60 mg/dL. Questionnaires based on the Edinburgh hypoglycemia scale were filled out by the participants. Glycemic parameters and gastrointestinal (GI) hormones were also investigated. Based on the questionnaires, five patients presented more than four symptoms that were highly indicative of PBH at 12 months. According to glucose values at 120 min, one patient experienced PBH at 6 months and four patients experienced it at 12 months. Postprandial insulin values at 30 min and 6 months seem to be a strong predictor for PBH ($p < 0.001$). GLP-1 and glucagon values were not significantly associated with PBH. PBH can affect patients with T2DM after MBS, reaching the edge of hypoglycemia. Postprandial insulin levels at 30 min and 6 months might predict the occurrence of PBH at 12 months, but this requires further validation with a larger sample size.

Keywords: bariatric surgery; post-bariatric hypoglycemia; late dumping; diabetes mellitus, type 2; Roux-en-Y gastric bypass

1. Introduction

Post-bariatric hypoglycemia (PBH) is defined as postprandial hyper-insulinemic hypoglycemia, which occurs 2–4 h after meal consumption, presenting with Whipple's triad criteria [1]. Since the implementation of metabolic bariatric surgery (MBS) unveiled the underlying mechanisms of hypoglycemia, the term PBH superseded the age-old term of late dumping syndrome [2]. The true prevalence of PBH is still unknown, fluctuating in the literature from 0.1 to 25%, due to the variation in diagnostic methods and hypoglycemia unawareness, which challenges the interpretation of symptoms. PBH is mainly associated with laparoscopic Roux-en-Y gastric bypass (LRYGBP), but it is also reported after sleeve gastrectomy (SG) and one-anastomosis gastric bypass (OAGB) [3]. With the advent of PBH, clinicians have been grappling with providing a common language, and, eventually, the American Society of Metabolic and Bariatric Surgery in 2017 and the European Society of Endocrinology in 2024 reached a consensus and suggested guidelines for the management of this complication. Hence, there are still severe drawbacks, such as the exact diagnostic criteria, the cut-off values for hypoglycemia, the type of provocative test, and the lack of diagnostic tools for evaluating hypoglycemia symptoms, leading to a non-standardized approach for PBH [4–6].

Metabolic bariatric surgery (MBS) is currently acknowledged as the most efficient method for achieving not only sustainable weight loss but also optimal glycemic control, radically changing the landscape and establishing the contemporary term of metabolic surgery [7]. The intriguing implicated pathophysiological alterations, after the changes in the gastrointestinal tract, have paved the way towards relentless research in order to elucidate the underlying mechanisms, which might serve as potential pharmaceutical targets. The gastric fundus, foregut–hindgut theory, gut microbiota, and bile acids are only some of these recognized mechanisms, while microRNAs have appeared recently as another potential mechanism [4,8,9]. Notwithstanding research endeavors that shed light on the realm of MBS, its increased prevalence has led clinicians to encounter more not-well-recognized complications, preserving the vicious cycle of obscurity and uncertainty.

Delving deeper into the pathophysiology of PBH, the exact mechanisms are still ambiguous, while it is an even more intriguing fact that patients with obesity and type 2 diabetes mellitus (T2DM) might develop postoperative hypoglycemia, reaching the opposite edge of hyperglycemia [10]. In the past, nesidioblastosis and the increased calculated β-cell area were considered the main culprits of PBH; however, partial pancreatectomies did not resolve this condition, excluding this potential mechanism [11,12]. Currently, incretins appear to have a pivotal role through positive feedback in β-cells, resulting in insulin hypersecretion, while the disruption of other counter-regulatory mechanisms such as glucagon might also be implicated in PBH occurrence [13,14].

Although PBH might be considered a rare complication, it is probably underreported, and, undoubtedly, severe PBH can have detrimental effects on quality of life, impairing cognitive function and increasing mortality. Therefore, elucidating the underlying mechanisms and implementing a standardized approach that will provide a more accurate diagnosis are mandatory necessities that will serve as a backbone for the development of targeted pharmaceutical agents, thereby providing more efficient treatment and prediction [5]. Findings from a previous randomized trial among patients with obesity and T2DM who underwent LRYGBP with or without gastric fundus resection suggested that fundus resection is not implicated in glycemic control, which was the primary outcome of the study [8]. Among the studied population, especially one year postoperatively, profound PBH was observed in some patients 2 h after the oral glucose tolerance test (OGTT), and they manifested neuroglycopenic symptoms. The aim of this study is to investigate this cohort in terms of factors associated with PBH in patients with obesity and T2DM and suggest mechanisms that might be implicated in this increasingly recognized complication.

2. Materials and Methods

2.1. Study Design

This is an observational cohort study with prospectively collected samples and a retrospective interview of the patients, which was conducted in the bariatric unit of the University Hospital of Patras in Greece and included patients with obesity and T2DM. Initially, these patients were enrolled in a randomized clinical trial forming two intervention arms: LRYGBP and LRYGBP with fundus resection [8]. The trial was registered at clinicaltrials.gov (NCT05854875), and the results of this study have been previously published. The total included 24 patients who were retrospectively investigated for PBH at 6 and 12 months postoperative. These patients were selected from the registry of the metabolic and bariatric unit and they signed informed consents. All procedures performed were in accordance with the 1964 Helsinki Declaration, and this study was approved by the local research and ethics committee (No. 730/10.12.2019) [15]. This cohort study was performed following the strengthening of the criteria for reporting cohort, cross-sectional, and case–control studies in surgery (STROCSS 2021) [16]. The primary outcome was postprandial glucose levels at 120 min during OGTT 12 months postoperatively. The secondary outcomes included insulin, glucagon, GLP-1 levels, calculated β-cell area, and insulinogenic index. Finally, a potential correlation of the aforementioned parameters at 6 and 12 months, with PBH at 12 months, was also investigated.

2.2. Patient Population

The studied cohort included 24 patients aged between 18 and 60 years old, with a BMI $\geq$40 kg/m^2 and T2DM defined by the criteria of the American Diabetes Association (ADA) [17]. The patients underwent LRYGBP and LRYGBP with fundus resection, and they were evaluated preoperatively and at 6 and 12 months postoperatively. The duration of T2DM was determined to be less than 8 years, since longer durations are related to irreversible β-cell function impairment and poorer postoperative recovery. All participants were evaluated by different specialties, and behavioral and anthropometric parameters and metabolic profiles were assessed. The exclusion criteria were gestation, diabetes mellitus type I, alcohol or drug abuse, major depressive disorder, non-compliance with the medical personnel's instructions, and previous abdominal surgeries with altered gastrointestinal anatomy.

All operations were completed laparoscopically by the same surgeon in the surgical department of the tertiary referral hospital. Both procedures included the creation of a small gastric pouch of 30 mL capacity, a very long biliopancreatic limb of 200 cm, and an alimentary limb of 150 cm. Gastrojejunal anastomosis was created with a circular stapler of 25 mm diameter after the transoral placement of the anvil with assistance from the anesthesiologist. In the fundus resection group, the gastric body and fundus were mobilized by dividing the gastrocolic ligament and short gastric vessels until exposing the angle of His. A gastric fundus with dimensions of approximately ±5.5 cm (width) and ±10 cm (vertical length) was removed with the use of a linear stapler [8].

One year after the end of the randomized clinical trial, these patients were contacted and responded to a questionnaire in order to evaluate symptoms of PBH. The questionnaire was adapted from the Edinburgh hypoglycemia scale, which consists of 11 key symptoms associated with hypoglycemia, and they are segregated into three categories: autonomic, neuroglycopenic, and malaise. Specifically, these symptoms include sweating, palpitation, shaking, hunger, confusion, drowsiness, odd behavior, speech difficulty, incoordination, nausea, and headache. This model has been externally validated and is suggested as a standardized approach for evaluating hypoglycemia symptoms [18]. Patients were considered arbitrarily highly suspicious for PBH if they exhibited more than 4 symptoms of the Edinburgh scale. The imposed question was "Did you feel any of the aforementioned symptoms 1 to 3 h postprandially?" The onset of symptoms and the random self-measurement of glucose levels during these episodes were also questioned and evaluated. All patients were postoperatively instructed by expert dietitians to follow a diet enriched in protein with low carbohydrates. However, the exact type of meal consumed before the occurrence of these symptoms was not reported due to the retrospective nature of the questionnaire and the inability of patients to reliably determine this.

2.3. Laboratory Measurements

As described in the previous publication, blood samples were collected during a 75 gr OGTT at 0, 30, 60, and 120 min. This procedure was repeated preoperatively at 6 and 12 months. The measurement of insulin and GLP-1 levels was explicitly described previously, while these prospectively collected stored samples were also utilized for the measurement of glucagon. These samples were in ethylene-diamine-tetra-acetic acid (EDTA) vials, which contained 1.8 TIU (trypsin inhibitor units) of proteinase inhibitor, aprotinin (Trasylol). They were centrifuged at 4 °C for 20 min and at 1600 RCF (relative centrifuge force), and they were stored at −70 °C. Glucagon was measured with commercial ELISA kits (Invitrogen, ThermoFisher Scientific, catalog number EHGCG), and the minimum detectable dose was 2.5 pg/mL. The aforementioned gastrointestinal (GI) hormones were all measured during the OGTT at 0, 30, 60, and 120 min preoperatively at 6 and 12 months. Fasting c-peptide was calculated preoperatively at 6 and 12 months with commercial ELISA kits and used for estimating the "calculated β-cell area" index.

2.4. Definitions and Criteria

For defining hypoglycemia, a cut-off value of 60 mg/dL was selected. Based on the recommendations from the American Diabetes Association (ADA) and the European Association for the Study of Diabetes (EASD), a cut-off value of 54 mg/dL is suggested since glucose levels below this threshold are related to impaired cognitive function and neuroglycopenic and autonomic symptoms [19]. However, we selected a slightly higher cut-off value because patients with T2DM were investigated. Beta-cell function was assessed with the use of the insulinogenic index, which was calculated as the ratio of insulin change to glucose change from 0 to 30 min. The insulinogenic index mainly describes the first phase of insulin secretion, which is remarkably associated with β-cell function [20].

The postprandial values of glucose, insulin, glucagon, and GLP-1 were estimated with area under the curve (AUC) using the trapezoidal method. Supposing that GI hormones are implicated in PBH, we particularly evaluated the postprandial levels of insulin and GLP-1 at different time points during the OGTT. Specifically, based on the literature, an abrupt postprandial increase in insulin and GLP-1 is observed at 30 and 60 min postprandially. Therefore, the postprandial levels of insulin and GLP-1 at these time points were investigated for a potential correlation with PBH. Finally, the ratio of fasting c-peptide to fasting glucose (ng/mL × mg/dL) was utilized to estimate the calculated β-cell area. This index was validated by Meier et al., and it exhibited a significant linear correlation with the histological assessment of the β-cell area [21,22].

2.5. Statistical Analysis

For statistical analyses, the SPSS version 20.0 statistics software package (Statistical Package for the Social Sciences, SPSS Inc., Chicago, IL, USA) was utilized, while graphs were generated using GraphPad Prism version 5.0 (Graph-Pad Software, Inc., San Diego, CA, USA). For continuous parameters, the mean ± standard error (SE) was utilized. The non-parametric Kruskal–Wallis test was used for comparing parameters at different time points (baseline, 6 months, and 12 months). Statistical significance was set at p T2DM0.05 and was adjusted using the Bonferroni correction.

For the correlation of different parameters with PBH, a biserial correlation was applied, where PBH was the dichotomous variable (0 for glucose above 60 mg/dL and 1 for glucose below 60 mg/dL). For assessing predictors of PBH, a stepwise binary regression analysis was used, and the aforementioned binary variable was included for PBH. Finally, receiver operating characteristic (ROC) curves were generated to assess the reliability of predictive factors for PBH diagnosis at 12 months.

3. Results

3.1. Baseline and Follow-Up Characteristics

Eleven male and thirteen female patients were enrolled in the cohort study, with a mean age of 46.75 ± 10.98 years. Preoperatively, the mean weight and BMI were 153.15 ± 36.8 kg and 53.2 ± 10.6 kg/m^2, respectively. Weight loss was remarkable postoperatively, and at 12 months, there was a significant decrease in terms of weight and BMI: 89.43 ± 18.6 kg ($p < 0.05$) and 30.62 ± 4.81 kg/m^2 ($p < 0.05$), respectively. EWL% was significantly increased between 6 and 12 months from 54.55 ± 7.66 to 70.33 ± 12.4 ($p < 0.05$).

Regarding T2DM, the patients had a mean HbA1c of 7.94 ± 1.74 and c-peptide of 4.42 ± 1.89 ng/mL, with a mean preoperative duration of 3.77 ± 2.3 years. At 6 months, both HbA1c and c-peptide significantly decreased ($p < 0.05$) and, at 12 months, they remained fairly constant at 5.36 ± 0.55 and 2.65 ± 1.96, respectively. Based on glucose measurement during the OGTT, preoperatively, none of the patients presented PBH. Conversely, at 6 months, one patient (4%) experienced glucose levels below 60 mg/dL, and at

12 months, the number of these patients quadrupled, reaching 16.6% (Table 1). Regarding the preoperative diabetes treatment, only one patient was completely off anti-diabetic medications. The other twenty-three patients were on oral medications, while seven took insulin and four GLP-1 analogs. Postoperatively, 95% (23/24) showed complete diabetes remission at one year without taking any medication. Only one patient from the LRYGBP with fundus resection group experienced relapse and was re-introduced to oral medications at one year. Finally, PBH was not associated with the type of surgery since PBH occurred in patients from both groups.

Table 1. Baseline and follow-up characteristics of the patients.

Parameters	Baseline	6 Months		12 Months		
	Mean ± SD	Mean ± SD	*p* 0–6	Mean ± SD	*p* 0–12	*p* 6–12
Age (year)	46.75 ± 10.98					
Gender (M) (F)	(11) (13)					
Weight (kg)	153.15 ± 36.8	104.62 ± 23.66	**<0.05**	89.43 ± 18.6	**<0.05**	0.173
BMI (kg/m^2)	53.2 ± 10.6	36.03 ± 6.05	**<0.05**	30.62 ± 4.81	**<0.05**	**<0.05**
EWL %		54.55 ± 7.66		70.33 ± 12.4		**<0.05**
HbA1c (%)	7.94 ± 1.74	5.31 ± 0.53	**<0.05**	5.36 ± 0.55	**<0.05**	0.909
c-peptide (ng/mL)	4.42 ± 1.89	2.77 ± 0.88	**<0.05**	2.65 ± 1.96	**<0.05**	0.503
T2DM duration (year)	3.77 ± 2.3					
Anti-diabetic medications (insulin) (GLP1 analogs)	23 (7) (4)	0 (0) (0)		1 (0) (0)		
Patients with symptoms of PBH (%)	1 (4)	3 (12.5)		5 (20.8)		
Patients with Glu at 120 min < 60 mg/dL (%)	0 (0)	1 (4)		4 (16.6)		

Values are expressed as mean ± SD; M (male); F (female); EWL (excess weight loss); T2DM (type 2 diabetes mellitus); PBH (post-bariatric hypoglycemia); *p* 0–6 (between baseline and 6 months); *p* 0–12 (between baseline and 12 months); *p* 6–12 (between 6 and 12 months); $p < 0.05$ bold for significance.

3.2. Hypoglycemia Symptoms and Edinburgh Questionnaire

The questionnaires regarding PBH were answered retrospectively by all 24 patients enrolled in the initial randomized controlled study. Five patients presented more than four symptoms on the Edinburgh scale and were considered highly suspicious for PBH.

Overall, the most common symptoms were autonomic, specifically sweating, palpitation, and shaking comprising 25%, 33%, and 21%, respectively. Regarding neuroglycopenic symptoms, drowsiness was the most common at 12.5%, followed by confusion at 8%, while hunger, odd behavior, speech difficulty, and incoordination were equally presented at 4%. Finally, as far as malaise is concerned, nausea comprised 21% and headache comprised 4%. Sweating, palpitation, shaking, and nausea were present in all five patients, which are symptoms highly indicative of PBH (Table 2).

Regarding the time of the presentation, only one patient reported these symptoms preoperatively; three patients reported these symptoms at 6 months, and five patients reported them during evaluation (Table 1). None of the patients who participated in the questionnaire reported any syncope or a random measurement of glucose value below 60 mg/dL.

Table 2. Patients with hypoglycemia symptoms based on the questionnaires adjusted for the Edinburgh scale. High clinical suspicion for patients presenting above 4 symptoms.

Symptoms	Overall Patients (n = 24) n (%)	Patients with High Clinical Suspicion (n = 5) n (%)
Autonomic		
Sweating	6 (25)	5 (100)
Palpitation	8 (33)	5 (100)
Shaking	5 (21)	5 (100)
hunger	1 (4)	1 (20)
Neuroglycopenic		
Confusion	2 (8)	2 (40)
Drowsiness	3 (12.5)	3 (60)
Odd behavior	1 (4)	0 (0)
Speech difficulty	1 (4)	1 (20)
Incoordination	1 (4)	1 (20)
Malaise		
Nausea	5 (21)	5 (100)
headache	1 (4)	1 (20)

3.3. *Glycemic Parameters and Calculated β-Cell Area*

Glycemic control was achieved from the 6th month, with patients demonstrating a significant decrease in glucose and insulin fasting levels (Table 3; Figure 1). Specifically, from baseline to 12 months postoperatively, glucose fasting declined from 130.54 ± 51.15 to 88.13 ± 21.52 mg/dL ($p < 0.05$), while insulin fasting remarkably decreased from 23.91 ± 13.6 to 9.83 ± 13.36 μIU/mL ($p < 0.05$). Along with the glycemic improvement, β-cell function also witnessed an outstanding enhancement, with the insulinogenic index increasing from 0.5052 ± 0.44 at baseline to 0.9862 ± 1 at 6 months ($p < 0.05$) and 1.483 ± 1.63 at 12 months ($p < 0.05$). Considering that, at 30 and 60 min postprandially, insulin demonstrates peak secretion, these time points were evaluated and exhibited an increase in mean values, not reaching statistical significance ($p > 0.05$). Based on the graph, the first and second phases of insulin secretion were improved (Figure 1).

Table 3. Glycemic parameters and calculated β-cell area at baseline and 6 and 12 months.

Parameters	Baseline	6 Months		12 Months		
	Mean ± SD	Mean ± SD	p 0–6	Mean ± SD	p 0–12	p 6–12
Glu fasting (mg/dL)	130.54 ± 51.15	85.08 ± 13.79	**<0.05**	88.13 ± 21.52	**<0.05**	0.885
Glu 120 min (mg/dL)	225.29 ± 76.88	103.87 ± 39.94	**<0.05**	89.04 ± 47.74	**<0.05**	0.597
Insulin fasting (μIU/mL)	23.91 ± 13.6	8.52 ± 5.77	**<0.05**	9.83 ± 13.36	**<0.05**	0.765
Insulin 30 min (μIU/mL)	55.8 ± 32.45	68.52 ± 57.56	0.680	99.63 ± 78.66	0.103	0.263
Insulin 60 min (μIU/mL)	75.36 ± 52.64	88.53 ± 110.4	0.588	99.87 ± 118	0.834	0.744
Insulin AUC	7927.5 ± 4530	6747.6 ± 6688	0.177	8030 ± 7550	0.836	0.433
Insulinogenic index	0.5052 ± 0.44	0.9862 ± 1	**<0.05**	1.483 ± 1.63	**<0.05**	0.352
Calculated β-cell area	0.035 ± 0.01	0.032 ± 0.012	0.869	0.03 ± 0.02	0.228	0.321

Values are expressed as mean ± SD; $p < 0.05$ bold for significance.

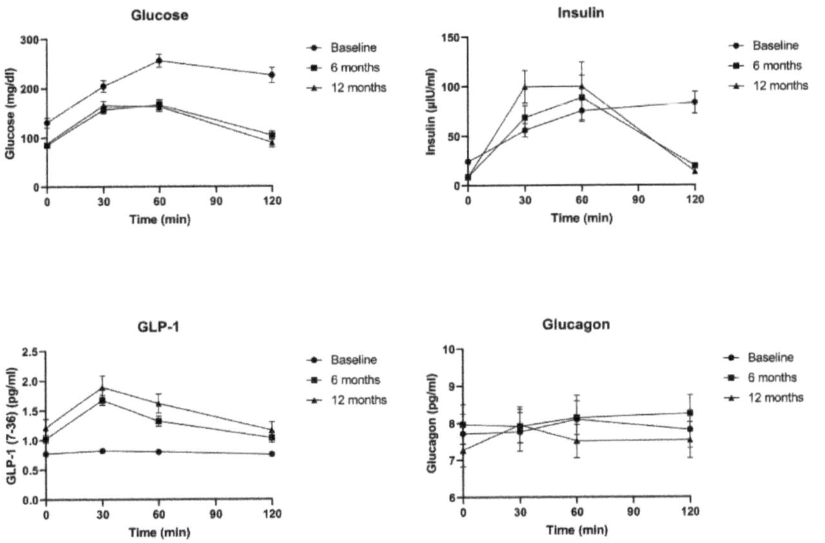

Figure 1. Graphs of glucose, insulin, and GI hormones during OGTT at baseline and 6 and 12 months.

In order to investigate the theory of nesidioblastosis, the calculated β-cell area was evaluated 6 and 12 months postoperatively. The mean values were comparable at all time points ($p < 0.05$) without showing changes in calculated β-cell area postoperatively (Table 3).

3.4. GLP-1 and Glucagon

GLP-1 demonstrated a significant increase postoperatively in both fasting and postprandial levels. Specifically, fasting levels increased from 0.78 ± 0.14 to 1.39 ± 0.58 pg/mL ($p < 0.05$), while GLP-1 improved its pattern secretion with peak release at 30 min postprandially compared with preoperatively ($p < 0.05$). GLP-1 AUC levels also significantly increased from 94.72 ± 19.63 to 182.77 ± 87.19 ($p < 0.05$) (Table 4, Figures 1 and 2).

Table 4. Gastrointestinal hormones glucagon and GLP-1 at baseline and 6 and 12 months.

Gastrointestinal Hormones	Baseline	6 Months		12 Months		
	Mean ± SD	**Mean ± SD**	***p* 0–6**	**Mean ± SD**	***p* 0–12**	***p* 6–12**
Glucagon fasting (pg/mL)	7.71 ± 2.62	7.96 ± 2.48	0.637	7.26 ± 2.05	0.502	0.266
Glucagon AUC	948.25 ± 307.9	971.19 ± 250.52	0.406	911.68 ± 252.5	0.933	0.375
GLP-1 fasting (pg/mL)	0.78 ± 0.14	1.14 ± 0.48	**<0.05**	1.39 ± 0.58	**<0.05**	0.184
GLP-1 AUC	94.72 ± 19.63	156.25 ± 43.1	**<0.05**	182.77 ± 87.19	**<0.05**	0.650

$p < 0.05$ bold for significance.

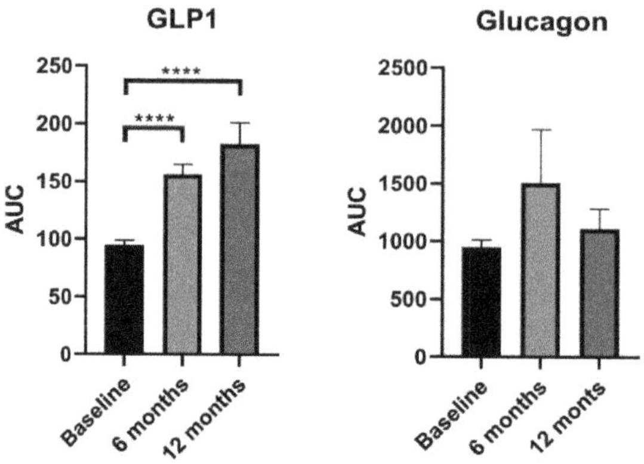

Figure 2. Bar graphs of GLP-1 and glucagon AUC levels at baseline and 6 and 12 months. **** $p < 0.0001$.

Glucagon fasting and postprandial levels during OGTT did not show a significant change from baseline to 6 or 12 months ($p > 0.05$). Based on the graphs, fasting and AUC levels followed the same pattern, experiencing a slight increase at 6 months and returning to preoperative levels without achieving statistical significance at 12 months ($p > 0.05$) (Table 4, Figures 1 and 2).

3.5. Correlations and Predictive Factors

According to the biserial correlation, postprandial insulin levels at 30 and 60 min—at 6 and 12 months postoperatively—were significantly positively related to the binary variable of glucose 120 min at 12 months (0 for glucose > 60 mg/dL and 1 for glucose < 60 mg/dL), meaning that increasing values at these time points were associated with PBH. Conversely, GLP-1 levels at these time points were not associated with PBH (Table 5).

The high correlation coefficient between the binary glucose variable at 12 months postoperatively and postprandial insulin at 30 and 60 min at 6 months postoperatively was an unexpected and interesting finding. In order to investigate whether the postprandial levels of insulin at 6 and 12 months could be a useful marker for PBH, a stepwise binary regression analysis was performed in order to determine the strongest predictive factor from the aforementioned parameters. The results of the analysis indicated that postprandial insulin levels at 30 min and 6 months might be a strong predictor for PBH at 12 months ($p < 0.001$). The rest of the tested variables did not show a similar potential and were excluded from the model (Table 6).

The final step was validating the accuracy of the postprandial insulin levels at 30 min and 6 months as a potential prognostic marker. The validation was assessed by generating ROC curves. The positive result was the occurrence of PBH. The ROC curves revealed that insulin at 30 min at 6 months was a sensitive and reliable biomarker since its calculated AUC value was the highest at 0.933 (Figure 3). The rest of the tested biomarkers showed lower values of AUC, as depicted in Figure 3. Therefore, this reinforces the potential use of insulin at 30 min and 6 months as a potential PBH prognostic biomarker.

Table 5. Biserial correlation of parameters with the binary variable of glucose at 120 min at 12 months.

		Cat_glu12_120	Insulin_6_30	Insulin_6_60	GLP1_6_30	GLP1_6_60	Insulin_12_30	Insulin_12_60	GLP1_12_30	GLP1_12_60
Cat_glu12_120	Pearson Correlation	1	0.709 **	0.600**	−0.063	−0.010	0.568**	0.694 **	0.083	−0.016
	Sig. (2-tailed)		0.000	0.002	0.775	0.962	0.005	0.000	0.706	0.944
	N	23	23	23	23	23	23	23	23	23
Insulin_6_30	Pearson Correlation	0.709 **	1	0.823 **	−0.172	−0.151	0.757 **	0.868 **	−0.070	−0.200
	Sig. (2-tailed)	0.000		0.000	0.422	0.480	0.000	0.000	0.751	0.359
	N	23	24	24	24	24	23	23	23	23
Insulin_6_60	Pearson Correlation	0.600 **	0.823 **	1	−0.210	−0.181	0.675 **	0.936 **	0.213	−0.182
	Sig. (2-tailed)	0.002	0.000		0.324	0.396	0.000	0.000	0.329	0.407
	N	23	24	24	24	24	23	23	23	23
GLP1_6_30	Pearson Correlation	−0.063	−0.172	−0.210	1	0.182	−0.085	−0.109	−0.004	0.197
	Sig. (2-tailed)	0.775	0.422	0.324		0.395	0.699	0.621	0.987	0.369
	N	23	24	24	24	24	23	23	23	23
GLP1_6_60	Pearson Correlation	−0.010	−0.151	−0.181	0.182	1	−0.163	−0.214	−0.269	0.162
	Sig. (2-tailed)	0.962	0.480	0.396	0.395		0.458	0.327	0.214	0.460
	N	23	24	24	24	24	23	23	23	23
Insulin_12_30	Pearson Correlation	0.568 **	0.757 **	0.675 **	−0.085	−0.163	1	0.827 **	−0.130	−0.335
	Sig. (2-tailed)	0.005	0.000	0.000	0.699	0.458		0.000	0.555	0.118
	N	23	23	23	23	23	23	23	23	23
Insulin_12_60	Pearson Correlation	0.694 **	0.868 **	0.936 **	−0.109	−0.214	0.827 **	1	0.125	−0.244
	Sig. (2-tailed)	0.000	0.000	0.000	0.621	0.327	0.000		0.570	0.261
	N	23	23	23	23	23	23	23	23	23
GLP1_12_30	Pearson Correlation	0.083	−0.070	0.213	−0.004	−0.269	−0.130	0.125	1	−0.075
	Sig. (2-tailed)	0.706	0.751	0.329	0.987	0.214	0.555	0.570		0.734
	N	23	23	23	23	23	23	23	23	23
GLP1_12_60	Pearson Correlation	−0.016	−0.200	−0.182	0.197	0.162	−0.335	−0.244	−0.075	1
	Sig. (2-tailed)	0.944	0.359	0.407	0.369	0.460	0.118	0.261	0.734	
	N	23	23	23	23	23	23	23	23	23

** Correlation is significant at the 0.01 level (2-tailed); cat_glu12_120 (dichotomous variable of glucose levels at 120 min at 12 months: 0 for above 60 mg/dL and 1 for below 60 mg/dL).

Table 6. Stepwise binary regression analysis and excluded variables.

Model Summary							
Model	R	R^2	Adj R^2	SEE	R^2 Change	F Change	Sig. F Change [a]
1	0.709 [a]	0.502	0.479	0.30454	0.502	21.193	0.000
Excluded Variables							
Model 1	Beta In	t	Sig.	Partial Correlation	Collinearity Statistics Tolerance		
Insulin_12_30	0.074 [b]	0.306	0.763 [b]	0.068	0.428		
Insulin_12_60	0.319 [b]	1.029	0.316 [b]	0.224	0.246		
Insulin_6_60	0.057 [b]	0.207	0.838 [b]	0.046	0.328		

The dependent variable is the categorical variable of postprandial glucose at 120 min and postoperative 12 months (Cat Glu12 120). Only postprandial insulin at 30 min and 6 months is calculated as a prognostic biomarker ([a]). The rest of the tested parameters have no prognostic potential ([b]).

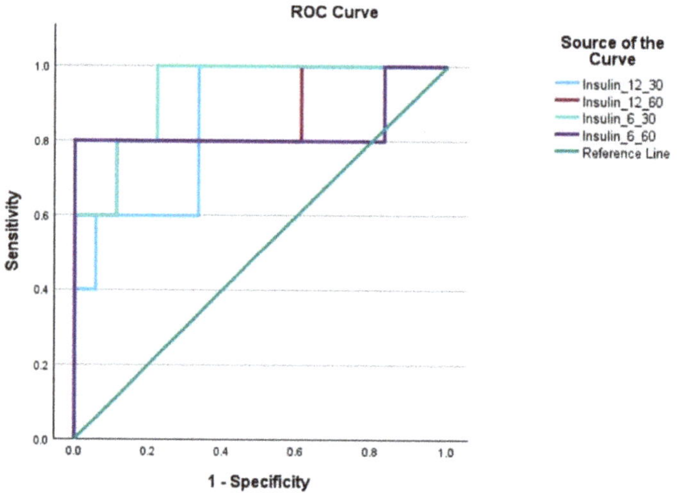

Area Under the ROC Curve	
Test Result Variable(s)	**Area**
Insulin_6_30	0.933
Insulin_6_60	0.833
Insulin_12_30	0.856
Insulin_12_60	0.856

Figure 3. ROC curves for postprandial insulin values and AUC levels. The proposed early PBH biomarker (Insulin_6_30) shows the highest AUC value. The rest of the postprandial insulin levels tested show lower values of AUC.

4. Discussion

The aim of this study was to investigate PBH in a cohort of patients with T2DM and obesity after LRYGBP and identify potentially involved mechanisms that could serve as tools for predicting the occurrence of this complication. Postprandial insulin levels are associated with the presence of PBH; in particular, insulin levels at 30 min during OGTT at

6 months might be used as a predictor for PBH. Conversely, postprandial levels of GLP-1 and glucagon, as well as the calculated β-cell area, are not significantly related to PBH. The type of surgery is not associated with PBH, further supporting our previous findings, which showed that fundus resection is not implicated in glycemic control [8].

Although PBH has been recognized as a complication of MBS for several years, its true incidence is not yet determined. From studies utilizing continuous glucose monitoring (CGM), this incidence increases from 25 to 75%, while after provocative tests, namely the OGTT and mixed meal test, it is estimated to be between 19 and 30% [23,24]. On the basis of our findings, 16% of the patients presented postprandial glucose levels below 60 mg/dl after 12 months, and 20% had symptoms highly indicative of PBH according to the retrospective questionnaire evaluation. However, it is interesting to note that only patients with T2DM were included, which contradicts some observational studies that propose preoperative T2DM as a protective factor for PBH [23]. The mean duration of preoperative T2DM in our cohort was 3.7 years, and, most probably, the irreversible damage of β-cells had not occurred. As a result, after LRYGBP and gastrointestinal anatomy alterations, β-cell function was restored, and glycemic control was achieved. In line with this notion, Raverdy et al. suggested that PBH after LRYGBP occurs in patients with higher pre-existing beta-cell functions, as estimated via the insulinogenic index, when insulin sensitivity is restored in relation to weight loss, which more succinctly explains our findings [22]. The mean preoperative insulinogenic index of the four patients of the cohort who presented PBH was 0.654, and it showed a remarkable four-fold increase at 12 months, reaching 2.5, which is far higher than the mean value of the insulinogenic index of the cohort, as depicted in Table 3. This indicates that after, achieving weight loss and improving insulin sensitivity, β-cell function is restored, and patients with an inherent increased β-cell function will demonstrate increased values of the insulinogenic index.

Another demanding part of PBH diagnosis is the objective report of the symptoms and the diagnostic methods used. It is well known that PBH can present without any symptoms, resulting in the term "hypoglycemia unawareness", as demonstrated mainly from studies using CGM [23,25]. Furthermore, the lack of clinical tools is a severe drawback for assessing PBH. Many studies investigating PBH have implemented the Sigstad score, which is a false approach because this score is used for detecting early dumping syndrome [26]. In line with this notion, a recently published study found that the Sigstad score is not a reliable or valid method for detecting late dumping syndrome after MBS [27]. Perhaps, the Edinburgh hypoglycemia scale test and instructions for patients with respect to measuring blood glucose levels whenever they present these symptoms would be a more rational approach.

The optimal diagnostic approach for the diagnosis of PBH has not yet been determined by clinicians. From provocative tests, the mixed meal test appears as a more preferred method because it resembles an ordinary meal. Conversely, OGTT, which was also used in this cohort, can result in PBH in 70% of RYGB patients, with small differences between symptomatic and asymptomatic patients, rendering OGTT less useful in confirming the diagnosis [5]. Although the documented glucose values in the studied cohort were after OGTT, the type of meal before the onset of symptoms was unknown when patients filled out the questionnaires. The lack of information was a major drawback because it can affect the occurrence of PBH. Specifically, meals with a high carbohydrate load are the main culprits for PBH and should be replaced with small meals enriched in protein and fiber [1]. Finally, CGM over the course of 3 days and during normal meals is more sensitive and is perhaps the most promising method [28]. Nevertheless, more evidence is required based on the recent guidelines of the European Society of Endocrinology [8].

Delving deeper into the pathophysiology, the most compelling theory revolving around PBH is the exaggerated insulinotropic response, resulting in overwhelming hypoglycemia [29]. This increased postprandial insulin secretion is attributed to elevated β-cell sensitivity during hyperglycemia, while concurrently blunted insulin suppression is witnessed when glucose falls below fasting levels [30–32]. In our study, postprandial insulin levels at 30 and 60 min and 6 months or 12 months were significantly associated with postprandial glucose values below 60 mg/dL. Specifically, postprandial insulin levels at 30 min at 6 months might be used as a predictive factor for PBH at 12 months, although this should be validated in a larger sample. Turning to details, the mean values of postprandial insulin levels at 30 min experienced by the four patients with PBH, at baseline, 6 months, and 12 months were 74.25, 164.82, and 209.25 μIU/mL, respectively, showing a remarkable postoperative increase when insulin sensitivity and glucose homeostasis were restored. Whether this is a result of an increase in pre-existing β-cell function that was restored after weight loss or dysregulation in β-cell response requires more investigation since many factors are implicated.

Apart from insulin's action, its secretion is also closely related to enteroinsular axis activity, which is mediated by incretins GLP-1 and GIP. Particularly, postprandial GLP-1 levels are significantly positively associated with insulin secretion, bolstering the fact that incretin contributes to enhanced β-cell function postoperatively [3,33]. Utilizing more evidence about PBH, patients who experience hypoglycemia after RYGBP are reported to have enhanced GLP-1 responses to meal ingestion compared with asymptomatic RYGB individuals [34]. In our study, fasting and postprandial GLP-1 levels were remarkably improved at 6 and 12 months, and they were most probably the main culprits that led to optimal glycemic control and T2DM remission in the study cohort. Supposing that GLP-1 contributes to insulin secretion, we hypothesized that postprandial GLP-1 levels at 30 min, where the maximum secretion is observed, depending on the values, could be involved in PBH at 12 months. Nevertheless, GLP-1 levels at 30 min and even at 60 min could not be used, surprisingly, as predictors for PBH at 12 months based on binary regression analysis. Furthermore, from the biserial correlation, the aforementioned parameters were not significantly related to PBH, creating controversy regarding their role in PBH. Therefore, according to our findings, an inherent pre-existing β-cell function with insulin hypersecretion seems to be a prerequisite for PBH rather than GLP-1 levels alone.

Apart from incretins and insulin, the disruption of counter-regulatory mechanisms, such as glucagon, might be implicated in PBH, increasing the frequency of these episodes [35]. While glucagon is normally released in response to hypoglycemia, stimulating hepatic glucose output, after RYGBP, the postprandial glucagon response among patients with and without hypoglycemia is identical, indicating a dysregulated a-cell response to hypoglycemia [36]. Particularly in T2DM patients, the paracrine control of a-cell glucagon is jeopardized, resulting in a-cell insensitivity, increased fasting glucagon levels, and blunted postprandial glucagon suppression [37]. In our study, postprandial glucagon levels did not significantly change. However, fasting and postprandial levels were slightly decreased at 12 months compared with 6 months, showing a gradual improvement in a-cell sensitivity. Moreover, from the biserial correlation, glucagon levels at any time point were not correlated with the PBH, exhibiting a more limited role. Hence, the attenuation of counter-regulatory mechanisms in T2DM patients, together with the significant changes that occurred after RYGBP, create complex interactions that require further investigation. Finally, based on a recently published study, glucagon's insulinotropic role is witnessed after MBS, which is mediated through the GLP-1 receptor on β-cells, further complicating glucagon action [38].

A while after the turn of the millennium, Service et al. published a landmark study in order to explain PBH, and they suggested the increased calculated β-cell area after RYGBP as the main culprit because nesidioblastosis characteristics were observed in specimens from patients undergoing partial pancreatectomy for PBH [12,39]. However, the theory of nesidioblastosis was steadily abandoned because the removal of islet cells via partial pancreatectomy did not entirely resolve hypoglycemia. On the other hand, it was observed that β-cell nuclear diameter was increased with respect to BMI, and this was preserved together with β-cell hyperfunction after RYGBP. In line with this notion, we evaluated calculated β-cell area, as indicated by Meier et al., and no significant changes were observed postoperatively. Moreover, the calculated β-cell area was not associated with PBH in the biserial correlation. Therefore, according to the literature and our findings, pre-existing β-cell hyperfunction, which persists after weight loss, is probably the key leverage point for PBH [40,41].

Although these findings can be considered intriguing, there are several major limitations, requiring a cautious interpretation of the results. First and foremost, PBH was not the primary endpoint or one of the secondary endpoints of the initially designed randomized controlled study. PBH was mainly observed at twelve months after RYGBP through patients reporting symptoms of hypoglycemia or low glucose values, and this guided us in retrospectively evaluating these patients even though the samples were prospectively collected. Regarding the provocative test used, OGTT might not be the most ideal because it overdiagnoses PBH. Furthermore, except for the small sample size of the study cohort, which severely weakens our findings, the postoperative time period of one year is also not the most appropriate, since the physiological changes after MBS stabilize after one year, enabling us to safely study the involved mechanisms. Another major limitation of this study was the lack of data regarding the type of meal these patients consumed when they completed the questionnaire; this is because the consumption of meals with low carbohydrate and high protein levels is the cornerstone for avoiding PBH. Hence, the laboratory values of glucose below 60 mg/dl were documented after OGTT for all patients. Other than these severe limitations, the study cohort only included patients with T2DM and investigated several mechanisms implicated in PBH. Despite the small sample size, the potential predictive value of postprandial insulin levels at 6 months for PBH and 12 months and the role of GLP-1 and glucagon revolving around PBH are valuable findings, providing insights in a not yet clearly elucidated field. In any case, PBH cannot be easily investigated due to hypoglycemia unawareness and the inability to objectively report patients' symptoms.

5. Conclusions

According to our findings, pre-existing β-cell hyperfunction, which persists postoperatively after weight loss and might lead to increased postprandial insulin levels, is associated with PBH. Moreover, the postprandial insulin levels at 30 min and 6 months might be used as a predictive factor for PBH at 12 months, while GLP-1 and glucagon levels are not associated with PBH among patients with diabetes after LRYGBP. The predictive role of insulin can raise awareness among clinicians to adequately prepare for and inform patients to avoid the devastating effects of PBH; this should be validated using a larger sample size. Future research should aim to investigate the implicated mechanisms with well-designed studies, while clinical tools for objectively assessing PBH should also be validated.

Author Contributions: Conceptualization, D.K. and C.L.; methodology, D.K. and S.-S.V.; software, S.-S.V.; validation, D.K., C.L. and S.-S.V.; formal analysis, D.K.; investigation, D.K.; resources, E.K.; data curation, E.K.; writing—original draft preparation, D.K.; writing—review and editing, C.L., N.G. and I.K.; visualization, S.-S.V.; supervision, I.K.; project administration, I.K.; funding acquisition, I.K. All authors have read and agreed to the published version of the manuscript.

Funding: The publication fees of this manuscript have been financed by the Research Council of the University of Patras, Greece.

Institutional Review Board Statement: This study was conducted in accordance with the Declaration of Helsinki and approved by the local Research and Ethics Committee (No 730/10.12.2019) of the University General Hospital of Patras.

Informed Consent Statement: Informed consent was obtained from all subjects involved in the study.

Data Availability Statement: The data presented in this study are available from the corresponding author upon request.

Conflicts of Interest: The authors declare no conflicts of interest.

References

1. Eisenberg, D.; Azagury, D.E.; Ghiassi, S.; Grover, B.T.; Kim, J.J. ASMBS Position Statement on Postprandial Hyperinsulinemic Hypoglycemia after Bariatric Surgery. *Surg. Obes. Relat. Dis.* **2017**, *13*, 371–378. [CrossRef]
2. Rossini, G.; Risi, R.; Monte, L.; Sancetta, B.; Quadrini, M.; Ugoccioni, M.; Masi, D.; Rossetti, R.; D'Alessio, R.; Mazzilli, R.; et al. Postbariatric surgery hypoglycemia: Nutritional, pharmacological and surgical perspectives. *Diabetes Metab. Res. Rev.* **2024**, *40*, e3750. [CrossRef] [PubMed]
3. Rheinwalt, K.P.; Plamper, A.; Rückbeil, M.V.; Kroh, A.; Neumann, U.P.; Ulmer, T.F. One Anastomosis Gastric Bypass-Mini-Gastric Bypass (OAGB-MGB) Versus Roux-en-Y Gastric Bypass (RYGB)-a Mid-Term Cohort Study with 612 Patients. *Obes. Surg.* **2020**, *30*, 1230–1240. [CrossRef]
4. Kehagias, D.; Georgopoulos, N.; Habeos, I.; Lampropoulos, C.; Mulita, F.; Kehagias, I. The role of the gastric fundus in glycemic control. *Hormones* **2023**, *22*, 151–163. [CrossRef] [PubMed]
5. Hazlehurst, J.; Khoo, B.; Lobato, C.B.; Ilesanmi, I.; Abbott, S.; Chan, T.; Pillai, S.; Maslin, K.; Purkayastha, S.; McGowan, B.; et al. Society for Endocrinology (SfE) guidelines for the diagnosis and management of post bariatric hypoglycaemia. *Endocr. Connect.* **2024**, *13*, e230285. [CrossRef]
6. Tripyla, A.; Ferreira, A.; Schönenberger, K.A.; Näf, N.H.; Inderbitzin, L.E.; Prendin, F.; Cossu, L.; Cappon, G.; Facchinetti, A.; Herzig, D.; et al. Relationship between Symptom Perception and Postprandial Glycemic Profiles in Patients with Postbariatric Hypoglycemia After Roux-en-Y Gastric Bypass Surgery. *Diabetes Care* **2023**, *46*, 1792–1798. [CrossRef] [PubMed]
7. Eisenberg, D.; Shikora, S.A.; Aarts, E.; Aminian, A.; Angrisani, L.; Cohen, R.V.; de Luca, M.; Faria, S.L.; Goodpaster, K.P.S.; Haddad, A.; et al. 2022 American Society of Metabolic and Bariatric Surgery (ASMBS) and International Federation for the Surgery of Obesity and Metabolic Disorders (IFSO) Indications for Metabolic and Bariatric Surgery. *Obes. Surg.* **2023**, *33*, 3–14. [CrossRef]
8. Kehagias, D.; Lampropoulos, C.; Georgopoulos, N.; Habeos, I.; Kalavrizioti, D.; Vamvakas, S.S.; Davoulou, P.; Kehagias, I. Diabetes Remission After LRYGBP with and without Fundus Resection: A Randomized Clinical Trial. *Obes. Surg.* **2023**, *33*, 3373–3382. [CrossRef]
9. Yeh, J.K.; Chen, C.C.; Liu, K.H.; Peng, C.C.; Lin, T.A.; Chang, Y.S.; Wen, M.S.; Yeh, T.S.; Wang, C.Y. Serum microRNA panels predict bariatric surgery outcomes. *Obesity* **2022**, *30*, 389–399. [CrossRef]
10. Lath, D.; Cherian, K.E.; Paul, T.V.; Kapoor, N. Beyond diabetes remission a step further: Post bariatric surgery hypoglycemia. *World J. Diabetes* **2022**, *13*, 278–281. [CrossRef]
11. Carpenter, T.; Trautmann, M.E.; Baron, A.D. Hyperinsulinemic hypoglycemia with nesidioblastosis after gastric-bypass surgery. *N. Engl. J. Med.* **2005**, *353*, 2192–2194. [CrossRef]
12. Service, G.J.; Thompson, G.B.; Service, F.J.; Andrews, J.C.; Collazo-Clavell, M.L.; Lloyd, R.V. Hyperinsulinemic hypoglycemia with nesidioblastosis after gastric-bypass surgery. *N. Engl. J. Med.* **2005**, *353*, 249–254. [CrossRef]
13. Alsayed Hasan, M.; Schwartz, S.; McKenna, V.; Ing, R. An Imbalance of Pathophysiologic Factors in Late Postprandial Hypoglycemia Post Bariatric Surgery: A Narrative Review. *Obes. Surg.* **2023**, *33*, 2927–2937. [CrossRef]
14. Jalleh, R.J.; Umapathysivam, M.M.; Plummer, M.P.; Deane, A.; Jones, K.L.; Horowitz, M. Postprandial plasma GLP-1 levels are elevated in individuals with postprandial hypoglycaemia following Roux-en-Y gastric bypass—A systematic review. *Rev. Endocr. Metab. Disord.* **2023**, *24*, 1075–1088. [CrossRef]
15. World Medical Association Declaration of Helsinki: Ethical principles for medical research involving human subjects. *JAMA* **2013**, *310*, 2191–2194. [CrossRef]
16. Mathew, G.; Agha, R.; Albrecht, J.; Goel, P.; Mukherjee, I.; Pai, P.; D'Cruz, A.K.; Nixon, I.J.; Roberto, K.; Enam, S.A.; et al. STROCSS 2021: Strengthening the reporting of cohort, cross-sectional and case-control studies in surgery. *Int. J. Surg.* **2021**, *96*, 106165. [CrossRef]
17. 2. Classification and Diagnosis of Diabetes: Standards of Medical Care in Diabetes-2021. *Diabetes Care* **2021**, *44*, S15–S33. [CrossRef]
18. Deary, I.J.; Hepburn, D.A.; MacLeod, K.M.; Frier, B.M. Partitioning the symptoms of hypoglycaemia using multi-sample confirmatory factor analysis. *Diabetologia* **1993**, *36*, 771–777. [CrossRef]
19. Hypoglycaemia, cardiovascular disease, and mortality in diabetes: Epidemiology, pathogenesis, and management. *Lancet Diabetes Endocrinol.* **2019**, *7*, 385–396. [CrossRef]
20. Tura, A.; Kautzky-Willer, A.; Pacini, G. Insulinogenic indices from insulin and C-peptide: Comparison of beta-cell function from OGTT and IVGTT. *Diabetes Res. Clin. Pract.* **2006**, *72*, 298–301. [CrossRef]
21. Meier, J.J.; Menge, B.A.; Breuer, T.G.; Müller, C.A.; Tannapfel, A.; Uhl, W.; Schmidt, W.E.; Schrader, H. Functional assessment of pancreatic beta-cell area in humans. *Diabetes* **2009**, *58*, 1595–1603. [CrossRef]
22. Raverdy, V.; Baud, G.; Pigeyre, M.; Verkindt, H.; Torres, F.; Preda, C.; Thuillier, D.; Gélé, P.; Vantyghem, M.C.; Caiazzo, R.; et al. Incidence and Predictive Factors of Postprandial Hyperinsulinemic Hypoglycemia After Roux-en-Y Gastric Bypass: A Five year Longitudinal Study. *Ann. Surg.* **2016**, *264*, 878–885. [CrossRef] [PubMed]
23. Lee, C.J.; Brown, T.T.; Schweitzer, M.; Magnuson, T.; Clark, J.M. The incidence and risk factors associated with developing symptoms of hypoglycemia after bariatric surgery. *Surg. Obes. Relat. Dis.* **2018**, *14*, 797–802. [CrossRef]
24. Goldfine, A.B.; Patti, M.E. How common is hypoglycemia after gastric bypass? *Obesity* **2016**, *24*, 1210–1211. [CrossRef] [PubMed]

25. Halperin, F.; Patti, M.E.; Skow, M.; Bajwa, M.; Goldfine, A.B. Continuous glucose monitoring for evaluation of glycemic excursions after gastric bypass. *J. Obes.* **2011**, *2011*, 869536. [CrossRef] [PubMed]
26. Scarpellini, E.; Arts, J.; Karamanolis, G.; Laurenius, A.; Siquini, W.; Suzuki, H.; Ukleja, A.; Van Beek, A.; Vanuytsel, T.; Bor, S.; et al. International consensus on the diagnosis and management of dumping syndrome. *Nat. Rev. Endocrinol.* **2020**, *16*, 448–466. [CrossRef] [PubMed]
27. Rieck, J.H.; Heidinger, H.; Schlöricke, E.; Schmidt, N.; Krause, S. Is Sigstad's score really capable of detecting post-surgical late dumping syndrome? *Langenbeck's Arch. Surg.* **2024**, *409*, 94. [CrossRef]
28. Malik, S.; Mitchell, J.E.; Steffen, K.; Engel, S.; Wiisanen, R.; Garcia, L.; Malik, S.A. Recognition and management of hyperinsulinemic hypoglycemia after bariatric surgery. *Obes. Res. Clin. Pract.* **2016**, *10*, 1–14. [CrossRef]
29. Goldfine, A.B.; Mun, E.C.; Devine, E.; Bernier, R.; Baz-Hecht, M.; Jones, D.B.; Schneider, B.E.; Holst, J.J.; Patti, M.E. Patients with neuroglycopenia after gastric bypass surgery have exaggerated incretin and insulin secretory responses to a mixed meal. *J. Clin. Endocrinol Metab.* **2007**, *92*, 4678–4685. [CrossRef]
30. Abrahamsson, N.; Börjesson, J.L.; Sundbom, M.; Wiklund, U.; Karlsson, F.A.; Eriksson, J.W. Gastric Bypass Reduces Symptoms and Hormonal Responses in Hypoglycemia. *Diabetes* **2016**, *65*, 2667–2675. [CrossRef]
31. Salehi, M.; Woods, S.C.; D'Alessio, D.A. Gastric bypass alters both glucose-dependent and glucose-independent regulation of islet hormone secretion. *Obesity* **2015**, *23*, 2046–2052. [CrossRef] [PubMed]
32. Ilesanmi, I.; Tharakan, G.; Alexiadou, K.; Behary, P.; Alessimii, H.; Bovill-Taylor, C.; Kenkre, J.; Choudhury, S.; Doyle, C.; Purkayastha, S.; et al. Roux-en-Y Gastric Bypass Increases Glycemic Variability and Time in Hypoglycemia in Patients with Obesity and Prediabetes or Type 2 Diabetes: A Prospective Cohort Study. *Diabetes Care* **2021**, *44*, 614–617. [CrossRef] [PubMed]
33. Salehi, M.; Gastaldelli, A.; D'Alessio, D.A. Blockade of glucagon-like peptide 1 receptor corrects postprandial hypoglycemia after gastric bypass. *Gastroenterology* **2014**, *146*, 669–680.e2. [CrossRef] [PubMed]
34. Tharakan, G.; Behary, P.; Wewer Albrechtsen, N.J.; Chahal, H.; Kenkre, J.; Miras, A.D.; Ahmed, A.R.; Holst, J.J.; Bloom, S.R.; Tan, T. Roles of increased glycaemic variability, GLP-1 and glucagon in hypoglycaemia after Roux-en-Y gastric bypass. *Eur. J. Endocrinol.* **2017**, *177*, 455–464. [CrossRef] [PubMed]
35. Salehi, M.; Vella, A.; McLaughlin, T.; Patti, M.E. Hypoglycemia After Gastric Bypass Surgery: Current Concepts and Controversies. *J. Clin. Endocrinol. Metab.* **2018**, *103*, 2815–2826. [CrossRef]
36. Salehi, M.; Gastaldelli, A.; D'Alessio, D.A. Altered islet function and insulin clearance cause hyperinsulinemia in gastric bypass patients with symptoms of postprandial hypoglycemia. *J. Clin. Endocrinol. Metab.* **2014**, *99*, 2008–2017. [CrossRef] [PubMed]
37. Omar-Hmeadi, M.; Lund, P.E.; Gandasi, N.R.; Tengholm, A.; Barg, S. Paracrine control of α-cell glucagon exocytosis is compromised in human type-2 diabetes. *Nat. Commun.* **2020**, *11*, 1896. [CrossRef]
38. Pérez-Arana, G.M.; Díaz-Gómez, A.; Bancalero-de Los Reyes, J.; Gracia-Romero, M.; Ribelles-García, A.; Visiedo, F.; González-Domínguez, Á.; Almorza-Gomar, D.; Prada-Oliveira, J.A. The role of glucagon after bariatric/metabolic surgery: Much more than an "anti-insulin" hormone. *Front. Endocrinol.* **2023**, *14*, 1236103. [CrossRef]
39. Honka, H.; Salehi, M. Postprandial hypoglycemia after gastric bypass surgery: From pathogenesis to diagnosis and treatment. *Curr. Opin. Clin. Nutr. Metab. Care* **2019**, *22*, 295–302. [CrossRef]
40. Meier, J.J.; Butler, A.E.; Galasso, R.; Butler, P.C. Hyperinsulinemic hypoglycemia after gastric bypass surgery is not accompanied by islet hyperplasia or increased beta-cell turnover. *Diabetes Care* **2006**, *29*, 1554–1559. [CrossRef]
41. Patti, M.E.; Li, P.; Goldfine, A.B. Insulin response to oral stimuli and glucose effectiveness increased in neuroglycopenia following gastric bypass. *Obesity* **2015**, *23*, 798–807. [CrossRef] [PubMed]

biomedicines

MDPI

Article

Nocturnal Glucose Profile According to Timing of Dinner Rapid Insulin and Basal and Rapid Insulin Type: An *Insulclock*® Connected Insulin Cap-Based Real-World Study

Fernando Gómez-Peralta [1,*], Xoan Valledor [2], Cristina Abreu [1], Elsa Fernández-Rubio [3], Laura Cotovad [4], Pedro Pujante [5], Sharona Azriel [6], Jesús Pérez-González [2], Alba Vallejo [2], Luis Ruiz-Valdepeñas [2] and Rosa Corcoy [7,8,9]

1 Endocrinology and Nutrition Unit, Hospital General de Segovia, Luis Erik Clavería Neurólogo S.N Street, 40002 Segovia, Spain; cabreupadin@gmail.com
2 Research and Development Unit, Insulcloud S.L., 28020 Madrid, Spain; xoan@insulcloud.com (X.V.); suso@insulclock.com (J.P.-G.); alba@insulcloud.com (A.V.); luis@insulcloud.com (L.R.-V.)
3 Endocrinology and Nutrition Service, Cruces University Hospital, 48903 Barakaldo, Spain; elsa.fernandezrubio@osakidetza.eus
4 Endocrinology and Nutrition Service, Hospital Arquitecto Marcide, 15405 Ferrol, Spain; lauracotovad@hotmail.com
5 Endocrinology and Nutrition Service, Hospital Universitario Central de Asturias, 33011 Oviedo, Spain; pedropujanteal@gmail.com
6 Endocrinology and Nutrition Service, Hospital Universitario Infanta Sofía, 28702 San Sebastián De Los Reyes, Spain; sharona.azriel@gmail.com
7 Endocrinology and Nutrition Service, Hospital de la Santa Creu i Sant Pau, Institut de Recerca, 08041 Barcelona, Spain; rcorcoy@santpau.cat
8 Departament de Medicina, Universitat Autònoma de Barcelona, 08193 Barcelona, Spain
9 CIBER-BBN, 28029 Madrid, Spain
* Correspondence: fgomezp@saludcastillayleon.es

Abstract: Background: A study to assess the glucose levels of people with type 1 diabetes (T1D) overnight, based on the insulin type and timing. Methods: A real-world, retrospective study of T1D, using multiple daily insulin injections. Continuous glucose monitoring and insulin injection data were collected for ten hours after dinner using the *Insulclock*® connected cap. Meal events were identified using the ROC detection methodology. The timing of the rapid insulin, second injections, and the type of insulin analogs used, were evaluated. Results: The nocturnal profiles (n = 775, 49 subjects) were analyzed. A higher glucose AUC of over 180 mg/dL was observed in subjects with delayed injections (number; %; mg/dL × h): −45–15 min (n = 136; 17.5%, 175.9 ± 271.0); −15–0 min (n = 231; 29.8%, 164.0 ± 2 37.1); 0 + 45 min (n = 408; 52.6%, 203.6 ± 260.9), (p = 0.049). The use of ultrarapid insulin (FiAsp®) (URI) vs. rapid insulin (RI) analogs was associated with less hypoglycemia events (7.1 vs. 13.6%; p = 0.005) and TBR70 (1.7 ± 6.9 vs. 4.6 ± 13.9%; p = 0.003). Users of glargine U300 vs. degludec had a higher TIR (70.7 vs. 58.5%) (adjusted R-squared: 0.22, p < 0.001). The use of a correction injection (n = 144, 18.6%) was associated with a higher number of hypoglycemia events (18.1 vs. 9.5%; p = 0.003), TBR70 (5.5 ± 14.2 vs. 3.0 ± 11.1%; p = 0.003), a glucose AUC of over 180 mg/dL (226.1 ± 257.8 vs. 178.0 ± 255.3 mg/dL × h; p = 0.001), and a lower TIR (56.0 ± 27.4 vs. 62.7 ± 29.6 mg/dL × h; p = 0.004). Conclusion: The dinner rapid insulin timing, insulin type, and the use of correction injections affect the nocturnal glucose profile in T1D.

Keywords: ultrarapid insulin; second-generation basal insulin; nocturnal hyperglycemia; nocturnal hypoglycemia; connected insulin pen cap

1. Introduction

Maintaining a safe and stable blood glucose level during the night is crucial for people with type 1 diabetes (T1D). Determining the appropriate pre-dinner rapid insulin and basal insulin to adequately control both postprandial and nocturnal glucose can be a daily challenge, with a high level of uncertainty. Many factors, which are difficult to measure and predict, can affect the nocturnal glycemic profile, one of them being exercise during the day [1]. The safety and quality of life of individuals with T1D are clearly impacted by these factors [2].

Insulin regimens requiring multiple daily injections (MDIs) impose a considerable burden on people with T1D [3]. Previous studies have shown that the timing of prandial insulin injection can affect postprandial glucose levels [4,5]. However, these studies were conducted in laboratory settings or relied on self-reported insulin injection times and doses. Notably, a large percentage of people with T1D do not follow the recommended prandial insulin injection timing, which can result in different glucose dynamics and increase both postprandial excursions and nocturnal hypoglycemia risk [6].

Manufacturers recommend injecting regular human insulin 30–45 min before starting a meal, 15 min in the case of rapid insulin (RI) analogs, and at the start of a meal or within 20 min for second-generation ("ultrarapid") insulin (URI) [7,8]. There is limited scientific evidence on the nocturnal glucose profile depending on the timing and type of pre-dinner rapid insulin injections. However, connected insulin pens and caps can now automatically track continuous glucose monitoring (CGM) data, as well as the dose and exact time of insulin injections [9]. This is a promising development, as it can help people with T1D to manage their blood sugar levels more effectively and, ultimately, reduce the risk of complications [10].

Insulin therapy adherence can be influenced by socioeconomic factors, treatment complexity, and fear of hypoglycemia [11,12]. Errors in insulin administration, such as bolus omissions and delays, can prevent optimal glycemic control [13]. This can negatively impact the quality of life of people with diabetes and increase the risk of morbidity, mortality, and hospitalization [14].

Although it is recommended to administer the prandial bolus injection at least 15 min before mealtimes [15], it may not always be feasible in real life. Fortunately, URI is available, which can improve postprandial dynamics, even when injected after the meal has started. Our previous study, which focused on postprandial glucose dynamics, confirmed a reduction in both immediate hyper- and late hypoglycemia by using URI in a real-life setting [6].

Second-generation basal insulin (BI) analogs have been developed to help people with T1D face daily challenges. These analogs, such as insulin glargine 300 U/mL (Gla-300) and insulin degludec (IDeg), have a longer and flatter profile, with less variability [16]. However, randomized clinical trials have not consistently detected significant differences between the two insulins, using the CGM methodology [17]. In an MDI regimen, the different effects on the glucose profile caused by the two basal insulins are more easily observed during the night [18].

People with diabetes often administer additional (correction) insulin doses to immediately offset postprandial peaks [19]. Excessive correction frequently leads to postprandial hypoglycemia due to the "stacking insulin effect" [20].

Insulclock® is an innovative small cap designed to be easily attached to disposable insulin pens. Its primary function is to accurately record crucial information, such as the date, time, duration, and dose of insulin injections [21]. This recorded data is seamlessly integrated with other pertinent health metrics, including glucose levels from CGM devices or glucometers, dietary intake, and physical activity, through the user-friendly *Insulclock*® app. Patients are able to access and review the comprehensive data collected, enabling them to effectively monitor their health trends and patterns. Moreover, this information can be securely shared with their healthcare providers, facilitating collaborative analysis and personalized treatment plans. Notably, a multicenter randomized controlled trial has demonstrated the positive impact of the system on glycemic control and variability, adherence to insulin treatment, and overall quality of life for individuals with T1D and inadequate control [10].

The current study aimed to analyze the nocturnal glucose profile in people with T1D using MDIs, according to the timing of dinner rapid insulin and the type of rapid and basal insulin used.

2. Materials and Methods

2.1. Design

A retrospective study was carried out using anonymous, real-world data from the *Insulclock*® electronic database, from six participating centers in Spain. These centers were the Hospital General de Segovia in Segovia, Cruces University Hospital in Barakaldo, Hospital Arquitecto Marcide in Ferrol (A Coruña), Hospital Universitario Central de Asturias in Oviedo, Hospital Universitario 12 de Octubre in Madrid, and Hospital Universitario Infanta Sofía in San Sebastián de los Reyes.

At the beginning of the *Insulclock*® use, all participants provided written informed consent, allowing Insulcloud S.L. to collect and use their anonymized and tabulated data for scientific purposes. The study adhered to the ethical principles in the Declaration of Helsinki and was approved by the Research Ethics Committee of the Hospital General de Segovia in Segovia, Spain, before any study-related activities were undertaken.

2.2. Population and Database

The study analyzed data from consecutive T1D participants, who started using the *Insulclock*® connected insulin pen cap [21] from January to June 2022. The type of insulin used was not an inclusion criterion. The analysis focused on overnight periods, consisting of ten hours starting at dinner time, and included data from continuous glucose monitoring (CGM) and insulin injections. Only dinner glycemic excursions, starting with a glucose level between 70 mg/dL (3.9 mmol/L) and 250 mg/dL (13.9 mmol/L), and with 10 h data after dinner initiation, were included in the analysis.

The Glucose Rate Increase Detector (GRID) algorithm was employed to identify dinner times, by analyzing excursions in glucose levels between 19 to 23:59 h [22]. The algorithm estimates the rate of change in glucose levels from CGM data. It identifies glucose excursions by looking for a gradient $\geq$ 95.4 mg/dL/h (5.3 mmol/L/h) for two consecutive readings within 30 min, or $\geq$90 mg/dL/h (5.0 mmol/L/h) for three consecutive readings within 45 min, when the CGM signal is >129.6 mg/dL/h (7.2 mmol/L). The GRID algorithm has high specificity to detect meal-related glucose excursions and has been clinically validated for use with Automated Insulin Delivery (AID) systems and MDIs [23].

It is worth noting that all patients had been previously using CGM (*Freestyle Libre2*®), as part of their usual diabetes care.

2.3. Outcomes

This study assessed the impact of the rapid insulin injection timing, by comparing three groups of nocturnal glucose profiles based on when the injection was administered in relation to the start of the post-dinner rise in glucose levels (PE). The groups were: injections 45 to 15 min before (−45/−15), injections within 15 min before the PE onset (−15/0), and injections given from the start of the rise to 45 min after (0/+45).

The glucometrics and thresholds used to describe the glycemic dynamics during the analyzed nighttime periods were in line with the recommendations in the "Continuous glucose monitoring and metrics for clinical trials: an international consensus statement" [24].

To assess the magnitude of overnight hyperglycemia, we conducted a calculation of the area under the curve (AUC) for glucose levels surpassing the recommended upper limit of 180 mg/dL (10 mmol/L).

Hypoglycemic events are defined as periods when glucose levels are below 70 mg/dL (3.9 mmol/L) for more than 15 min. Two variables are used to quantify hypoglycemia: the percentage of overnight periods with a hypoglycemic event, and the time spent below the range of 70 mg/dL (3.9 mmol/L) (TBR70) in regard to glucose.

The time spent within the recommended target range of 70–180 mg/dL (3.9–10.0 mmol/L) (TIR) during the nighttime period was also assessed.

The differences in nocturnal glycemic profiles, according to the insulin type used, were evaluated. The study compared the two second-generation BI analogs, glargine 300 U/mL vs. insulin degludec, and the first-generation rapid insulin analogs (lispro, aspart, and glulisine) (RI) vs. second-generation "ultrarapid" insulin (URI) analogs (Fiasp®, Novo Nordisk, Denmark).

Additionally, the administration of a second injection (correction dose) 1–5 h after the first rapid insulin dose at dinner was also evaluated.

2.4. Statistical Analyses

Statistical analyses were performed using SPSS software, version 25.0 (Chicago, IL, USA). The level of statistical significance was set at a bilateral $p < 0.05$. Continuous variables were described by the mean and standard deviation (SD), when normally distributed, or by the median, interquartile range (IQR), when not normally distributed. Categorical variables were described by the number of valid cases and percentages. Comparisons of the proportions and/or frequency distributions were performed with the Chi-square test, Mann–Whitney, Kruskal–Wallis, or the ANOVA test, as appropriate, with the post-hoc Bonferroni correction.

Logistic and linear regression models were used to assess predictors of events of glucose under 70 mg/dL (3.9 mmol/L), time below the range of glucose 70 mg/dL (3.9 mmol/L) (TBR70), glucose AUC over 180 mg/dL, and time in range 70–180 mg/dL (3.9–10.0 mmol/L) (TIR), depending on timing of injection, use of a second injection, rapid and basal insulin type and pre-dinner glucose level. Simple regression models were first performed, and those variables reaching statistical significance were included in the multivariable regression models (forward selection). In the multivariable model, a p-value < 0.05 was considered significant. Those variables with a variance inflation factor >5 were removed from the models.

3. Results

3.1. Population

A total of 775 night periods were included, for 49 participants, 45.51 ± 13.2 years old, 28 of whom were women (57.1%).

Table 1 summarizes the clinical characteristics and baseline glucometrics of the included population, both overall and according to the type of rapid and basal insulin used.

Table 1. Demographic and clinical characteristics and glucometrics data of study participants.

	All	Glargine U300	Degludec	p	URI	RI	p	−45/−15 min	−15/−0 min	0/+45 min	p
N (%)	49	16 33%	33 67%		22 45%	27 55%					
Events	775	273 35.2%	502 64.8%		306 39.5%	469 60.5%		136 17.5%	231 29.8%	408 52.6%	
TIR (%)	63.4 ± 28	70.7 ± 25	58.5 ± 30	<0.001	61.1 ± 30	61.7 ± 28	0.96	61.9 ± 29	64.2 ± 27	59.7 ± 30	0.26
TBR70 (%)	3.3 ± 11.8	3.55 ± 12	3.38 ± 12	0.81	1.7 ± 7	4.6 ± 14	0.003	4.2 ± 14	3.0 ± 11	3.4 ± 11	0.67
Low glucose events (%)	11.1	10.62	11.35	0.75	7.1	13.6	0.005	11.0	9.5	12.0	0.63
AUC70 (mg/dL × h)	119 ± 496	134 ± 526	112 ± 486	0.49	41 ± 200	171 ± 640	0.04	148 ± 540	96 ± 435	124 ± 552	0.34
AUC180 (mg/dL × h)	186 ± 256	134 ± 218	215 ± 270	<0.001	204 ± 266	175 ± 248	0.36	176 ± 271	164 ± 237	204 ± 260	0.049
Average glucose value	165 ± 42	154 ± 38	159 ± 44	<0.001	170 ± 42	162 ± 43	0.01	163 ± 44	162 ± 40	167 ± 43	0.38

AUC70, a glucose area under the curve under 70 mg/dL (3.8 mmol/L); AUC180, a glucose area under the curve over 180 mg/dL (10 mmol/L); RI, rapid insulin analogs; TBR, time below range; TIR, time in range; URI, second-generation ("ultrarapid") analog; second-generation basal insulin (BI), insulin glargine 300 U/mL (glargine U300) and insulin degludec.

3.2. Nocturnal Glucose Dynamics Depending on the Rapid Insulin Injection Timing

The distribution of the analyzed night times, according to the dinner rapid insulin injection times, was as follows: −45/−15 injections accounted for 17.5% (n = 136), −15/0 injections for 29.8% (n = 231), and 0/+45 injections for 52.6% (n = 408).

Figure 1 displays the nocturnal glucose dynamics, depending on the dinner prandial insulin injection time.

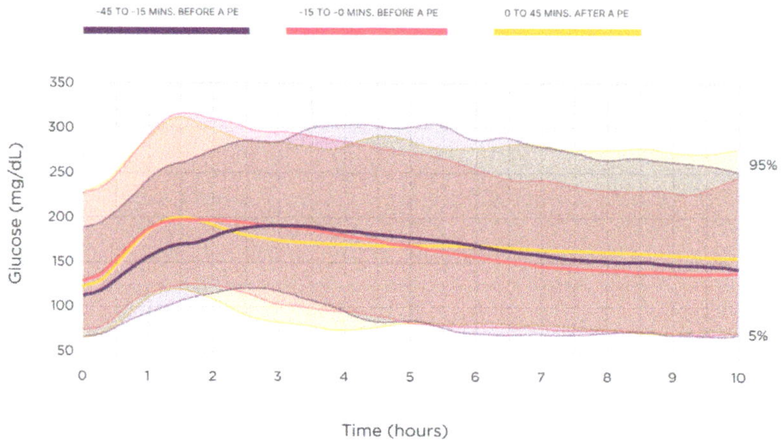

Figure 1. Nighttime glucose dynamics depending on the rapid insulin injection time.

The nocturnal high glucose excursion (glucose AUC of over 180 mg/dL [10 mmol/L]) results showed statistically significant differences between the groups, being higher in subjects with delayed rapid insulin injections 0/+45 min, (number, %, mg/dL × h): –45–15 min (n = 136, 17.5%, 175.96 ± 271.0); −15–0 min (n = 231, 29.8%,164.0 ± 237.1); 0+45 min (n = 408, 52.6%, 203.6 ± 260.9); overall $p = 0.049$ (Figure 2).

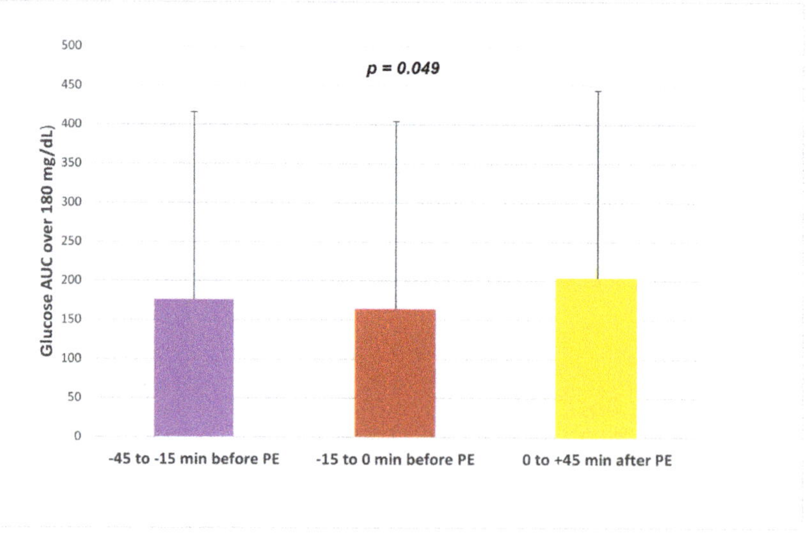

Figure 2. Nighttime glucose AUC of over 180 mg/dL [10 mmol/L] depending on the rapid insulin injection time.

The rate of nocturnal hypoglycemic events did not differ according to the timing of the rapid insulin injection, mean ± SD: -45–15 min, 11.0 ± 0.3; -15–0 min, 9.5 ± 0.3; 0 + 45 min, 12.0 + 0.3 (p = 0.630).

The time below the glucose range of 70 mg/dL (3.9 mmol/L) (TBR70) showed similar results (mean ± SD): −45–15 min, 4.2 ± 13.7%; −15–0 min, 3.0 ± 10.7%; 0 + 45 min, 3.4 ± 11.7% (p = 0.674).

3.3. Analysis According to Dinner Ultrarapid Insulin Use

The nocturnal glucose AUC of over 180 mg/dL and TIR 70–180 did not reach statistically significant differences between URI vs. RI use (mean ± SD): 175.3 ± 248 vs. 204 ± 266 mg/dL × h (p = 0.366) and 61.7 ± 28.3 vs. 61.1 ± 30.8 mg/dL × h (p = 0.968).

The use of URI vs. RI was associated with a lower TBR70 (1.7 ± 6.9 vs. 4.6 ± 13.9%; p = 0.003) (Figure 3) and less hypoglycemia events (7.1 vs. 13.6; p = 0.005) (Supplementary Figure S1).

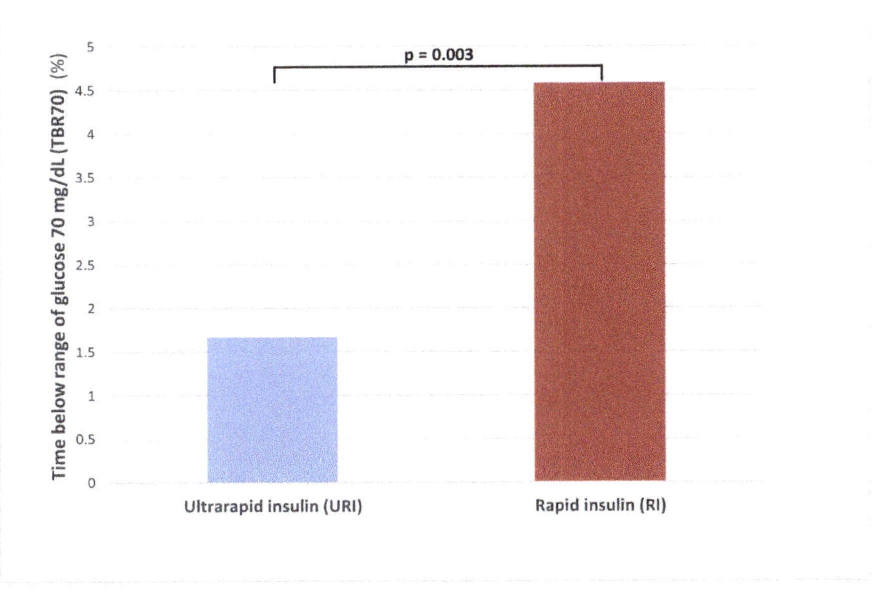

Figure 3. Time below the range of glucose 70 mg/dL (3.9 mmol/L) (TBR70) according to the use of ultrarapid insulin (URI) vs. rapid insulin (RI) analogs.

3.4. Analysis According to the Second-Generation Basal Insulin Type

Figure 4 describes the post-dinner and nocturnal glucose dynamics depending on the second-generation BI type.

Statistically significant differences were not detected regarding the type of second-generation BI used on the unadjusted glucometrics describing the nocturnal high glucose excursions (glucose AUC of over 180 mg/dL [10 mmol/L]), nocturnal hypoglycemic events, the time below the range of 70 mg/dL (3.9 mmol/L) (TBR70) in regard to glucose, nor the time in range 70–180 mg/dL (3.9–10.0 mmol/L) (TIR).

However, the multivariable logistic regression model, which included the timing of the injection, the BI type, and the pre-dinner glucose level, identified the use of Gla-300 as independently associated with a higher TIR 70–180 during the night (adjusted R-squared: 0.22, $p < 0.001$).

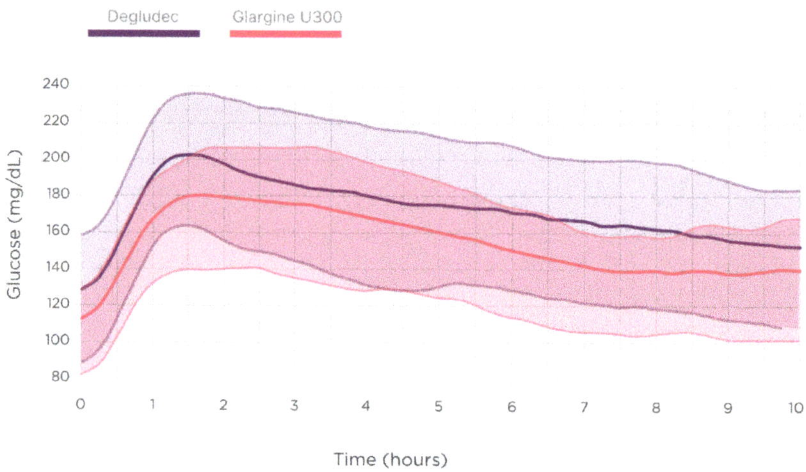

Figure 4. Nighttime glucose dynamics depending on the second-generation basal insulin type used (degludec vs. glargine U300).

3.5. Analysis According to the Use of a Second Insulin Injection (Correction Dose)

A second (correction) injection 1–5 h after the first rapid insulin dose at dinner was detected in 18.6% of the analyzed overnight periods (n = 144). This practice was associated with a higher number of hypoglycemia events (18.1 vs. 9.5%; $p = 0.003$), TBR70 (5.5 ± 14.2 vs. 3.0 ± 11.1%; $p = 0.003$), a glucose AUC of over 180 mg/dL (226.1 ± 257.8 vs. 178.0 ± 255.3 mg/dL × h; $p = 0.001$), and a lower TIR (56.0 ± 27.4 vs. 62.7 ± 29.6 mg/dL × h; $p = 0.004$).

3.6. Multivariable Analysis

The multivariable logistic regression model (Supplementary Table S1), which included the timing of the injection, the use of a second injection, and the rapid and basal insulin type, confirmed the following:

- The use of a URI was independently associated with a reduced risk (−52%) of glucose events < 70 mg/dL (3.9 mmol/L) (adjusted R-squared: 0.017; $p = 0.003$), and with a lower (−64%) TBR70 (adjusted R-squared: 0.016; $p = 0.003$);
- Not adding a second (correction) injection after dinner was independently associated with:
    - A reduction in overnight hypoglycemia: −47% glucose events < 70 mg/dL), adjusted R-squared: 0.017, $p = 0.003$, and −61% TBR70 (adjusted R-squared: 0.016; $p = 0.003$);
    - A reduction in overnight hyperglycemia: −21% glucose AUC of over 180 mg/dL (adjusted R-squared: 0.017; $p < 0.001$);
    - More time in the recommended glucose range 70–180 mg/dL (TIR): +6.7% (62.7 ± 29.6 mg/dL vs. 56.0 ± 27.4) (adjusted R-squared: 0.048; $p < 0.001$).

Additionally, using glargine U300 instead of degludec was associated with a higher TIR (70.7 vs. 58.5%, +12.2%) after adjustment according to the baseline glucose before dinner (adjusted R-squared: 0.22; $p < 0.001$).

4. Discussion

Individuals diagnosed with T1D are advised to maintain a stable and safe blood glucose level during nocturnal hours, striving to avoid both hyperglycemia and hypoglycemia. The timing of prandial pre-dinner rapid insulin administration and the use of an 'ultrarapid' insulin analog have been identified in our study as factors contributing to improved glucose control overnight. Additionally, our findings suggest that the use of Gla-300, a second-generation basal insulin, as opposed to degludec, is associated with a greater likelihood of achieving the recommended glucose levels during the nocturnal period.

Several studies have been conducted to determine the effect of prandial insulin timing on postprandial glucose dynamics [4,15]. However, less scientific evidence is available evaluating the relationship between the recommended timing for pre-dinner prandial insulin injections and the nocturnal glucose profile beyond the postprandial period. A study comparing preprandial vs. postprandial insulin glulisine in patients initiating a basal–bolus regimen for type 2 diabetes showed that nocturnal hypoglycemia rates were higher in the postprandial administration group [19]. Another randomized, open-labeled, cross-over trial found no statistically significant differences in nighttime hypoglycemic episodes between insulin aspart administered before or after meals in children and adolescents with T1D [25]. The PRONTO-T1D study in patients with type 1 diabetes showed that the rate of hypoglycemia was significantly lower for mealtime ultrarapid lispro (URLi) compared to post-meal URLi in the late postprandial period (>4 h after the meal) [26]. The data presented in this report showed higher nocturnal glucose (AUC of over 180 mg/dL) in subjects with delayed pre-dinner rapid insulin injections.

The use of second-generation rapid insulins, also known as 'ultrarapid' insulins, such as fast-acting insulin aspart (Fiasp©) and insulin ultra-rapid lispro (URLi), has been shown to improve postprandial glucose dynamics [27,28]. There is limited scientific evidence on how the type of rapid insulin injection before dinner affects the overall nighttime glucose profile, especially in people with T1D who are following an MDI regime. In the PRONTO-T1D CGM substudy, mealtime URLi decreased the nighttime TBR70 mg/dl compared with mealtime lispro [24]. However, the same study pointed out increasing glucose levels from evening to early morning in the group administered with mealtime URLi [24]. A meta-analysis of randomized controlled trials comparing faster-acting insulin aspart (Fiasp) to insulin aspart in people with diabetes mellitus showed that the nocturnal hypoglycemic episodes were not different [29].

Similarly, second-generation BI analogs, with longer, flatter, and less variable profiles, are currently available for use in the T1D population [16]. The studies comparing insulin degludec and insulin glargine 300 U/mL have shown conflicting results regarding their stability, variability, and clinical outcomes in the T1D population [17,30]. The present results indicate that, after adjusting according to the baseline glucose before dinner, using glargine U300 instead of degludec was associated with a higher TIR (70.7 vs. 58.5%, +12.2%). Our recently published study showed improved nocturnal CGM glucometrics with glargine 300 in comparison to IDeg-100 in patients with T1D in a real-world setting [18]. The present analysis supports these results.

According to a research study, a substantial number of individuals with T1D add a corrective insulin injection at least once a week, with 57% of adults and 65% of children reporting the need for it [3]. In the present study, 18.6% of the participants administered a corrective insulin dose following their evening meal. However, refraining from this practice could have a substantial impact on reducing overnight hypoglycemia and hyperglycemia, consequently leading to enhanced safety, glycemic control, and overall quality of life.

The necessity to validate and quantify the impact of insulin injection timing and type on glycemic control in real-world scenarios using CGM data, alongside the automatically recorded insulin dose and timing information, is crucial. Connected insulin pens and caps provide an opportunity to assemble this information and provide a more accurate picture of nocturnal glucose levels [9]. This study's main strengths lie in its real-world nature and the methodology used, which includes CGM and connected insulin pen cap data. However, its limitations include the fact that the meal content was not analyzed, which could have influenced the results. Additionally, it is important to note that the detection of glucose excursions relied on CGM data obtained from sensors in interstitial fluid, rather than on direct capture in relation to the beginning of the action of ingestion. There is a delay in detecting increases in glucose levels in interstitial fluid compared to glucose levels in the blood, especially during periods of rapid change [31]. Additionally, there is a delay between food ingestion and the appearance of glucose in the bloodstream. Previous studies have indicated that both delays typically average around ten minutes each [32]. Therefore, to calculate the actual time at which intake began based on the hyperglycemic excursion data from CGM data used in the present study, at least 10–20 min should be added. The absence of analysis according to the insulin dose could be taken as a limitation. However, the study research work hypothesis starts by assuming that the dose selection is made depending on the carbohydrate counting and carbohydrate/insulin ratio and insulin sensitivity factor previously set for every subject, as per the standard of care.

5. Conclusions

Delayed rapid insulin injection before dinner is frequent and causes hyperglycemia overnight. A considerable number of people with T1D add a second (correction) rapid insulin injection after dinner. It significantly increases both overnight hypoglycemia and hyperglycemia. The utilization of 'ultrarapid' insulin has shown promise in reducing the risk of nocturnal hypoglycemia. It is recommended that second-generation 'ultrarapid' insulins for individuals with T1D are considered to potentially optimize glucose control. However, further research is required to determine the optimal timing of insulin injections and the impact of different insulin types on nighttime glucose levels.

Supplementary Materials: The following supporting information can be downloaded at: https://www.mdpi.com/article/10.3390/biomedicines12071600/s1, Figure S1: Rate of hypoglycemia events < 70 mg/dL; Table S1, Multivariable regression model results.

Author Contributions: F.G.-P. designed and supervised the study, researched the data, analyzed the data, and wrote the manuscript. X.V. and C.A. supervised the study, researched the data, analyzed the data, and reviewed the manuscript. E.F.-R., L.C., P.P. and S.A. researched the data and reviewed the manuscript. A.V., J.P.-G., L.R.-V. and R.C. analyzed the data and reviewed the manuscript. All authors have read and agreed to the published version of the manuscript.

Funding: The study concept and design were developed, and the data collection, analysis, and interpretation performed, thanks to the unconditional efforts of all the investigators. No funding from the companies producing the mentioned products was received. The APC was funded by Insulcloud S.L.

Institutional Review Board Statement: The Research Ethics Committee at the Hospital General de Segovia, Segovia, Spain, approved the study (REC code 22-0252, 15 September 2022).

Informed Consent Statement: Informed consent was obtained from all the subjects involved in the study.

Data Availability Statement: The raw data supporting the conclusions in this article will be made available by the authors on request.

Acknowledgments: The authors acknowledge the editorial assistance of Nicole Quinn, Always English S.L.

Conflicts of Interest: Fernando Gómez-Peralta has taken part in advisory panels for Insulcloud S.L., Sanofi, and Novo Nordisk; has received research support from Sanofi, Novo Nordisk, Boehringer Ingelheim Pharmaceuticals, and Eli Lilly; and has acted as a speaker for Sanofi, Novo Nordisk, Boehringer Ingelheim Pharmaceuticals, AstraZeneca Pharmaceuticals LP, Bristol-Myers Squibb Co., and Eli Lilly. Cristina Abreu has received research support from Sanofi, Novo Nordisk, Boehringer Ingelheim Pharmaceuticals, and Eli Lilly, and has acted as a speaker for Sanofi, Novo Nordisk, Boehringer Ingelheim Pharmaceuticals, AstraZeneca Pharmaceuticals LP, and Bristol-Myers Squibb Co. Elsa Fernández-Rubio has acted as a speaker for Novo Nordisk, Lilly, and AstraZeneca Pharmaceuticals. Laura Cotovad has acted as a speaker for Sanofi, Novo Nordisk, Boehringer Ingelheim Pharmaceuticals, AstraZeneca Pharmaceuticals LP, and Eli Lilly. Pedro Pujante has received research support from Novo Nordisk, and has acted as a speaker for Sanofi, Novo Nordisk, Boehringer Ingelheim Pharmaceuticals, AstraZeneca Pharmaceuticals LP, and Eli Lilly. Sharona Azriel has acted as a speaker for Amgen, Abbott, Dexcom, Sanofi, Novo Nordisk, Novartis, Roche, Boehringer Ingelheim

Pharmaceuticals, AstraZeneca Pharmaceuticals LP, and Eli Lilly. Rosa Corcoy declares that she has received consultancy fees from Novo Nordisk and speakers' fees or support for attending meetings or taking part in research from Novo Nordisk, Lilly, Sanofi, Roche, Medtronic, and Novalab-Air liquide. The remaining authors have no conflicts of interest to disclose.

References

1. Campbell, M.D.; Walker, M.; Bracken, R.M.; Turner, D.; Stevenson, E.J.; Gonzalez, J.T.; Shaw, J.A.; West, D.J. Insulin Therapy and Dietary Adjustments to Normalize Glycemia and Prevent Nocturnal Hypoglycemia after Evening Exercise in Type 1 Diabetes: A Randomized Controlled Trial. *BMJ Open Diabetes Res. Care* **2015**, *3*, e000085. [CrossRef] [PubMed]
2. Jennum, P.; Stender-Petersen, K.; Rabøl, R.; Jørgensen, N.R.; Chu, P.-L.; Madsbad, S. The Impact of Nocturnal Hypoglycemia on Sleep in Subjects With Type 2 Diabetes. *Diabetes Care* **2015**, *38*, 2151–2157. [CrossRef]
3. Lane, W.; Lambert, E.; George, J.; Rathor, N.; Thalange, N. Exploring the Burden of Mealtime Insulin Dosing in Adults and Children With Type 1 Diabetes. *Clin. Diabetes* **2021**, *39*, 347–357. [CrossRef] [PubMed]
4. Mozzillo, E.; Franceschi, R.; Di Candia, F.; Ricci, A.; Leonardi, L.; Girardi, M.; Rosanio, F.M.; Marcovecchio, M.L. Optimal Prandial Timing of Insulin Bolus in Youths with Type 1 Diabetes: A Systematic Review. *J. Pers. Med.* **2022**, *12*, 2058. [CrossRef]
5. Slattery, D.; Amiel, S.A.; Choudhary, P. Optimal Prandial Timing of Bolus Insulin in Diabetes Management: A Review. *Diabet. Med.* **2018**, *35*, 306–316. [CrossRef] [PubMed]
6. Gómez-Peralta, F.; Valledor, X.; López-Picado, A.; Abreu, C.; Fernández-Rubio, E.; Cotovad, L.; Pujante, P.; García-Fernández, E.; Azriel, S.; Corcoy, R.; et al. Ultrarapid Insulin Use Can Reduce Postprandial Hyperglycemia and Late Hypoglycemia, Even in Delayed Insulin Injections: A Connected Insulin Cap-Based Real-World Study. *Diabetes Technol. Ther.* **2024**, *26*, 1–10. [CrossRef]
7. EMA Humalog. Available online: https://www.ema.europa.eu/en/medicines/human/EPAR/humalog (accessed on 16 January 2023).
8. EMA Fiasp. Available online: https://www.ema.europa.eu/en/medicines/human/EPAR/fiasp (accessed on 1 April 2023).
9. Tejera-Pérez, C.; Chico, A.; Azriel-Mira, S.; Lardiés-Sánchez, B.; Gomez-Peralta, F. Área de Diabetes-SEEN Connected Insulin Pens and Caps: An Expert's Recommendation from the Area of Diabetes of the Spanish Endocrinology and Nutrition Society (SEEN). *Diabetes Ther. Res. Treat. Educ. Diabetes Relat. Disord.* **2023**, *14*, 1077–1091. [CrossRef]
10. Gomez-Peralta, F.; Abreu, C.; Fernández-Rubio, E.; Cotovad, L.; Pujante, P.; Gaztambide, S.; Bellido, D.; Menéndez Torre, E.; Ruiz-Valdepeñas, S.; Bello, H.; et al. Efficacy of a Connected Insulin Pen Cap in People With Noncontrolled Type 1 Diabetes: A Multicenter Randomized Clinical Trial. *Diabetes Care* **2023**, *46*, 206–208. [CrossRef]
11. Martyn-Nemeth, P.; Schwarz Farabi, S.; Mihailescu, D.; Nemeth, J.; Quinn, L. Fear of Hypoglycemia in Adults with Type 1 Diabetes: Impact of Therapeutic Advances and Strategies for Prevention—A Review. *J. Diabetes Complicat.* **2016**, *30*, 167–177. [CrossRef]
12. Datye, K.A.; Boyle, C.T.; Simmons, J.; Moore, D.J.; Jaser, S.S.; Sheanon, N.; Kittelsrud, J.M.; Woerner, S.E.; Miller, K.M. Timing of Meal Insulin and Its Relation to Adherence to Therapy in Type 1 Diabetes. *J. Diabetes Sci. Technol.* **2018**, *12*, 349–355. [CrossRef]
13. Peyrot, M.; Rubin, R.R.; Kruger, D.F.; Travis, L.B. Correlates of Insulin Injection Omission. *Diabetes Care* **2010**, *33*, 240–245. [CrossRef] [PubMed]
14. Robinson, S.; Newson, R.S.; Liao, B.; Kennedy-Martin, T.; Battelino, T. Missed and Mistimed Insulin Doses in People with Diabetes: A Systematic Literature Review. *Diabetes Technol. Ther.* **2021**, *23*, 844–856. [CrossRef] [PubMed]
15. Cobry, E.; McFann, K.; Messer, L.; Gage, V.; VanderWel, B.; Horton, L.; Chase, H.P. Timing of Meal Insulin Boluses to Achieve Optimal Postprandial Glycemic Control in Patients with Type 1 Diabetes. *Diabetes Technol. Ther.* **2010**, *12*, 173–177. [CrossRef] [PubMed]
16. Bolli, G.B.; DeVries, J.H. New Long-Acting Insulin Analogs: From Clamp Studies to Clinical Practice. *Diabetes Care* **2015**, *38*, 541–543. [CrossRef]
17. Battelino, T.; Edelman, S.V.; Nishimura, R.; Bergenstal, R.M. Comparison of Second-Generation Basal Insulin Analogs: A Review of the Evidence from Continuous Glucose Monitoring. *Diabetes Technol. Ther.* **2021**, *23*, 20–30. [CrossRef]
18. Gomez-Peralta, F.; Chico Ballesteros, A.; Marco Martínez, A.; Pérez Corral, B.; Conget Donlo, I.; Fuentealba Melo, P.; Zaragozá Arnáez, F.; Matabuena Rodríguez, M. Insulin Glargine 300 U/Ml versus Insulin Degludec 100 U/Ml Improves Nocturnal Glycaemic Control and Variability in Type 1 Diabetes under Routine Clinical Practice: A Glucodensities-Based Post Hoc Analysis of the OneCare Study. *Diabetes Obes. Metab.* **2024**, *26*, 1993–1997. [CrossRef]
19. Pettus, J. Time to get serious about insulin timing. *Endocr. Pract. Off. J. Am. Coll. Endocrinol. Am. Assoc. Clin. Endocrinol.* **2017**, *23*, 503–505. [CrossRef]
20. McCall, A.L. Insulin Therapy and Hypoglycemia. *Endocrinol. Metab. Clin. North Am.* **2012**, *41*, 57–87. [CrossRef]
21. Gomez-Peralta, F.; Abreu, C.; Gomez-Rodriguez, S.; Ruiz, L. Insulclock: A Novel Insulin Delivery Optimization and Tracking System. *Diabetes Technol. Ther.* **2019**, *21*, 209–214. [CrossRef]
22. Harvey, R.A.; Dassau, E.; Zisser, H.; Seborg, D.E.; Doyle, F.J. Design of the Glucose Rate Increase Detector: A Meal Detection Module for the Health Monitoring System. *J. Diabetes Sci. Technol.* **2014**, *8*, 307–320. [CrossRef]
23. Danne, T.P.A.; Joubert, M.; Hartvig, N.V.; Kaas, A.; Knudsen, N.N.; Mader, J.K. Association Between Treatment Adherence and Continuous Glucose Monitoring Outcomes in People With Diabetes Using Smart Insulin Pens in a Real-World Setting. *Diabetes Care* **2024**, *47*, 995–1003. [CrossRef]

24. Battelino, T.; Alexander, C.M.; Amiel, S.A.; Arreaza-Rubin, G.; Beck, R.W.; Bergenstal, R.M.; Buckingham, B.A.; Carroll, J.; Ceriello, A.; Chow, E.; et al. Continuous Glucose Monitoring and Metrics for Clinical Trials: An International Consensus Statement. *Lancet Diabetes Endocrinol.* **2023**, *11*, 42–57. [CrossRef]
25. Danne, T.; Axel Schweitzer, M.; Keuthage, W.; Kipper, S.; Kretzschmar, Y.; Simon, J.; Wiedenmann, T.; Ziegler, R. Impact of Fast-Acting Insulin Aspart on Glycemic Control in Patients with Type 1 Diabetes Using Intermittent-Scanning Continuous Glucose Monitoring Within a Real-World Setting: The GoBolus Study. *Diabetes Technol. Ther.* **2021**, *23*, 203–212. [CrossRef] [PubMed]
26. Klaff, L.; Cao, D.; Dellva, M.A.; Tobian, J.; Miura, J.; Dahl, D.; Lucas, J.; Bue-Valleskey, J. Ultra Rapid Lispro Improves Postprandial Glucose Control Compared with Lispro in Patients with Type 1 Diabetes: Results from the 26-Week PRONTO-T1D Study. *Diabetes Obes. Metab.* **2020**, *22*, 1799–1807. [CrossRef] [PubMed]
27. Chow, E.; Chan, J.C.N. Targeting Postprandial Glucose Control Using Ultra-Rapid Insulins: Is Faster Better? *Sci. Bull.* **2022**, *67*, 2392–2394. [CrossRef]
28. Heise, T.; Piras de Oliveira, C.; Juneja, R.; Ribeiro, A.; Chigutsa, F.; Blevins, T. What Is the Value of Faster Acting Prandial Insulin? Focus on Ultra Rapid Lispro. *Diabetes Obes. Metab.* **2022**, *24*, 1689–1701. [CrossRef] [PubMed]
29. Pal, R.; Banerjee, M.; Bhadada, S.K. Glycaemic Efficacy and Safety of Mealtime Faster-Acting Insulin Aspart Administered by Injection as Compared to Insulin Aspart in People with Diabetes Mellitus: A Meta-Analysis of Randomized Controlled Trials. *Diabet. Med. J. Br. Diabet. Assoc.* **2021**, *38*, e14515. [CrossRef]
30. Owens, D.R.; S Bailey, T.; Fanelli, C.G.; Yale, J.-F.; Bolli, G.B. Clinical Relevance of Pharmacokinetic and Pharmacodynamic Profiles of Insulin Degludec (100, 200 U/mL) and Insulin Glargine (100, 300 U/mL)—A Review of Evidence and Clinical Interpretation. *Diabetes Metab.* **2019**, *45*, 330–340. [CrossRef]
31. Schmelzeisen-Redeker, G.; Schoemaker, M.; Kirchsteiger, H.; Freckmann, G.; Heinemann, L.; Del Re, L. Time Delay of CGM Sensors: Relevance, Causes, and Countermeasures. *J. Diabetes Sci. Technol.* **2015**, *9*, 1006–1015. [CrossRef]
32. Rossetti, P.; Quirós, C.; Moscardó, V.; Comas, A.; Giménez, M.; Ampudia-Blasco, F.J.; León, F.; Montaser, E.; Conget, I.; Bondia, J.; et al. Closed-Loop Control of Postprandial Glycemia Using an Insulin-on-Board Limitation Through Continuous Action on Glucose Target. *Diabetes Technol. Ther.* **2017**, *19*, 355–362. [CrossRef]

biomedicines

MDPI

Article

A Pilot Study on the Proteomics Profile of Serum Exosome-Enriched Extracellular Vesicles from Normal versus Individuals with Obesity-Related Insulin Resistance

Viswanathan Saraswathi [1,2], Weilun Ai [1,2], Vikas Kumar [3], Kanika Sharma [3], Thiyagarajan Gopal [1,2], Narendra Kumar [1,2], Harmeet Malhi [4], Tejasav Sehrawat [4] and Cyrus V. Desouza [1,2,*]

1 VA Nebraska-Western Iowa Health Care System, Omaha, NE 68105, USA; s.viswanathan@unmc.edu (V.S.); weilun.ai@unmc.edu (W.A.); thiyagarajan.clatr@sathyabama.ac.in (T.G.); narendra@dr.du.ac.in (N.K.)

2 Department of Internal Medicine, Division of Diabetes, Endocrinology, and Metabolism, University of Nebraska Medical Center, Omaha, NE 68198, USA

3 Department of Genetics Cell Biology & Anatomy, University of Nebraska Medical Center, Omaha, NE 68198, USA; vikas.kumar@unmc.edu (V.K.); kasharma@unmc.edu (K.S.)

4 Department of Internal Medicine, Division of Gastroenterology and Hepatology, Mayo Clinic College of Medicine, Rochester, MN 55905, USA; tejasav@gmail.com (T.S.)

* Correspondence: cdesouza@unmc.edu; Tel.: +1-402-995-5506; Fax: +1-402-449-0604

Abstract: Objective: Circulating exosome-enriched extracellular vesicles (EVs) have drawn considerable importance in obesity-related insulin-resistance (IR). We sought to compare the proteomics profile of serum exosomes from normal individuals and those with obesity and IR. Methods: We isolated serum exosomes from male subjects with obesity and insulin resistance (Ob-IR, HOMA-IR > 2.0) and lean/overweight insulin-sensitive (Normal (N), HOMA-IR < 2.0) individuals. The differential protein expression between the two groups was detected by a label-free quantitative mass spectrometry analysis followed by GO annotation and ingenuity pathway analysis (IPA). Results: We identified 23 upregulated and 46 downregulated proteins between Ob-IR and N groups. Some of these proteins are involved in altering insulin signaling (VPS13C, TBC1D32, TTR, and ADIPOQ), inflammation (NFκB and CRP), and B-cell proliferation/activation (IGLV4-69, IGKV1D-13, and IGHV4-28). GO analysis revealed that the differentially expressed proteins (DEPs) are mainly involved in regulating immune cell activation and are located in extracellular space. IPA analysis showed that top molecules mediating IR, inflammation and B-cell activation were upregulated in Ob-IR subjects compared to N subjects. Conclusions: Serum exosomal proteins can be used as biomarkers to identify the future risk of diabetes and a therapeutic target to prevent or slow down the progression of diabetes in high-risk individuals.

Keywords: obesity; insulin resistance; diabetes; proteomics

1. Introduction

The ever-rising worldwide prevalence of obesity and endocrine co-morbidities like insulin resistance (IR) makes it a public health problem [1,2]. Obesity-related IR has been a great challenge to clinicians and researchers due to the multifactorial nature of its pathogenesis affecting early diagnosis and effective therapeutic interventions [3]. Given that obesity and IR are vastly studied, it is known that multiple integrative approaches are needed to understand their complex biochemical and pathophysiological mechanisms. Obesity-related IR is a major risk factor for the development of type 2 diabetes (T2D), but the underlying mechanisms by which obesity-related IR progresses to T2D remains unclear. Moreover, glucose tolerance tests and hyperinsulinemic and euglycemic clamp studies are needed to confirm IR. However, these tests are not performed routinely to identify individuals with a high risk for developing T2D.

Recently, exosomes or extracellular vesicles (EVs) have been proven to act as paracrine communicators between cells, which has attracted the attention of many scientists. Exosomes play important roles in cell–cell communication and participate in several pathophysiological processes [4]. Exosomes are small extracellular membrane vesicles that are secreted by cells and contain proteins, lipids, and nucleic acids that can be taken up by other cells. They have been widely studied for their role as biomarkers or in the pathogenesis of various diseases.

Regarding obesity and its co-morbidities, several lines of evidence suggest that exosomal cargos, in particular, microRNAs, are altered in the plasma and/or adipose tissue (AT) of humans and are shown to participate in the development of IR (reviewed in [5]). However, only a few studies have shown that the protein cargo of exosomes are also altered in obesity. For example, Ge et al. have shown that circulating exosomes from non-diabetic individuals with obesity showed lower levels of omentin 1 which has been shown to be a mediator linking IR with β-cell function [6]. Another study has shown that transforming growth factor beta 1 (TGFBI) in circulating EVs may facilitate monitoring the T2D status in obese patients, and EV-mimecan (*aka* osteoglycin) may be useful to track visceral obesity [7]. Proteomics analysis of exosomes from mouse plasma has revealed an upregulation of two proteins (immunoglobulins) and downregulation of 10 proteins (14-3-3 protein isoforms, proteasome subunits, and others) in mice with diet-induced obesity [8]. Proteomics analysis has also been performed in adipocytes of human subjects which revealed that changes in proteins related to lipid metabolism and unfolded protein response discriminate insulin-resistant and insulin-sensitive individuals with unequal adiposity [9]. In addition to serving as a biomarker, the exosomal proteomics profile may also reveal the therapy response. For example, in a recent study, plasma exosomal proteomics cargo has been shown to alter in response to lifestyle interventions in adolescents with hepatic steatosis [10].

Research on exosome proteomes in obesity-related IR is still in its early stages, and more studies are needed to fully understand the role of exosomal cargo proteins as biomarkers or therapeutic targets to prevent/manage T2D in humans. Our study aims to investigate the differential expression of serum exosomal proteins in normal subjects (N) and individuals with obesity and IR. Using the label-free quantitative mass spectrometry (MS)-based proteomic approach, we analyzed the differential expression of serum exosomal proteins in N and Ob-IR groups.

2. Methodology

2.1. Study Design and Subjects

In this study, serum samples from 4 male subjects with obesity and IR and 4 lean/overweight insulin-sensitive men were used for exosome isolation. All blood samples for serum isolation were obtained while subjects were in a fasting state. The following inclusion and exclusion criteria were applied while choosing the subjects for the study. *Inclusion criteria.* (1) Age 19 to 75; (2) lean/Over-weight insulin sensitive: BMI between 20–29.9 kg/m^2 and no insulin resistance (HOMA-IR < 2.0); obesity and insulin resistance: BMI 30–55 kg/m^2 and with HOMA-IR $\geq$ 2; and (3) subjects should be on a stable dose of any medications for at least two months. *Exclusion Criteria.* (1) Patients currently taking NSAIDs more than 3/week on a prescription basis or taking a daily dose of NSAID; (2) history of diabetes and patients taking diabetes medications as these drugs may alter adipose tissue metabolic functions; (3) history of uncontrolled hypertension defined as >160 systolic and 95 diastolic on medication; (4) history of renal disease with GFR < 60; (5) history of hepatic failure or AST/ALT > three times the normal range; (6) patients with active cancer within the last 2 years except for skin cancers; (7) patients with acute illness needing hospitalization within the last 2 months; (8) patients with acute inflammation; (9) patients with cardiovascular events such as myocardial infarction, stroke, amputation, unstable angina within the last six months; (10) pregnancy; and (11) presence of psychosis, suicidal ideations, untreated major depression, dementia and history of stimulant dependence/substance abuse. The study was approved by the Institutional Review Board at the VA Nebraska-Western Iowa Health Care System (NWIHCS). All participants gave informed consent.

2.2. Isolation of Exosomes

The ultracentrifugation (UC) method has been widely used for proteomics analysis of exosomes because it provides high-purity exosomes. We isolated exosomes using the UC method as reported earlier with slight modifications [11]. Briefly, 1.5 mL of the serum samples was centrifuged at 2000× *g* for 15 min at 4 °C. Supernatant was diluted 1:3 volumes in sterile phosphate-buffered saline (PBS) and centrifuged at 2000× *g* for 30 min at 4 °C. The supernatants were centrifuged at 10,000× *g* for 45 min at 4 °C to remove larger vesicles. Prior to ultrafiltration, samples were filtered through a 0.45 µm filter. The supernatant was centrifuged at 100,000× *g* for 2 h at 4 °C using a Beckman ultracentrifuge. The pellet was resuspended in PBS, filtered again (0.45 µm) and centrifuged at 100,000× *g* for 2 h at 4 °C. The pellet (containing exosomes) was resuspended in PBS, aliquoted and kept at −80 °C until further use.

2.3. Nanoparticle Tracking Analysis

An aliquot of freshly isolated exosomes or samples stored at 4 °C overnight was used for nanoparticle tracking analysis (NTA) to determine the size distribution of exosomes using the NanoSight NS300 (Malvern, Malvern, UK) with a 405 nm laser instrument. Samples were analyzed using the basic control settings: infusion Rate, 20 µL/min; detection threshold, 5; and camera level, 10–15. Data were analyzed using the NTA 3.0 software.

2.4. Electron Microscopic Imaging of Exosomes

Morphologies of exosomes were determined using the transmission electron microscopy (TEM) Electron microscopic studies were carried out at the University of Nebraska Medical Center's electron microscopy core facility using FEI Tecnai G2 Spirit transmission electron microscope (Field Electron and Ion Company, Hillsboro, OR, USA) operated at 80 kv.

2.5. Label-Free Quantitative Mass Spectrometry and Data Analysis

Serum exosomes were lysed using the RIPA buffer (J62524.AE, Thermo Fisher Scientific, Waltham, MA, USA) containing protease and a phosphatase inhibitor cocktail (78444, Thermo Fisher Scientific). For proteomics analysis, 50 µg of protein per sample from four biological replicates per group was taken and the detergent was removed by chloroform/methanol extraction. The protein pellet was re-suspended in 100 mM ammonium bicarbonate and digested with MS-grade Pierce trypsin (Thermo Fisher scientific, Waltham, MA, USA) overnight at 37 °C following reduction with 10 mM DTT at 56 °C for 30 min and alkylation using 50 mM iodoacetamide at RT for 25 min. Peptides were cleaned with PepClean C18 spin columns (Thermo) and were re-suspended in 2% acetonitrile (ACN) and 0.1% formic acid (FA). Each sample containing 500 ng of protein was loaded onto trap column Acclaim PepMap 100 75 µm × 2 cm C18 LC columns (Thermo Scientific™) at a flow rate of 4 µL/min and then separated with a Thermo RSLC Ultimate 3000 (Thermo Scientific™) on a Thermo Easy-Spray PepMap RSLC C18 75 µm × 50 cm C-18 2 µm column (Thermo Scientific™). A step gradient of 4–25% solvent B (0.1% FA in 80% ACN) from 10 to 100 min and 25–45% solvent B for 100 to 130 min at 300 nL/min was used at 50 °C with a 155 min total run time. Eluted peptides were analyzed using a Thermo Orbitrap Exploris 480 (Thermo Scientific™) mass spectrometer in a data-dependent acquisition mode. A survey full scan MS (from m/z 350–1200) was acquired in the Orbitrap with a resolution of 60,000. The Normalized AGC target for MS1 was set as 300% and the ion filling time as 25 ms. The most intense ions with charge states 2–6 were isolated in 3 s cycle and fragmented using the higher-energy collisional dissociation (HCD) fragmentation method with a 30% normalized collision energy detected at a mass resolution of 15,000 at 200 m/z. The AGC target for MS/MS was set as 50% and the ion filling time set to auto for 30 s with a 10 ppm mass window. Protein identification was performed by searching MS/MS data against the swiss-prot Homo sapiens protein database downloaded in December 2022 using the in-house PEAKS X + DB search engine. The search was set up for full tryptic peptides with a maximum of two missed cleavage sites. Acetylation of protein N-terminus and oxidized methionine were included as variable modifications and carbamidomethylation of cysteine was set as fixed modification. The precursor mass tolerance threshold was set at 10 ppm and the maximum fragment mass error was 0.02 Da. The significance threshold of the ion score was calculated based on a false discovery rate of $\leq$1%. Quantitative data analysis was performed using progenesis QI proteomics 4.2 (Nonlinear Dynamics, Waters Corporation, Milford, MA, USA). Proteomics data have been deposited to the MassIVE repository, a member of the ProteomeXchange Consortium (PXD045735).

2.6. Western Blot Analysis

Exosome lysates were subjected to SDS-PAGE under reducing and heat-denaturing conditions using Bis-Tris Plus Mini Protein Gels (4–12%, NW04125BOX, Thermo Fisher Scientific) and MOPS SDS Running Buffer (B000102, Thermo Fisher Scientific). Then, the proteins were transferred to the 0.2 μm PVDF membrane (ISEQ00010, Millipore, Burlington, MA, USA) using the transfer buffer (BT0006, Thermo Fisher Scientific) containing 10% methanol. After transferring, the membrane was incubated with 5% fat-free milk powder for 1 h at room temperature. After blocking by 5% fat-free milk powder, membranes were incubated in appropriate primary antibodies overnight at 4 °C to detect target proteins. The primary antibodies against CD9 (10626D, Invitrogen, Waltham, MA, USA), flotillin 1 (18634, Cell Signaling Technology, Danvers, MA, USA), GM130 (12480, Cell Signaling Technology), Calnexin (2433S, Cell Signaling Technology), VPS13C (28676-1-AP, Proteintech, Rosemont, IL, USA), adiponectin (21613-1-AP, Proteintech), and immunoglobulin κ light chain (14678-1-AP), were used for immuno-detection at 1:1000 dilution. After washing three times with TBS buffer containing 0.5% Tween-20 (TBST), membranes were incubated with anti-rabbit (7074, Cell Signaling) or anti-mouse (7076, Cell Signaling) secondary antibody conjugated to HRP-linked antibody at 1:5000 dilution or 1 h at room temperature. Secondary antibody signals were revealed by enhanced chemiluminescence reagent (1705062, Biorad, Hercules, CA, USA). To normalize the protein bands with total protein, exosome samples were run on a gel. The gel was fixed in 50% methanol containing 10% acetic acid for 1 h. Then, the protein gel was subjected to staining with 0.1% Coomassie Brilliant Blue R-250 (1610400, Biorad, Hercules, CA, USA) for 3 h. The gel was then de-stained using 50% methanol plus 10% acetic acid for 2 h.

2.7. Statistical Analysis

Statistical analysis was performed using the one-way ANOVA and the Benjamini-Hochberg (BH) method was used to adjust the p values for multiple-testing-caused false discovery rate (FDR). The adjusted $p \leq 0.05$ was considered significant. Various plots such as PCA, Venn diagram, and volcano plot were generated using Partek Genomics Suite 7.0. GO pathway enrichment was used to analyze the proteins involved in the biological process, cellular component, and molecular function. Western blot data were analyzed by one-tailed Student's t-test.

3. Results

3.1. Characteristics of Study Groups

The anthropometric and clinical characteristics of the study subjects are summarized in Table 1. As expected, the BMI and HOMA-IR used in the selection of the two groups are different between the two groups. In addition, body weight, diastolic blood pressure, glucose, insulin, and alanine aminotransferase (ALT) were significantly higher in Ob-IR versus N subjects. No change in other variables including total cholesterol, triglycerides, LDL cholesterol, and HDL cholesterol were noted.

Table 1. Baseline characteristics of study participants.

Measurement	Normal (n = 4)	Obese-IR (n = 4)	p Value
Age (years)	44 ± 4.2	44 ± 6.2	0.9745
Height (in)	98 ± 26.6	71 ± 0.7	0.3337
Weight (lb)	176 ± 29.5	283 ± 15.1 *	0.0179
Body mass index (kg/m^2)	28 ± 0.6	40 ± 2.4 **	0.0026
Systolic BP (mmHg)	121± 7.5	134 ± 4.7	0.2181
Diastolic BP (mmHg)	77 ± 2.3	88 ± 3.1 *	0.0296
Insulin (µIU/mL)	5 ± 0.4	18 ± 2 ***	0.0008
Glucose (mg/dL)	91 ± 2.7	114 ± 6.5 *	0.0178
HOMA-IR	1 ± 0.1	5 ± 0.6 ***	0.0009
Total cholesterol (mg/dL)	179 ± 9.7	194 ± 11.7	0.3618
Triglycerides (mg/dL)	128 ± 28.1	136 ± 11.4	0.3618
LDL cholesterol (mg/dL)	107 ± 11.1	118 ± 10.6	0.7947
HDL cholesterol (mg/dL)	46 ± 6.3	49 ± 2	0.5003
BUN (mg/dL)	15 ± 0.8	16 ± 2.3	0.6932
Creatinine (mg/dL)	1 ± 0.1	1 ± 0.1	0.5601
Sodium (mmol/L)	139 ± 0.5	139 ± 0.5	0.4881
Potassium (mmol/L)	4 ± 0.1	4 ± 0.1	0.4842
Calcium (mg/dL)	9 ± 0.1	9 ± 0.3	>0.9999
CO2 (mmol/L)	28 ± 0.5	26 ± 1.1	0.1055
Chloride (mmol/L)	103 ± 0.6	104 ± 1.4	0.5334
Alkaline phosphatase (U/L)	59 ± 5.	80 ± 9.5	0.1016
ALT (U/L)	32 ± 2.4	57 ± 10 *	0.0474
AST (U/L)	33 ± 1.8	43 ± 9	0.2940
Bilirubin (mg/dL)	2 ± 0.7	1 ± 0	0.1908

Values are mean ± SEM. BP, blood pressure; HOMA-IR, Homeostatic Model Assessment for Insulin Resistance; ALT, alkaline phosphatase; AST, acid phosphatase. * $p < 0.05$, ** $p < 0.01$, *** $p < 0.001$ vs. normal subjects.

3.2. Isolation and Characterization of Serum Exosomes in Obesity-Related IR

The exosomes were isolated from the serum samples by ultracentrifugation. NTA was used to measure the size and concentration based on the tracking of Brownian movement. The mean size (196 ± 33.7 and 228 ± 35.7 in N and Ob-IR groups, respectively) and concentration ($4.78 \times 10^8 \pm 2.66 \times 10^8$ and $1.68 \times 10^7 \pm 3.91 \times 10^6$ in N and Ob-IR groups, respectively) did not vary significantly between groups. A representative NTA plot for each group is shown in Figure 1A. TEM was utilized to further characterize the morphology of the exosomes. The exosomes appeared as round vesicles of heterogenous sizes (Figure 1B). Next, we performed the Western blot analysis to detect exosome markers. The exosome markers including CD9 and flotillin 1 were detected in our samples. On the other hand, calnexin and GM130, a marker of endoplasmic reticulum and Golgi, respectively, were not altered, indicating that our samples mostly contained EVs (Figure 1C). Taken together, these results demonstrated that the exosomes were successfully isolated from the serum with high purity and well-characterized by various methods.

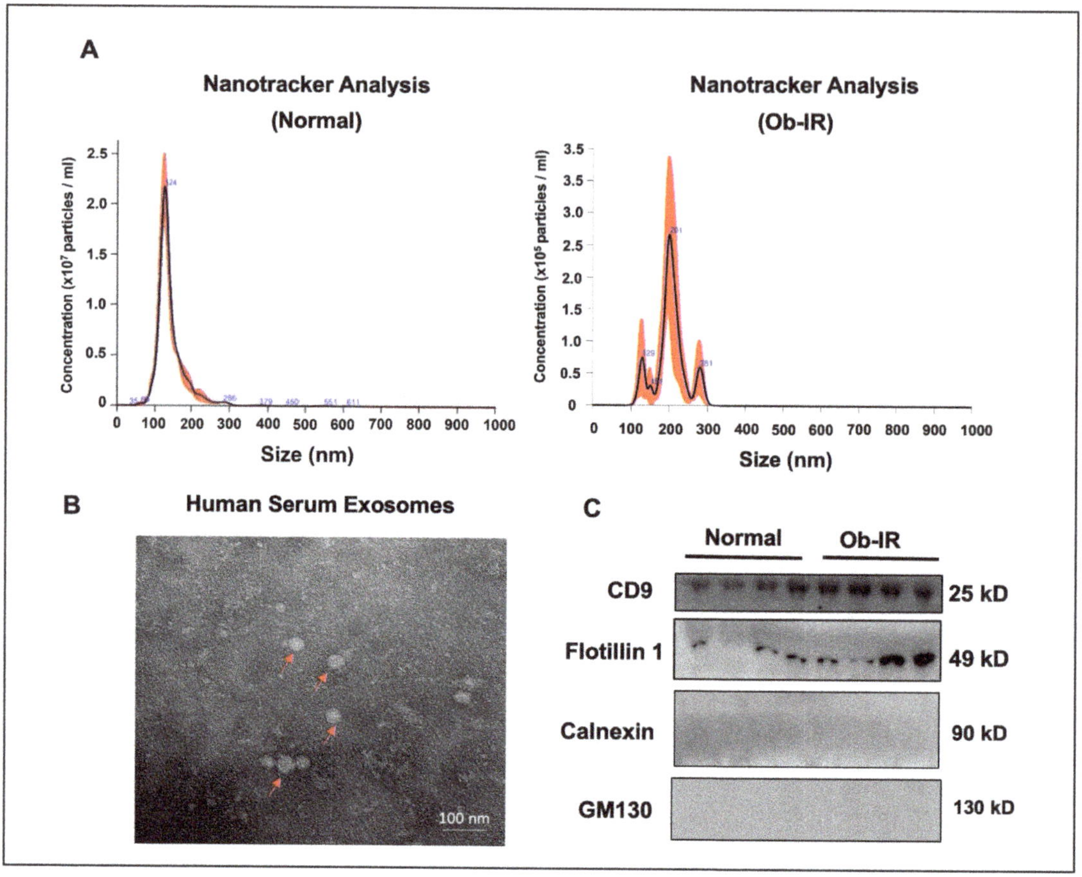

Figure 1. Characterization of exosome-enriched extracellular vesicles (EVs) isolated from human serum. (**A**) Representative histogram of particle concentration and size distribution profile of EVs determined by the nanotracker analysis (NTA). (**B**) Electron microscopic picture of serum exosomes. (**C**) Western blot analysis showing exosome markers.

3.3. Identification of DEPs between Ob-IR and N Groups

We next performed the proteomics analysis on the exosome samples. The principal component analysis (PCA) was performed for assessing the quality of data which shows distinct clustering of the proteome between groups (Figure 2A). A total of 503 and 504 proteins were profiled in N and Ob-IR groups, respectively. The Venn diagram shows that 108 proteins are present only in the normal group and 109 proteins are found only in the Ob-IR group whereas 395 proteins are present in both groups (Figure 2B). Only proteins detected in both groups were used for further analysis. We noted that 69 exosomal proteins were differentially expressed (23 upregulated and 46 downregulated) at an adjusted $p < 0.05$. The DEPs are depicted in a volcano plot (Figure 2C).

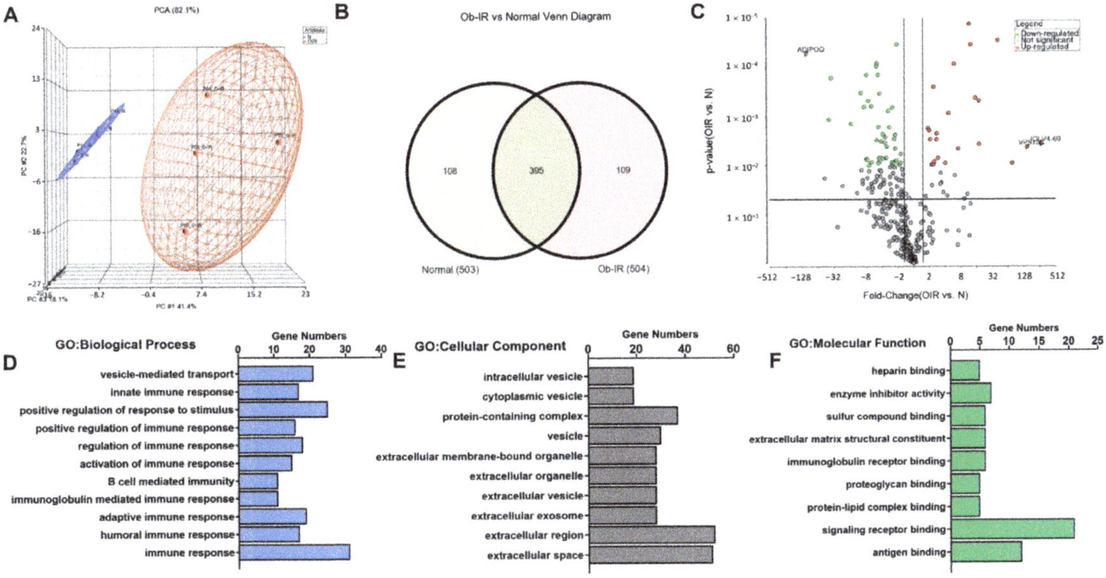

Figure 2. Proteomic analysis of serum-derived exosomes. (**A**) Principle Component Analysis plot. (**B**) The Venn diagram displays the distribution of exosomal proteins between normal subjects (N) and individuals with obesity and insulin resistance (Ob-IR). (**C**) Volcano plot showed the significantly altered proteins between the N and Ob-IR groups. The ratio of expression of these proteins in Ob-IR vs. N are plotted against the p value. The red and green dots indicate the up- and downregulated proteins, respectively. The gray dots indicate proteins that had no significant difference. (**D–F**) The gene ontology (GO) enrichment analyses of differentially expressed proteins (DEPs). GO enrichment analysis of DEPs in the (**D**) biological process, (**E**) cellular component, and (**F**) the molecular function categories. All significantly enriched GO terms ($p < 0.05$) involving DEPs are displayed.

3.4. GO Enrichment Analysis

All the DEPs were subjected to GO enrichment analysis which shows the enrichment of genes in three categories: (1) biological processes, (2) cellular component, and (3) molecular function (Figure 2D–F). Regarding biological processes, most of the DEPs were enriched in the humoral and adaptive immune response, immune system process, and B-cell-mediated immunity. DEPs enriched in the cellular component were those present in the extracellular region, extracellular space, extracellular vesicle, extracellular exosome, and cell periphery, indicating that the DEPs are present mainly in the exosome fraction. DEPs regulating the molecular functions are mostly enriched in signaling receptor binding, antigen binding, and immunoglobulin receptor binding, suggesting an altered immune response between groups. Together the GO enrichment analysis shows that DEPs are mostly enriched in exosomes and modulate processes regulating the immune response.

A detailed list of DEPs with fold changes and p-values are shown in Table 2. Regarding specific markers associated with IR and T2D risk, we noted a striking increase in the vacuolar protein-sorting 13 homolog C (VPS13C, 152-fold, $p = 4.23 \times 10^{-3}$) in Ob-IR subjects compared to N individuals. In addition, the levels of TBC1 Domain Family Member 32 (TBC1D32, 17.75-fold, $p = 4.84 \times 10^{-4}$) and transthyretin (TTR, 1.9-fold, $p = 1.75 \times 10^{-3}$) were increased in the Ob-IR group. On the other hand, a profound reduction in proteins improving insulin sensitivity, in particular, adiponectin, an insulin-sensitizing adipokine, was seen in Ob-IR compared to N subjects (ADIPOQ, −101.996-fold, $p = 5.14 \times 10^{-5}$). Further, we noted a reduction in the levels of ficolin 3 (FCN3, −1.86-fold, $p = 9.7 \times 10^{-3}$) and zinc-α2 glycoprotein (AZGP1, −1.74-fold, $p = 6.0 \times 10^{-3}$) which are known for their role in promoting insulin sensitivity. We have also shown the abundance of these proteins in individual samples in Figure 3.

Table 2. Differentially expressed proteins in exosomes.

Accession	Gene Names	p Value	Log Fold Change (OIR vs. N)	Log2 Protein Abundance (N)	Log2 Protein Abundance (Ob-IR)
Q15848	ADIPOQ	5.14×10^{-5}	−101.996	20.3359	13.6635
P04114	APOB	0.00264854	−3.43471	27.3783	25.5981
P02655	APOC2	0.00779055	−7.66736	26.2571	23.3183
P02656	APOC3	9.54×10^{-5}	−5.07365	28.3374	25.9944
P02649	APOE	0.00325172	−4.16134	25.9174	23.8604
P29972	AQP1	0.00884853	−6.3104	18.9832	16.3254
P25311	AZGP1	0.00600575	−1.74242	24.1581	23.3571
P06276	BCHE	0.0030989	−5.01385	22.5725	20.2466
P02747	C1QC	0.00909716	−1.75507	26.6362	25.8247
P07358	C8B	0.00922879	−2.36558	23.9494	22.7072
O43866	CD5L	0.00802754	−4.32778	27.1963	25.0827
P00751	CFB	0.00724882	−3.33718	26.8489	25.1102
Q92496	CFHR4	0.007138	−3.31359	20.048	18.3196
Q9BXR6	CFHR5	0.000347282	−4.41694	17.1679	15.0249
P49747	COMP	0.0101491	−7.1216	17.3908	14.5586
Q96IY4	CPB2	0.000335808	−9.83874	22.2431	18.9446
Q9NQ79	CRTAC1	0.000143608	−7.74126	18.6834	15.7309
P00748	F12	0.000142249	−4.73022	24.3553	22.1134
P12259	F5	0.000641014	−8.68021	21.7898	18.6721
Q15485	FCN2	0.00739225	−3.87146	21.6952	19.7424
O75636	FCN3	0.00974348	−1.8598	24.6062	23.7111
P02671	FGA	0.0034269	−3.49751	23.4074	21.6011
P02751	FN1	0.00461717	−2.20996	26.129	24.985
P69905	HBA2	0.00166529	−2.87522	29.2208	27.6971
P68871	HBB	0.00415203	−3.23454	30.1874	28.4938
A0A0C4DH39	IGHV1-58	8.15×10^{-5}	−4.95533	20.0733	17.7643
A0A0B4J2H0	IGHV1-69D	3.37×10^{-5}	−2.08215	21.1561	20.098
P0DP01	IGHV1-8	0.00231204	−3.85637	19.9576	18.0103
A0A0C4DH32	IGHV3-20	0.000622795	−6.30424	21.2174	18.5611
P0DP08	IGHV4-38-2	0.00806797	−2.13237	19.4472	18.3548
P01824	IGHV4-39	0.00806797	−2.13237	23.1349	22.0425
P01834	IGKC	0.00290762	−2.3229	31.4403	30.2244
P01699	IGLV1-44	0.00116193	−38.3801	22.3701	17.1078
P01718	IGLV3-27	0.00911879	−4.65614	21.3846	19.1654
P19652	ORM2	0.00876663	−2.49516	27.8332	26.514
P0DOX7	P0DOX7	0.00290762	−2.3229	30.8636	29.6477
P01833	PIGR	0.00921069	−2.57522	20.6286	19.2639
Q01970	PLCB3	0.000474843	−7.22989	24.0273	21.1733
P00747	PLG	0.000771804	−2.99473	26.7129	25.1304
P55058	PLTP	0.0071463	−4.47115	21.9089	19.7483
P08185	SERPINA6	0.00140644	−14.7621	24.3355	20.4517
Q13103	SPP2	0.00746342	−7.86724	18.2868	15.311
P27105	STOM	0.00238428	−2.2169	19.9259	18.7774
P02787	TF	0.000659321	−2.53408	31.079	29.7375
P02786	TFRC	0.00163401	−4.66298	20.696	18.4747
P07996	THBS1	0.000165745	−35.3192	21.977	16.8346
P02652	APOA2	0.00926537	78.3317	20.577	26.8685
P02748	C9	0.00195931	2.01393	23.9378	24.9478
P15169	CPN1	0.000251491	2.4278	21.0871	22.3667
P22792	CPN2	0.00984944	2.22805	24.357	25.5128

Table 2. *Cont.*

Accession	Gene Names	*p* Value	Log Fold Change (OIR vs. N)	Log2 Protein Abundance (N)	Log2 Protein Abundance (Ob-IR)
P02741	CRP	0.000866202	4.71278	19.7541	21.9907
Q4L180	FILIP1L	1.32×10^{-5}	11.5713	20.4921	24.0246
P62805	H4C16	0.00372999	17.8419	13.495	17.6522
A0A0B4J1V6	IGHV3-73	0.00917639	4.07111	20.1666	22.192
A0A0C4DH34	IGHV4-28	8.56×10^{-5}	6.05381	18.8953	21.4932
A0A0B4J2D9	IGKV1D-13	3.45×10^{-5}	12.4358	21.8398	25.4763
A0A0C4DH24	IGKV6-21	0.00225202	2.80145	21.107	22.5931
P01706	IGLV2-11	0.00978276	2.39056	22.1182	23.3756
A0A075B6H9	IGLV4-69	0.00365724	280.396	10.7438	18.8752
A0A0B4J1Y8	IGLV9-49	0.00467814	7.21009	16.4558	19.3058
Q06033	ITIH3	0.00727725	2.96715	25.4247	26.9938
P19838	NFKB1	0.000426808	15.1041	22.7597	26.6766
O60313	OPA1	2.83×10^{-5}	40.72	13.8771	19.2248
P22891	PROZ	0.00859579	2.50669	17.3095	18.6352
P20742	PZP	0.00298606	2.1067	23.7413	24.8163
Q96NH3	TBC1D32	0.000483639	17.7464	14.9629	19.1124
P02766	TTR	0.00174771	1.90673	27.9756	28.9067
Q709C8	VPS13C	0.004229	152.354	15.4026	22.6539
P04275	VWF	0.00300269	2.78745	20.2546	21.7336

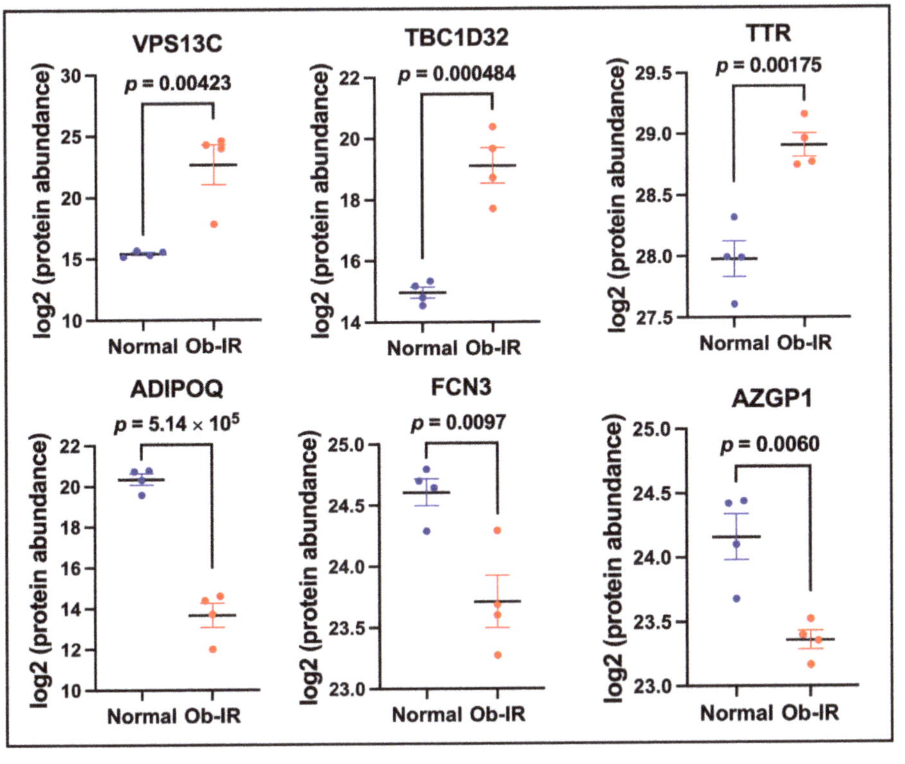

Figure 3. Markers of insulin resistance in exosomes. Proteins altering insulin signaling and/or glucose uptake in exosomes from normal and Ob-IR subjects. Values are mean ± SEM of 4 samples per group.

Inflammatory pathways play an important role in the development of T2D. Accordingly, we noted an increase in the levels of nuclear factor κB1 (NFκB1, 15-fold, $p = 4.3 \times 10^{-4}$), C-reactive protein (CRP, 4.4-fold, $p = 8.66 \times 10^{-4}$), and complement 9 (C9, 2.01-fold, 2.0×10^{-3}) in EVs from Ob-IR compared to N subjects. As shown in Figure 4, the abundance of these proteins is higher in Ob-IR subjects compared to N subjects.

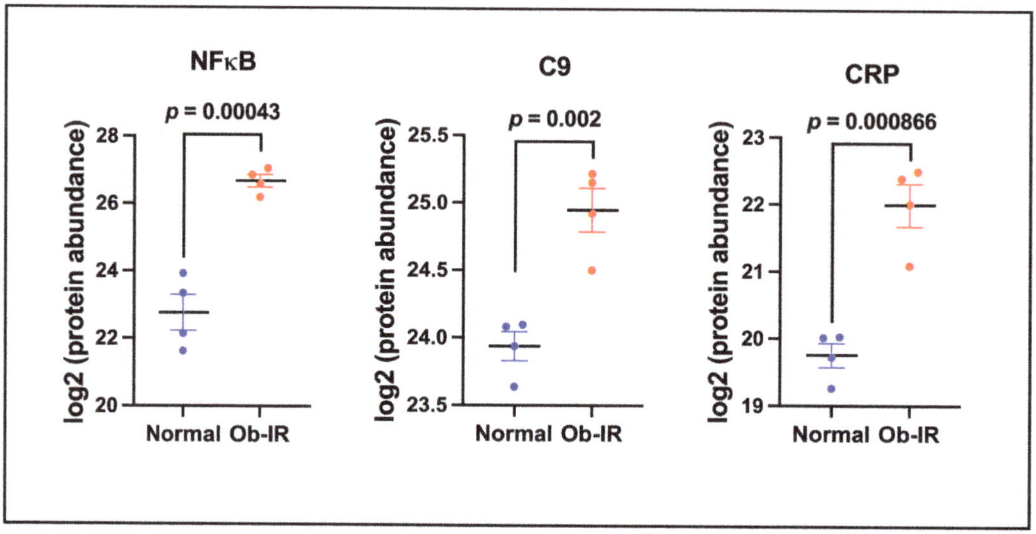

Figure 4. Markers of inflammatory response in exosomes. Proteins altering inflammation in exosomes from normal and Ob-IR subjects. Values are mean ± SEM of 4 samples per group.

Intriguingly, markers of immune cell development/activation showed a prominent increase in EVs from Ob-IR individuals compared to controls. In particular, proteins involved in B-cell development/B-cell receptor signaling were significantly higher in Ob-IR subjects compared to N individuals. For example, immunoglobulin lambda variable 4-69 (IGLV4-69) showed a 280-fold increase in Ob-IR subjects compared to the control ($p = 3.66 \times 10^{-3}$). Moreover, the levels of many other immunoglobulin chains including IGLV9-49 (7.2-fold, $p = 4.7 \times 10^{-3}$), immunoglobulin kappa variable 1D-13 (IGKV1D-13, 12.4-fold, $p = 3.45 \times 10^{-5}$), IGKV6-21 (2.8-fold, $p = 2.25 \times 10^{-3}$), immunoglobulin heavy variable 3-73 (IGHV3-73, 4.1-fold, $p = 9.2 \times 10^{-3}$) and IGHV4-28 (6.1-fold, $p = 8.56 \times 10^{-5}$) were significantly upregulated in the Ob-IR group compared to the N group. We also noted a decrease in the levels of some immunoglobulin chains including IGLV1-44 (−38.38-fold, $p = 1.16 \times 10^{-3}$) and IGHV1-58 (−4.95533-fold, $p = 8.15 \times 10^{-5}$). The distribution of protein abundance for these markers among different samples in each group is shown in Figure 5. Together, these data show that several markers involved in B-cell development/activation are significantly altered between N and Ob-IR subjects, providing evidence for the role of a novel player in obesity-related IR.

The protein levels of top-altered markers were confirmed by Western blot analyses (Figure 6A). These data show that VPS13C was upregulated in Ob-IR subjects compared to the N group. For B-cell activation, we performed the Western blot analysis for immunoglobulin κ light chain which also showed an upregulation in Ob-IR subjects. In line with our proteomics data, our Western blot analysis showed a decrease in adiponectin in the exosomes derived from Ob-IR subjects compared to N subjects. The proteins detected by Western blot analysis were normalized to total protein in each lane measured by the Coomassie brilliant blue staining of gels (Figure 6B) and the quantification data is shown in Figure 6C.

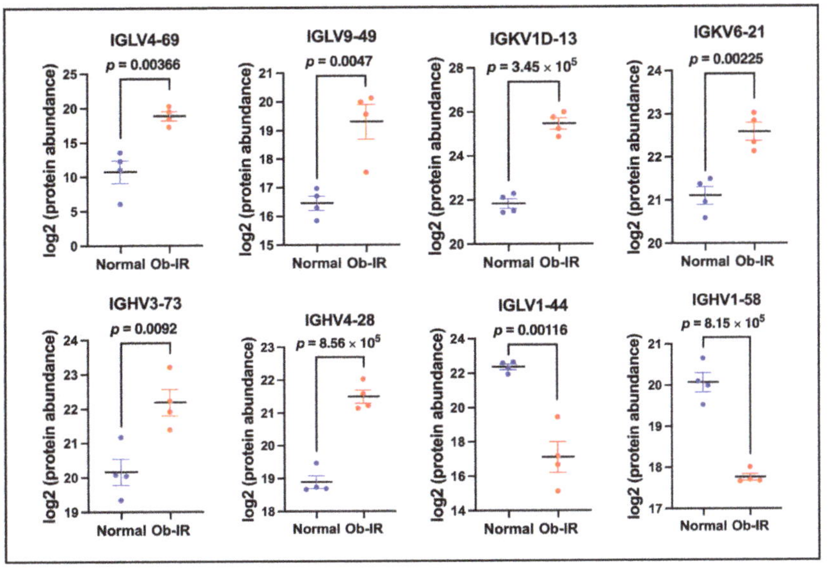

Figure 5. Markers of B cell proliferation/activation. Proteins representing markers of B-cell development and/or activation in exosomes from normal and Ob-IR subjects. Values are mean ± SEM of 4 samples per group.

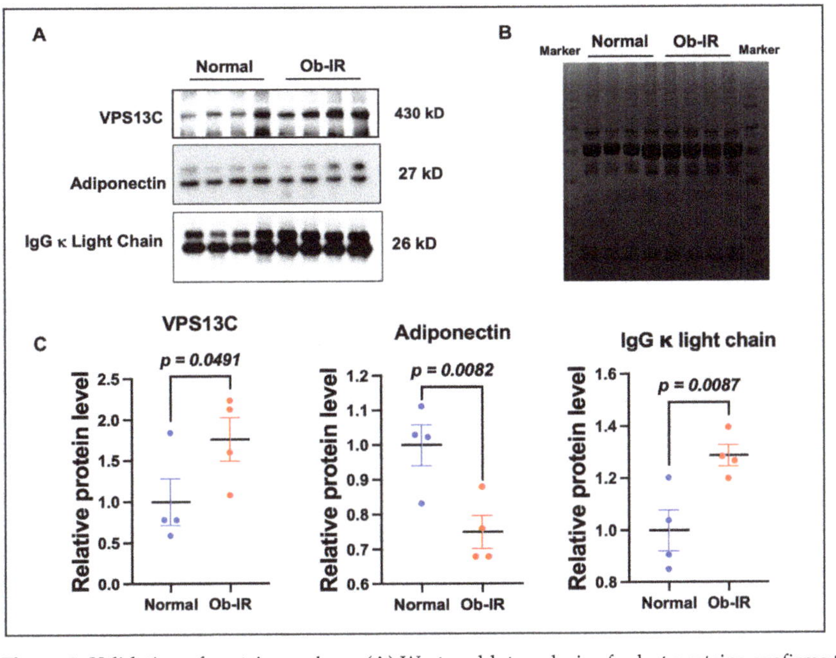

Figure 6. Validation of protein markers. (A) Western blot analysis of select proteins confirms the proteomics data. (B) Coomassie blue staining of protein bands. (C) Densitometric analysis of protein bands normalized to total protein. Values are mean ± SEM of 4 samples per group.

3.5. Ingenuity Pathway Analysis

Next, all the differential proteins were used for pathway analysis using the Ingenuity Pathway Analysis (IPA) software (version: 111725566). The corresponding Swissport accession numbers were accessed from the human Swiss-Prot database and uploaded to IPA software. The proteins were mapped to disease and function categories and canonical pathways available in IPA databases. The annotated pathways were ranked by the *p*-value.

The IPA analysis of DEPs revealed that the significantly affected pathways include the acute phase response signaling ($p = 1.09 \times 10^{16}$) (Figure 7A) and PI3K signaling in B lymphocytes ($p = 5.25 \times 10^{12}$) (Figure 7B). The significantly altered canonical pathways include the B-cell development and/or B-cell receptor signaling. The DEPs identified in the top network are associated with humoral immune response, inflammatory response, and hematological system development and function, with a score of 41, indicating a strong association. This is consistent with the GO analysis which also showed that DEPs are enriched mostly in the immune response and immune system process.

The top upregulated molecules include the DEPs promoting B-cell development/activation (IGLV4-69, IGKV1D-13, IGLV9-49), inflammation (NF-κB), and insulin resistance (VPS13C, TBC1D32). The downregulated molecules include DEPs improving insulin resistance, in particular, ADIPOQ. Together, these data show that B-cell proliferation/activation are altered between N and Ob-IR subjects along with markers of insulin resistance and inflammation. Further, the top-altered proteins, VPS13C, IGKV1D-13, and ADIPOQ can be used as biomarkers to detect high risk individuals or develop therapeutic targets to prevent the development of T2D in Ob-IR subjects.

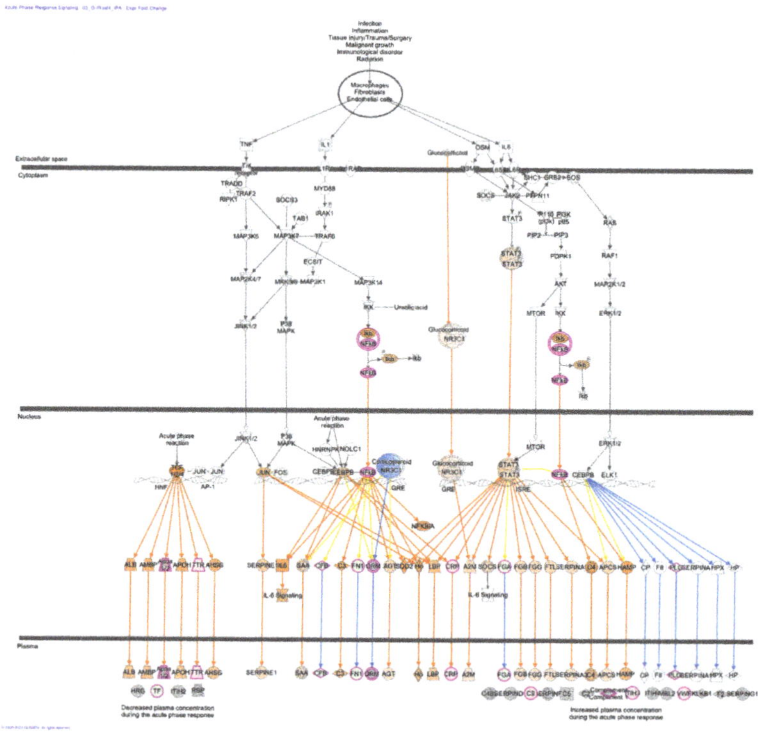

(A)

Figure 7. *Cont.*

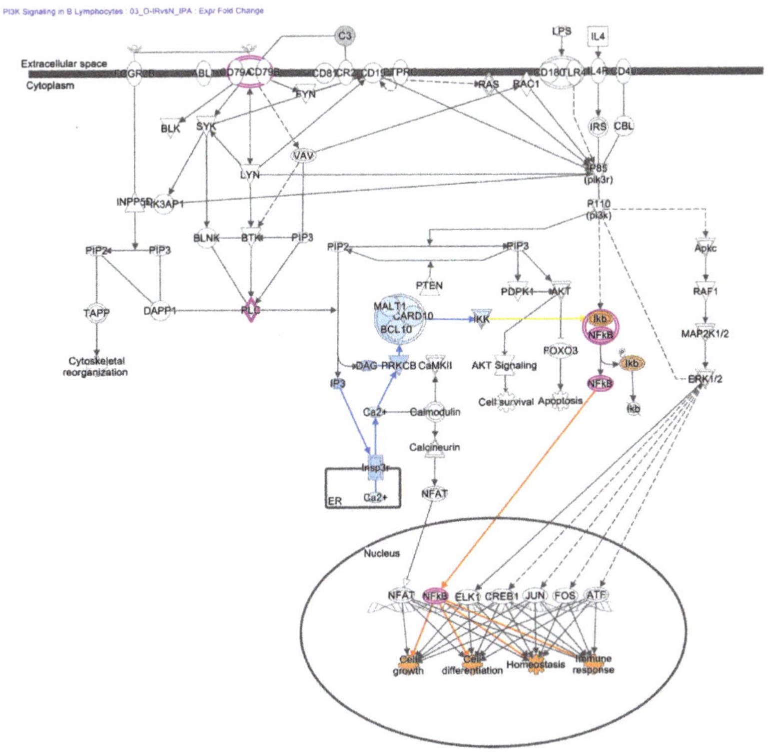

(B)

Figure 7. Two of the significantly enriched canonical pathways in Ob-IR group. (**A**) PI3 Kinase signaling in B lymphocytes in Ob-IR group overlapped with DEPs. (**B**) Acute phase reactant signaling in Ob-IR overlapped with DEPs. Red: proteins upregulated in our data set; the intensity of the color indicates the degree of upregulation. The upregulated proteins are highlighted with purple borders. Orange: proteins predicted to be upregulated in our data set; blue: proteins predicted to be downregulated in our data set; and white: proteins not specific to our data set but incorporated as part of the network.

4. Discussion

We have identified 23 upregulated and 46 downregulated proteins in serum exosomes of Ob-IR subjects compared to lean/overweight normal (N) subjects. The DEPs are mainly involved in regulating insulin signaling, inflammation, and B-cell proliferation/activation. GO analysis revealed that the DEPs are mainly located in the extracellular space and regulate immune cell activation. IPA analysis further showed that the top molecules altering between the N and Ob-IR subjects are those regulating insulin signaling, inflammation and B-cell proliferation/activation. Together, our data show that markers of insulin signaling, inflammation, and B-cell activation are altered in the exosomal cargo between N and Ob-IR subjects. These data suggest that exosomal proteins could be used as a biomarker to identify high-risk individuals for T2D and a therapeutic target to prevent T2D in this population (Figure 8).

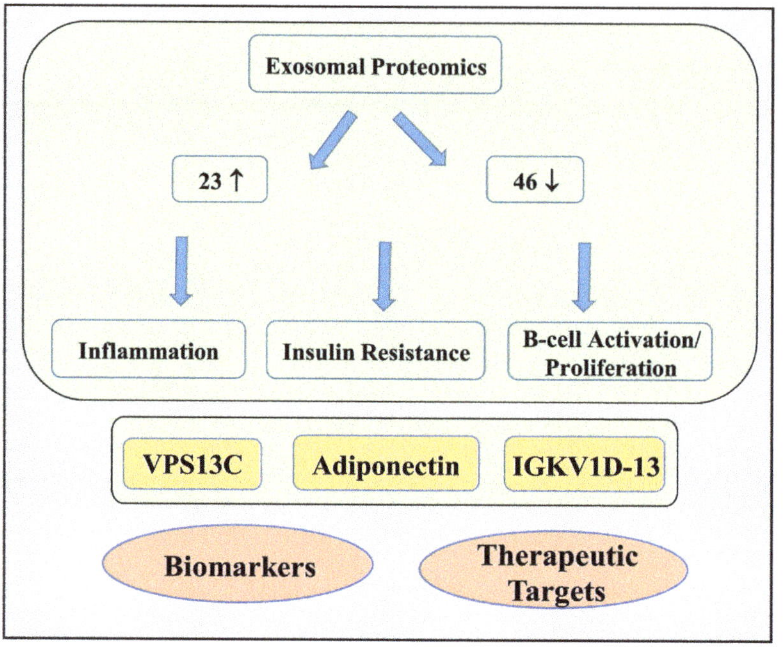

Figure 8. Schematic picture depicting the differentially expressed proteins in exosomes from normal subjects and individuals with obesity and insulin resistance. Proteomics analysis revealed that markers of insulin resistance, inflammation, and B cell activation are increased in exosomes from Ob-IR subjects. The top-altered molecules including VPS13C, adiponectin, and IGKV1D-13 can be considered as biomarkers or therapeutic targets to block the progression of T2D in patients with obesity and insulin resistance.

Exosomes are increasingly recognized as an important tool to identify biomarkers or understand the pathogenesis of a wide variety of diseases, in particular, obesity-related diseases. With regard to its role as a biomarker, the miRNA cargo of EVs has been frequently studied. For example, a clinical study by Jones et al. (in 2017) showed that circulating extracellular miRNAs secreted by the plasma EVs could be predictive biomarkers for obesity-related IR phenotypes [12]. Another clinical study showed that circulating miRNAs in the exosomes could be a futuristic biomarker for T2D in individuals with obesity [13]. However, very little is known regarding the proteomics profile of exosomes in obesity-related IR. Ge et al. showed that plasma exosomes from subjects with obesity and IR had lower levels of omentin compared to exosomes derived from normal subjects [6]. The top-altered proteins in our study include VPS13C, ADIPOQ, and IGKV1D-13 which can be used as biomarkers for obesity-related IR and to identify individuals with a future risk for T2D. Of note, the VPS13C locus was previously linked to T2D and glycemic traits in a GWAS published earlier [14,15]. Another study has shown that the depletion of VPS13C caused a post-transcriptional increase in the cellular GLUT4 protein and enhanced the cell surface GLUT4 levels in C2C12 myotubes, a process critical for glucose uptake [16]. These reports suggest that a link exists between VPS13C and T2D and our data provide further evidence that VPS13C is increased in serum exosomes from Ob-IR subjects. In addition, our data show that TBC1D32 levels were higher in exosomes from Ob-IR subjects compared to N subjects. Another TBC1D family member, TBC1D1, has been reported to interact with VPS13C and regulate GLUT4-mediated glucose transport in C2C12 myotubes [16]. Our data suggest that TBC1D32 may also have a role in regulating glucose uptake. Indeed, TBC1D32 is known to interact with PPARγ (which plays an important role in regulating glucose uptake in adipocytes) [17]. We also noted a significant increase in TTR, another protein, mediating IR [18].

In addition to an increase in the levels of proteins mediating IR, we also noted a decrease in the levels of some proteins which are known to improve insulin sensitivity. As mentioned, we noted a dramatic decrease in adiponectin in exosomes from Ob-IR subjects. Adiponectin is a well-known adipokine, which is considered a biomarker for obesity-related IR [19]. We provide evidence that not only the plasma level, but also the exosome level of adiponectin was lower in subjects with Ob-IR. In addition, the levels of FCN3 and AZGP1, the other proteins improving insulin sensitivity [20–22], were lower in exosomes from Ob-IR subjects compared to N subjects. Taken together, the proteomics analysis of serum exosomes revealed markers of IR and future risk of T2D in Ob-IR subjects.

Although obesity is a strong risk factor for T2D, the mechanisms by which obesity leads to the development of IR remains unclear. Obesity-related inflammation is an important risk factor for the development of IR [23,24]. Accordingly, we noted an increase in inflammatory proteins including NF-κB, CRP, and C9 in Ob-IR subjects. In addition to the inflammatory response, changes in immune cell activation/proliferation which, in turn, alter the immune response, also plays a role in the development of IR. In fact, the most striking finding of our study is that several markers of B cell activation/proliferation were significantly altered between the Ob-IR and N groups. Of note, aberrant B cell activation can result in autoantibody production which, in turn, can promote the development of IR. While type 1 diabetes is an autoimmune disease, accumulating evidence suggests that the activation of B-cells plays a role in the pathogenesis of T2D as well. For example, B cell antibody secretion was higher in patients with obesity and diabetes, compared to patients with obesity and no diabetes [25]. IR in individuals with obesity was associated with a unique profile of IgG autoantibodies [26]. The percentage of B lymphocytes was positively associated with IR, and this was proposed to serve as an appropriate predictor of IR in women with gestational diabetes mellitus [27]. The circulating levels of B2 B cells, a subset of B cells, is positively correlated with hemoglobin A1C in T2D patients [28]. The finding that several markers of antibody fragments were higher in exosomes from Ob-IR subjects, suggests that B cell activation is an important mediator for the development of IR in obesity, and that exosomal B cell activation markers may serve as a therapeutic target to slow down the progression of T2D in obese-IR subjects.

Our study has many strengths. First, the serum samples from age- and gender-matched subjects from N and Ob-IR groups were used for exosome isolation. Second, we were able to identify several proteins that differentially altered between the N and Ob-IR groups. This could be due to the fact that we used serum samples as opposed to plasma samples which were used in other studies. Finally, we were able to validate the proteomics data by the Western blot analysis which increases the confidence and reliability of the data. Regarding limitations, the sample number is low in our study. However, it is a pilot study, and our future studies will involve a larger number of samples from both male and female subjects. Another limitation of this study and any study assessing the circulating exosomes is that the exosomes preparations include some lipoproteins due to the overlap in their size [29]. Therefore, the changes in DEPs could be partly attributed to the levels of lipoproteins in exosomes. However, the DEPs highlighted in this report do not include any proteins associated with lipoproteins.

5. Conclusions

Taken together, our study suggests that the exosomal proteomics profile is differentially altered between normal subjects and individuals with obesity and IR. These studies highlight the importance of exosomal proteins as biomarkers to identify individuals with a future risk for developing T2D. Our findings are also relevant when considering the targeting of B cell activation to prevent or delay the progression of T2D in high-risk individuals. Future studies are warranted to understand the mechanisms by which these DEP contribute to the pathogenesis of IR in humans.

Author Contributions: Conceived and designed the study (V.S. and C.V.D.), established methods (H.M., T.S., V.K. and K.S.), acquired samples and data (C.V.D., W.A., T.G., N.K., V.K. and K.S.), analyzed data and constructed figures (W.A., V.S. and V.K.), wrote the manuscript (V.S.), interpreted results (V.S., C.V.D., H.M. and T.S.), reviewed the manuscript (W.A., V.K., K.S., T.G., N.K., H.M., T.S. and C.V.D.). All authors have read and agreed to the published version of the manuscript.

Funding: The work was supported by a Merit Award from the Department of Veterans Affairs (I01CX002084) and a pilot award from the Great Plains Institutional Development Award (IDeA) Networks for Clinical and Translational Research.

Institutional Review Board Statement: The study was conducted in accordance with the Declaration of Helsinki, and approved by the Institutional Review Board of the VA Nebraska-Western Iowa Heath Care System (protocol code 1137 and date of approval 1 May 2018).

Informed Consent Statement: Informed consent was obtained from all subjects involved in the study.

Data Availability Statement: The proteomics data presented in the study are openly available in [MassIVE Repository (MSV000092982)]. The other raw data supporting the conclusions of this article will be made available by the authors on request.

Acknowledgments: This paper is the result of work conducted with the resources and the facilities at the VA Nebraska-Western Iowa Health Care System, Omaha.

Conflicts of Interest: The authors declared no conflicts of interest.

References

1. Saklayen, M.G. The Global Epidemic of the Metabolic Syndrome. *Curr. Hypertens. Rep.* **2018**, *20*, 12. [CrossRef] [PubMed]
2. Neeland, I.J.; Poirier, P.; Despres, J.P. Cardiovascular and Metabolic Heterogeneity of Obesity: Clinical Challenges and Implications for Management. *Circulation* **2018**, *137*, 1391–1406. [CrossRef] [PubMed]
3. Tong, Y.; Xu, S.; Huang, L.; Chen, C. Obesity and insulin resistance: Pathophysiology and treatment. *Drug Discov. Today* **2022**, *27*, 822–830. [CrossRef] [PubMed]
4. Kalluri, R.; LeBleu, V.S. The biology, function, and biomedical applications of exosomes. *Science* **2020**, *367*, eaau6977. [CrossRef]
5. Pan, S.; Chen, Y.; Yan, J.; Li, F.; Chen, X.; Xu, X.; Xing, H. The emerging roles and mechanisms of exosomal non-coding RNAs in the mutual regulation between adipose tissue and other related tissues in obesity and metabolic diseases. *Front. Endocrinol.* **2022**, *13*, 975334. [CrossRef] [PubMed]
6. Ge, Q.; Xie, X.; Chen, X.; Huang, R.; Rui, C.X.; Zhen, Q.; Hu, R.; Wu, M.; Xiao, X.; Li, X. Circulating exosome-like vesicles of humans with nondiabetic obesity impaired islet beta-cell proliferation, which was associated with decreased Omentin-1 protein cargo. *Genes Dis.* **2022**, *9*, 1099–1113. [CrossRef] [PubMed]
7. Camino, T.; Lago-Baameiro, N.; Bravo, S.B.; Molares-Vila, A.; Sueiro, A.; Couto, I.; Baltar, J.; Casanueva, E.F.; Pardo, M. Human obese white adipose tissue sheds depot-specific extracellular vesicles and reveals candidate biomarkers for monitoring obesity and its comorbidities. *Transl. Res.* **2022**, *239*, 85–102. [CrossRef] [PubMed]
8. Baptista Pereira, P.; Torrejon, E.; Ferreira, I.; Carvalho, A.S.; Teshima, A.; Sousa-Lima, I.; Beck, H.C.; Costa-Silva, B.; Matthiesen, R.; Macedo, M.P.; et al. Proteomic Profiling of Plasma- and Gut-Derived Extracellular Vesicles in Obesity. *Nutrients* **2024**, *16*, 736. [CrossRef]
9. Xie, X.; Yi, Z.; Sinha, S.; Madan, M.; Bowen, B.P.; Langlais, P.; Ma, D.; Mandarino, L.; Meyer, C. Proteomics analyses of subcutaneous adipocytes reveal novel abnormalities in human insulin resistance. *Obesity* **2016**, *24*, 1506–1514. [CrossRef] [PubMed]
10. DiStefano, J.K.; Piras, I.S.; Wu, X.; Sharma, R.; Garcia-Mansfield, K.; Willey, M.; Lovell, B.; Pirrotte, P.; Olson, M.L.; Shaibi, G.Q. Changes in proteomic cargo of circulating extracellular vesicles in response to lifestyle intervention in adolescents with hepatic steatosis. *Clin. Nutr. ESPEN* **2024**, *60*, 333–342. [CrossRef]
11. Nakao, Y.; Fukushima, M.; Mauer, A.S.; Liao, C.Y.; Ferris, A.; Dasgupta, D.; Heppelmann, C.J.; Vanderboom, P.M.; Saraswat, M.; Pandey, A.; et al. A Comparative Proteomic Analysis of Extracellular Vesicles Associated With Lipotoxicity. *Front. Cell Dev. Biol.* **2021**, *9*, 735001. [CrossRef] [PubMed]
12. Jones, A.; Danielson, K.M.; Benton, M.C.; Ziegler, O.; Shah, R.; Stubbs, R.S.; Das, S.; Macartney-Coxson, D. miRNA Signatures of Insulin Resistance in Obesity. *Obesity* **2017**, *25*, 1734–1744. [CrossRef] [PubMed]
13. Catanzaro, G.; Conte, F.; Trocchianesi, S.; Splendiani, E.; Bimonte, V.M.; Mocini, E.; Filardi, T.; Po, A.; Besharat, Z.M.; Gentile, M.C.; et al. Network analysis identifies circulating miR-155 as predictive biomarker of type 2 diabetes mellitus development in obese patients: A pilot study. *Sci. Rep.* **2023**, *13*, 19496. [CrossRef] [PubMed]
14. Dupuis, J.; Langenberg, C.; Prokopenko, I.; Saxena, R.; Soranzo, N.; Jackson, A.U.; Wheeler, E.; Glazer, N.L.; Bouatia-Naji, N.; Gloyn, A.L.; et al. New genetic loci implicated in fasting glucose homeostasis and their impact on type 2 diabetes risk. *Nat. Genet.* **2010**, *42*, 105–116. [CrossRef] [PubMed]

15. Grarup, N.; Overvad, M.; Sparso, T.; Witte, D.R.; Pisinger, C.; Jorgensen, T.; Yamauchi, T.; Hara, K.; Maeda, S.; Kadowaki, T.; et al. The diabetogenic VPS13C/C2CD4A/C2CD4B rs7172432 variant impairs glucose-stimulated insulin response in 5722 non-diabetic Danish individuals. *Diabetologia* **2011**, *54*, 789–794. [CrossRef] [PubMed]
16. Hook, S.C.; Chadt, A.; Heesom, K.J.; Kishida, S.; Al-Hasani, H.; Tavare, J.M.; Thomas, E.C. TBC1D1 interacting proteins, VPS13A and VPS13C, regulate GLUT4 homeostasis in C2C12 myotubes. *Sci. Rep.* **2020**, *10*, 17953. [CrossRef] [PubMed]
17. Calvier, L.; Chouvarine, P.; Legchenko, E.; Hoffmann, N.; Geldner, J.; Borchert, P.; Jonigk, D.; Mozes, M.M.; Hansmann, G. PPARgamma Links BMP2 and TGFbeta1 Pathways in Vascular Smooth Muscle Cells, Regulating Cell Proliferation and Glucose Metabolism. *Cell Metab.* **2017**, *25*, 1118–1134.e7. [CrossRef] [PubMed]
18. He, Y.; Qiu, R.; Wu, B.; Gui, W.; Lin, X.; Li, H.; Zheng, F. Transthyretin contributes to insulin resistance and diminishes exercise-induced insulin sensitivity in obese mice by inhibiting AMPK activity in skeletal muscle. *Am. J. Physiol. Endocrinol. Metab.* **2021**, *320*, E808–E821. [CrossRef] [PubMed]
19. Frithioff-Bojsoe, C.; Lund, M.A.V.; Lausten-Thomsen, U.; Hedley, P.L.; Pedersen, O.; Christiansen, M.; Baker, J.L.; Hansen, T.; Holm, J.C. Leptin, adiponectin, and their ratio as markers of insulin resistance and cardiometabolic risk in childhood obesity. *Pediatr. Diabetes* **2020**, *21*, 194–202. [CrossRef] [PubMed]
20. Chen, H.; Lu, J.; Chen, X.; Yu, H.; Zhang, L.; Bao, Y.; Lu, F.; Tang, J.; Gu, C.; Jia, W. Low serum levels of the innate immune component ficolin-3 is associated with insulin resistance and predicts the development of type 2 diabetes. *J. Mol. Cell Biol.* **2012**, *4*, 256–257. [CrossRef] [PubMed]
21. Pearsey, H.M.; Henson, J.; Sargeant, J.A.; Davies, M.J.; Khunti, K.; Suzuki, T.; Bowden-Davies, K.A.; Cuthbertson, D.J.; Yates, T.E. Zinc-alpha2-glycoprotein, dysglycaemia and insulin resistance: A systematic review and meta-analysis. *Rev. Endocr. Metab. Disord.* **2020**, *21*, 569–575. [CrossRef] [PubMed]
22. Lei, L.; Li, K.; Li, L.; Fang, X.; Zhou, T.; Zhang, C.; Luo, Y.; Liu, H.; Li, X.; Zheng, H.; et al. Circulating zinc-alpha2-glycoprotein levels are low in newly diagnosed patients with metabolic syndrome and correlate with adiponectin. *Nutr. Metab.* **2017**, *14*, 53. [CrossRef] [PubMed]
23. Xu, H.; Barnes, G.T.; Yang, Q.; Tan, G.; Yang, D.; Chou, C.J.; Sole, J.; Nichols, A.; Ross, J.S.; Tartaglia, L.A.; et al. Chronic inflammation in fat plays a crucial role in the development of obesity-related insulin resistance. *J. Clin. Investig.* **2003**, *112*, 1821–1830. [CrossRef] [PubMed]
24. Weisberg, S.P.; McCann, D.; Desai, M.; Rosenbaum, M.; Leibel, R.L.; Ferrante, A.W., Jr. Obesity is associated with macrophage accumulation in adipose tissue. *J. Clin. Investig.* **2003**, *112*, 1796–1808. [CrossRef] [PubMed]
25. Zhai, X.; Qian, G.; Wang, Y.; Chen, X.; Lu, J.; Zhang, Y.; Huang, Q.; Wang, Q. Elevated B Cell Activation is Associated with Type 2 Diabetes Development in Obese Subjects. *Cell Physiol. Biochem.* **2016**, *38*, 1257–1266. [CrossRef] [PubMed]
26. Winer, D.A.; Winer, S.; Shen, L.; Wadia, P.P.; Yantha, J.; Paltser, G.; Tsui, H.; Wu, P.; Davidson, M.G.; Alonso, M.N.; et al. B cells promote insulin resistance through modulation of T cells and production of pathogenic IgG antibodies. *Nat. Med.* **2011**, *17*, 610–617. [CrossRef] [PubMed]
27. Zhuang, Y.; Zhang, J.; Li, Y.; Gu, H.; Zhao, J.; Sun, Y.; Wang, R.; Zhang, C.; Chen, W.; Weng, J.; et al. B Lymphocytes Are Predictors of Insulin Resistance in Women with Gestational Diabetes Mellitus. *Endocr. Metab. Immune Disord. Drug Targets* **2019**, *19*, 358–366. [CrossRef] [PubMed]
28. Hammad, R.H.; El-Madbouly, A.A.; Kotb, H.G.; Zarad, M.S. Frequency of Circulating B1a and B2 B-cell Subsets in Egyptian Patients with Type 2 Diabetes Mellitus. *Egypt. J. Immunol.* **2018**, *25*, 71–80. [PubMed]
29. Thery, C.; Witwer, K.W.; Aikawa, E.; Alcaraz, M.J.; Anderson, J.D.; Andriantsitohaina, R.; Antoniou, A.; Arab, T.; Archer, F.; Atkin-Smith, G.K.; et al. Minimal information for studies of extracellular vesicles 2018 (MISEV2018): A position statement of the International Society for Extracellular Vesicles and update of the MISEV2014 guidelines. *J. Extracell. Vesicles* **2018**, *7*, 1535750. [CrossRef] [PubMed]

biomedicines

MDPI

Article

Insulin and Metformin Administration: Unravelling the Multifaceted Association with Mortality across Various Clinical Settings Considering Type 2 Diabetes Mellitus and COVID-19

Łukasz Lewandowski [1,†], Agnieszka Bronowicka-Szydełko [1,†], Maciej Rabczyński [2,*], Dorota Bednarska-Chabowska [2], Joanna Adamiec-Mroczek [3], Adrian Doroszko [4], Małgorzata Trocha [2], Krzysztof Kujawa [5], Agnieszka Matera-Witkiewicz [6], Edwin Kuźnik [2], Paweł Lubieniecki [2], Marcin Madziarski [7], Janusz Sokołowski [8], Ewa A. Jankowska [9,‡] and Katarzyna Madziarska [2,‡]

1 Department of Biochemistry and Immunochemistry, Wroclaw Medical University, Chałubińskiego Street 10, 50-368 Wroclaw, Poland; lukasz.lewandowski@umw.edu.pl (Ł.L.); agnieszka.bronowicka-szydelko@umw.edu.pl (A.B.-S.)

2 Clinical Department of Diabetology and Internal Disease, Wroclaw Medical University, Borowska Street 213, 50-556 Wroclaw, Poland; dorota.bednarska-chabowska@umw.edu.pl (D.B.-C.); malgorzata.trocha@umw.edu.pl (M.T.); edwin.kuznik@usk.wroc.pl (E.K.); pawel.lubieniecki@usk.wroc.pl (P.L.); katarzyna.madziarska@umw.edu.pl (K.M.)

3 Clinical Department of Ophthalmology, Wroclaw Medical University, Borowska Street 213, 50-556 Wroclaw, Poland; joanna.adamiec-mroczek@umw.edu.pl

4 Department of Cardiology, Faculty of Medicine, 4th Military Hospital, Wroclaw University of Science and Technology, Weigla 5 Street, 50-981 Wroclaw, Poland; adrian.doroszko@pwr.edu.pl

5 Statistical Analysis Centre, Wroclaw Medical University, K. Marcinkowski Street 2–6, 50-368 Wroclaw, Poland; krzysztof.kujawa@umw.edu.pl

6 Screening of Biological Activity Assays and Collection of Biological Material Laboratory, Wroclaw Medical University Biobank, Faculty of Pharmacy, Wroclaw Medical University, Borowska Street 221A, 50-556 Wroclaw, Poland; agnieszka.matera-witkiewicz@umw.edu.pl

7 Clinical Department of Rheumatology and Internal Medicine, University Hospital, Borowska Street 213, 50-556 Wroclaw, Poland; marcin.madziarski@usk.wroc.pl

8 Department of Emergency Medicine, Wroclaw Medical University, Borowska Street 213, 50-556 Wroclaw, Poland; janusz.sokolowski@umw.edu.pl

9 Institute of Heart Diseases, Wroclaw Medical University, Borowska Street 213, 50-556 Wroclaw, Poland; ewa.jankowska@umw.edu.pl

* Correspondence: maciej.rabczynski@umw.edu.pl; Tel.: +48-71-733-22-50

† These authors contributed equally to this work.

‡ These authors contributed equally to this work.

Abstract: Due to the molecular mechanisms of action of antidiabetic drugs, they are considered to be effective in the treatment of both COVID-19 and the post-COVID-19 syndromes. The aim of this study was to determine the effect of administering insulin and metformin on the mortality of patients with type 2 diabetes (T2DM) with symptomatic COVID-19 with the use of logistic regression models. The association between death and insulin and metformin was weak and could not be included in the multivariate model. However, the interaction of both drugs with other factors, including remdesivir and low-molecular-weight heparin (metformin), age and hsCRP (insulin), modulated the odds of death. These interactions hint at multifaceted (anti-/pro-) associations of both insulin and metformin with the odds of death, depending on the patient's characteristics. In the multivariate model, RDW-SD, adjusted with low-molecular-weight heparin treatment, age, sex and K^+, was associated with mortality among patients with COVID-19 and T2DM. With a 15% increase in RDW-SD, the risk of death increased by 87.7%. This preliminary study provides the foundations for developing further, more personalized models to assess the risk of death in T2DM patients, as well as for identifying patients at an increased risk of death due to COVID-19.

Keywords: COVID-19; diabetes; mortality

1. Introduction

According to the WHO, the prevalence of *SARS-CoV-2* reached approximately 662 million cases on the day of 16 January 2023, leading to 6 million deaths due to the development of the COVID-19 syndrome [1]. Although the pandemic has already passed, some people, especially those who suffered from full-blown COVID-19, may experience acute consequences of COVID-19, the so-called long COVID or post-COVID-19 syndrome (PCS), recognized by the WHO as the next epidemic of the 21st century [2]. This term refers to symptoms persisting for more than 3 months after COVID-19, causing long-term changes in single organs or multi-organ changes [1]. It is predicted that PCS may affect millions of people worldwide [1], mainly people with comorbidities [3], e.g., type 2 diabetes mellitus (2TDM). The symptoms of PCS are difficulty with concentration, cognitive dysfunction, amnesia, depression, fatigue and anxiety [3], and the risk factors for the persistence of neuropsychiatric symptoms in PCS are older age, female sex and the severity of comorbidities, e.g., diabetes [4], which is often associated with tachycardia, sarcopenia, microcirculatory dysfunction or organ damage [5]. PCS is therefore a phenomenon that affects life expectancy.

The study reported in this manuscript focuses on diabetes, which was shown to develop de novo in patients suffering from COVID-19 [4]. Diabetes is estimated to be associated with approximately 15% of patients suffering from severe COVID-19. The mortality rate in COVID-19-positive diabetic patients was reported to be 2- to 3-fold higher compared to COVID-19-negative diabetic patients [5]. The literature (studies and meta-analyses) shows higher mortality in the COVID-19-positive diabetic population compared to the COVID-19-positive non-diabetic population [6–9]. Moreover, optimal diabetic control (in the case of T1DM/T2DM) was associated with better outcomes and fewer comorbidities among COVID-19-positive patients [10]. Such statistics account for the urge to partake in therapeutic intervention [5]. However, the information on the COVID-19-associated diabetic cases and their responses to drug treatment are scarce. Research into new strategies in its treatment and prevention may improve the quality of medical decisions in terms of mortality, exacerbation and optimal response to drugs [11], and shed some light on the metabolic alterations in these patients.

A handful of clinical studies aimed to combine the classic anti-viral and anti-inflammatory drugs in one treatment scheme in order to combat COVID-19 [11]. However, since the molecular action of agents used in antidiabetic treatment is multidimensional and may possibly modulate the course of COVID-19 and its related oxidative stress and cytokine storm [12–15], interactions with antidiabetic treatments ought to be taken into account when analyzing multidimensional models used in more complex studies. To our knowledge, no studies analyzed the difference in the odds of mortality associated with antidiabetic treatment in the context of the simultaneous effects of the coexisting covariates (comorbidities, patient characteristics and demography, and biochemical parameters). The lack of such an investigation renders the one-dimensional studies prone to generate false assumptions, owing to the aforementioned multifaceted action of antidiabetic drugs and the *SARS-CoV-2* affinity towards cell membrane proteins [5,13,15–18], often acting as intrinsic cell-to-cell messengers.

The aim of this preliminary study was to explore the mortality-wise effect of insulin and metformin administration in the European (Polish) model of the COVID-19-positive diabetic population sample composed of all patients admitted to the Temporary COVID-19 Hospital in Wroclaw, Poland. Typically, patients transferred to this specific hospital were characterized by an increased risk of in-hospital mortality due to increased COVID-19 severity. Along with the estimated effect of insulin and metformin on survival, their interactions with other factors (including other agents) were studied (in the form of second- or third-degree interactions) to check for synergies in modulating the mortality rate. Only significant interactions were reported and further analyzed, as opposed to the less optimal process of adjusting the findings with a pre-assumed set of patient features. This study design was chosen so as to give a foundation for future, more patient- and treatment-oriented risk assessment models that would be validated on bigger, stratified, diabetic population samples. These tools would enable the identification of patients with a higher risk of death from COVID-19. This targets those for whom analysis of the values of the selected laboratory and demographic parameters, and taking into account the treatment methods for both T2DM and COVID-19, would prove to be at-risk in the context of assessment of the outcome of the disease.

2. Materials and Methods

2.1. Inclusion/Exclusion Criteria and the Population from Which the Sample Was Taken

A retrospective analysis was performed on 430 medical records of patients with type 2 diabetes and *SARS-CoV-2* infection (the total number included data from 2151 patients) hospitalized between February 2020 and June 2021 at the University and Temporary COVID-19 Hospital organized by the University Medical Hospital in Wroclaw (Poland), which were collected as part of the COLOS registry (COronavirus in LOwer Silesia). All patients admitted at the hospital due to COVID-19 symptoms tested positive for the presence of *SARS-CoV-2* in nasopharyngeal swab specimens using the RT-PCR method (via reverse transcription and polymerase chain reaction), which was recommended by the World Health Organization (WHO) [19]. The tests were performed using the two-gene test (ORF1ab, N) SARS-CoV-2 Real Time PCR LAB-KIT (BIOMAXIMA, Lublin, Poland), using the QuantStudio 6 Flex device (Applied Biosystems, Warsaw, Poland). Isolation of nukelic acids was performed on a Magna Pure 96 apparatus (Roche, Basel, Switzerland). The observation period lasted from the day of hospital admission to the day of discharge or death. The study protocol was approved by the Bioethical Committee and Ethics Committee of the Medical University in Wroclaw, Poland (No: KB-444/2021), and permission was granted for the publication of anonymized data. All patients provided written consent for admission into the study, which stipulated that the results may be used for research purposes. This study was in accordance with Helsinki declaration.

The dataset included demographic information (sex, age), concurrent conditions, performed procedures, vital signs and laboratory test results during hospitalization. This study accounted for the following variables determined before hospital admission: gender; type 2 diabetes therapies used before hospital admission, including metformin, insulin, metformin and insulin, insulin and another oral antidiabetic drug, GLP agonists (semiglutide or dulaglutide injected subcutaneously) or metformin and another oral antidiabetic drug (SGLT-2 inhibitors); the Glasgow Coma Scale (GCS) ≤ 14; oxygen saturation without respiratory support $SpO_2 \leq 94\%$; lung lesions (typical of *SARS-CoV-2* infection, observed under the CT scan); dyspnea; chest pain; cough; smell disorders; taste disorders; diarrhea, vomiting or abdominal pain; hypertension; hemorrhage (gastrointestinal, respiratory, intracranial, genital, urinary); myocardial infraction; heart failure; prehospitalization oxygen therapy; chronic kidney; atrial fibrillation or flutter; asthma; chronic obstructive pulmonary disease (COPD); sleep apnea syndrome; stroke; dialysis; red cell distribution width—standard deviation (RDW-SD); concentration of lymphocyte (LYMPH), interleukin 6 (IL-6), procalcitonin (PCT), albumin, ferritin, C-reactive protein, sodium, potassium, glucose, D-dimers, fibrinogen, uric acid, bilirubin, diacylglycerides (TG), glycated hemoglobin (HbA1c), low-density lipoprotein (LDL), high-density lipoprotein (HDL), urea, creatinine, troponin and lactate dehydrogenase (LDH); and estimated glomerular filtration rate (eGFR) calculated based on the Modification of Diet in Renal Disease (MDRD) Study Equation [20]. The analysis also took into account features that were observed upon clinical assessment or introduced (in the case of iatrogenic factors) during the hospitalization. Apart from antidiabetic agents for which the administration was continued during the hospitalization, therapeutic agents were introduced in the treatment upon admission of the study participants to the Temporary COVID-19 Hospital. The initial dataset included variables such as stroke, revascularization (PCI or CABG), features of pulmonary obstruction or pneumonia, shock (hypovolemic, cardiogenic, septic), hemorrhage (gastrointestinal, respiratory, intracranial, genital, urinary), myocardial infarction, venous thromboembolism (embolism, deep vein thrombosis, embolism and thrombosis), new neurological disorders, smell disorders and taste disorders, convalescent plasma, remdesivir and acetylsalicylic acid. The study group was divided based on survival during the hospitalization. The study participants were not further monitored in terms of mortality after their hospitalization had ended. In each of these two groups, the method of treating type 2 diabetes (T2DM) was identified, according to Figure 1.

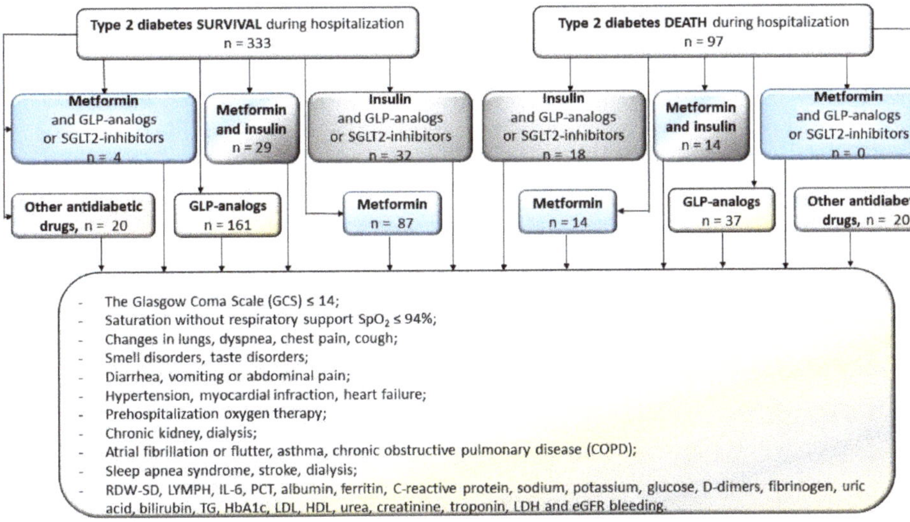

Figure 1. Diagram illustrating the frequency of drug use in regard to antidiabetic treatment in the diabetic patients with COVID-19. A set of features that were analyzed among the two survival statuses is given as a reference.

2.2. Statistical Methods

Data preprocessing and visualization were performed with Python 3.10.7 (packages: pandas 1.4.4, numpy 1.21.4, matplotlib 3.5.3, seaborn 0.11.2). Statistics were employed with use of Statistica 13.3 on license by Wroclaw Medical University. Characteristics of the population sample were performed with use of the Mann–Whitney U and χ^2 tests. In case of low (<5) estimated count in any contingency table cell, Yates correction for continuity was applied. The normality assumption was checked with use of the Q–Q plots and the Shapiro–Wilk test.

Odds of death were analyzed with use of logistic regression models. Expert analysis of the dataset by a multidisciplinary team (consisting of medical doctors, biochemists, laboratory medicine professionals, statisticians and a data scientist) led to drawing candidates to be featured in the initial set used for deriving the optimal multivariate model. A subsequent analysis of the % of missing data led to obtaining the initial set of effects (variables) used for modeling. Some continuous effects were log-transformed so as to meet the assumption of linearity vs. log(Odds) tested with the Box-Tidwell test. To make the intercepts from the model resemble real-life conditions, continuous variables were centered at selected, typical values of the entire population sample from which the data used in this study was extracted. At the beginning of the analysis, univariate odds ratios (ORs) were analyzed (Table A1). Subsequently, the optimal model was derived from the initial set of the variables with use of the stepwise elimination (p cut-off for inclusion/exclusion: 0.05) iterative process (Table A2). Interaction analysis was the final part of the study, in which significant interactions (Table A3) and the effects that took part in them were incorporated into the models, based on the type 1 likelihood ratio (LR) test aimed to assess whether any interaction would be more explanatory in the context of the odds of death, compared to the naïve model which was not based on any variables. The interactions that were significant were incorporated in models reported in this manuscript. The mentioned models contained the intercepts, interaction terms and the features (effects) taking place in these interactions—as per the good practice in data modeling.

3. Results

3.1. Characteristics of the Population Sample Used in this Study

Among patients with T2DM hospitalized due to symptomatic COVID-19, significant differences affecting survival were observed among the following criteria described upon hospital admission: sex (women survival: 48.35%, women death: 34.58%), $SpO_2 \leq 94\%$ (survival: 51.04%, death: 67.39%), hemorrhage (survival: 5.41%, death: 14.95%), myocardial infarction (survival: 14.11%, death: 28.97%), heart failure (survival: 21.62%, death: 28.97%), prehospitalization oxygen therapy (survival: 47.75%, death: 64.49%), chronic kidney diseases, CKDs (survival: 18.02%, death: 29.91%). Furthermore, the type of therapy used in type 2 diabetes also influenced the differences in patient survival: using only metformin (survival: 26.13%, death: 13.08%) versus insulin and other antidiabetic drugs (survival: 9.61%, death: 16.82%) had different results, which, of course, stemmed from the stage of advancement of T2DM. Table 1 shows the baseline demographic and clinical characteristics of the study participants. Non-survivors differed from the survivors in terms of the following laboratory-measured parameters: RDW-SD, LYMPH, IL-6, PCT, albumin, ferritin, hsCRP, potassium, glucose, eGFR, urea, creatinine, LDH and troponin, as shown in Table 1.

Table 1. Baseline characteristics of COVID-19 patients at admission to the hospital and during the hospitalization.

Variable		Category	Survivors (N = 333)	Non-Survivors (N = 107)	p
Demographic Variables (upon Hospital Admission)					
Sex		Female	161 (48.35%)	37 (34.58%)	0.0127
Age [years]	Me (1Q–3Q)	-	70 (64–76)	75 (67–83)	0.0001
Clinical Variables (upon Hospital Admission)					
Variable		**Category**	**Survivors (N = 333)**	**Non-Survivors (N = 107)**	p
Metformin only		YES	87 (26.13%)	14 (13.08%)	0.0053
Insulin and other antidiabetic drugs		YES	32 (9.61%)	18 (16.82%)	0.0410
$SpO_2 \leq 94\%$		YES	98 (51.04%)	31 (67.39%)	0.0456
Hemorrhage		YES	18 (5.41%)	16 (14.95%)	0.0013
Myocardial infarction		YES	47 (14.11%)	31 (28.97%)	<0.001
Heart failure		YES	72 (21.62%)	34 (31.78%)	0.0326
Prehospitalization oxygen therapy		YES	159 (47.75%)	69 (64.49%)	0.002
CKD		YES	60 (18.02%)	32 (29.91%)	0.0085
Clinical Variables (after the Hospital Admission)					
Variable		**Category**	**Survivors (N = 333)**	**Non-Survivors (N = 107)**	p
Revascularization: PCI or CABG		YES	6 (1.80%)	7 (6.54%)	0.0118
Features of pulmonary obstruction or pneumonia		YES	186 (55.86%)	85 (79.44%)	<0.001
Shock: hypovolemic, cardiogenic, septic		YES	13 (3.90%)	45 (42.06%)	<0.001
Hemorrhage: gastrointestinal, respiratory, intracranial, genital, urinary		YES	18 (5.41%)	16 (14.95%)	0.0013
Myocardial infarction		YES	6 (1.80%)	6 (5.61%)	0.0355
Acetylsalicylic acid		YES	89 (26.73%)	41 (38.32%)	0.022

Table 1. *Cont.*

Variable	Laboratory Variables (upon Hospital Admission)	Survivors	Non-Survivors	p
	n	324	106	
RDW-SD [fL]	Me (1Q–3Q)	45.0 (41.60–49.10)	47.85 (43.40–52.40)	<0.001
	n	224	97	
LYMPH [count/μL]	Me (1Q–3Q)	1.11 (0.755–1.565)	0.76 (0.54–1.24)	<0.001
	n	105	29	
IL-6 [pl/mL]	Me (1Q–3Q)	15.3 (7.16–32.20)	56.3 (22.40–144.00)	<0.001
	n	242	103	
PCT [pg/mL]	Me (1Q–3Q)	0.10 (0.04–0.25)	0.31 (0.15–1.10)	<0.001
	n	101	76	
Albumin [mg/dL]	Me (1Q–3Q)	3.20 (2.90–3.60)	2.90 (2.50–3.20)	<0.001
	n	160	59	
Ferritin [μg/L]	Me (1Q–3Q)	507.40 (238.45–834.30)	850.00 (423.10–1368.10)	<0.001
	n	324	105	
CRP [mg/dL]	Me (1Q–3Q)	52.76 (12.85–112.45)	93.07 (0.62–487.40)	<0.001
	n	322	106	
K [mmol/L]	Me (1Q–3Q)	4.17 (3.70–4.62)	4.50 (4.10–4.80)	<0.001
	n	297	100	
Glucose [mg/dL]	Me (1Q–3Q)	152 (112.00–225.00)	196.50 (131.00–189.00)	0.0035
	n	323	106	
eGFR [mL/min/1.73 m^2]	Me (1Q–3Q)	62.00 (41.00–81.00)	47.00 (26.00–69.00)	<0.001
	n	303	105	
Urea [mg/dL]	Me (1Q–3Q)	48.00 (34.00–78.00)	76.00 (52.00–113.00)	<0.001
	n	323	106	
Creatinine [mg/dL]	Me (1Q–3Q)	1.10 (0.84–1.52)	1.47 (0.98–2.32)	<0.001
	n	201	80	
LDH [U/L]	Me (1Q–3Q)	322.00 (244.00–438.00)	494.00 (328.50–665.50)	<0.001
	n	206	79	
Troponin [ng/L]	Me (1Q–3Q)	18.65 (7.30–67.90)	61.90 (21.30–275.50)	<0.001

Abbreviations: CABG, coronary artery bypass grafting; CKD, chronic kidney disease; CRP, C-reactive protein concentration; eGFR, estimated glomerular filtration rate; IL-6, interleukin 6; LDH, lactate dehydrogenase activity; LYMPH, lymphocyte count; Me, median value; PCI, percutaneous coronary intervention; PCT, procalcitonin concentration; Q, quartile.

Among patients who died during hospitalization, there were more frequent occurrences of hypovolemic shock, cardiogenic shock or sepsis (survival: 3.90%, death: 42.06%). Hemorrhagic episodes were more common (survival: 5.41%, death: 14.95%). Moreover, non-survivors showed/underwent the following features more frequently: pulmonary obstruction or pneumonia (survival: 55.86%, death: 79.44%), myocardial infarction (survival: 1.80%, death: 5.61%) and revascularization procedures such as percutaneous coronary intervention (PCI) or coronary artery bypass grafting (CABG) (survival: 1.80%, death: 5.61%). As per treatment-wise choices, non-survivors were characterized with higher intakes of acetylsalicylic acid, most presumably as a result of the more severe course of COVID-19 (survival: 26.73%, death: 38.32%), as shown in Table 1. There were no statistically significant differences in the administration of convalescent plasma or remdesivir between the two groups.

3.2. Univariate Modulation of the Odds of Death

According to the univariate analysis (Figure 2), 10 out of 15 variables proved to have significant influence on the odds of death. Having the SpO_2 lower than 94 increased the odds of death by 98.2% ($p \approx 0.048$). Male individuals were 77.1% more likely to die compared to female ($p \approx 0.013$). Each one-year increase in age would increase these odds by 3.8% ($p < 0.001$). Among the used drugs analyzed in this study, two out of six proved to be associated with higher odds of death: LMWH (by 3.506-fold, $p < 0.001$) and acetylsalicylic acid (by 70.3%, $p \approx 0.023$). The administration with other agents (remdesivir, convalescent plasma, metformin, insulin) was found to be, per se, insignificant in terms of modulation of these odds. Each subsequent increase in hsCRP (by 1 mg/L) and potassium (by 1 mmol/L) increased the odds by 0.4% ($p \approx 0.001$) and 88.6% ($p < 0.001$), respectively. Each 15% increase in RDW-SD increased the odds by 53.8% ($p < 0.001$), while each 2-fold increase in creatinine and urea increased these odds by 53.7% ($p \approx 0.001$) and 87.7% ($p < 0.001$), respectively.

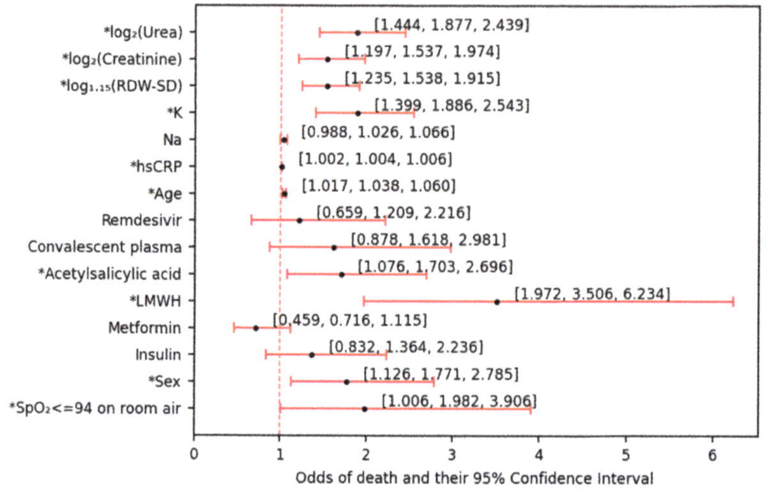

Figure 2. Univariate odds ratios (ORs) of death, associated with the analyzed set of effects (variables). These ORs show the fold change in odds of death associated with each effect, individually (e.g., the baseline odds for each effect would refer solely to this effect), * significant results ($p < 0.05$).

Although the calculated odds ratios (ORs) for administration with metformin and insulin were 0.716 and 1.364, respectively, these insights were insignificant in relation to the entire population ($p > 0.05$, as the confidence interval exceeded the OR = 1 line shown in Figure 2).

3.3. Multi-Effect Modulation of the Odds of Death According to the Model Derived with the Stepwise Elimination Model

The derived multi-effect model (Table 2) consisted of the following effects: potassium ($p < 0.001$), sex ($p \approx 0.014$), RDW-SD ($p \approx 0.002$), age ($p \approx 0.002$) and LMWH treatment ($p \approx 0.002$).

Table 2. The derived multi-effect model for estimating the odds of death in type 2 diabetic, COVID-19-positive patients.

Iteration: Stepwise Elimination (*p* Cut-Off for Inclusion/Exclusion: 0.05); Baseline Group: Female. No LMWH. K: 4.10 mmol/L. RDW-SD: 45.78. Aged 64 Years											
Effect/Interaction	**Analyzed Cat.**	**Reference Cat.**	**β**	**β SE**	**Wald Stat.**	**β −95% CI**	**β 95% CI**	**Est. Effect**	**Est. Effect −95% CI**	**Est. Effect 95% CI**	***p***
Intercept (baseline odds)	-	-	−4.768	0.738	41.783	−6.213	−3.322	0.009	0.002	0.036	<0.001
K. centered at 4.10 mmol/L (OR)	-	-	0.683	0.254	7.257	0.186	1.180	1.980	1.205	3.255	0.007
Sex (OR)	Male	Female	1.029	0.417	6.090	0.212	1.846	2.798	1.236	6.337	0.014
$\log_{1.15}$(RDW-SD). centered at 27.36 (OR)	-	-	0.629	0.207	9.216	0.223	1.036	1.877	1.250	2.817	0.002
Age. centered at 64 years old (OR)	-	-	0.067	0.021	10.065	0.025	0.108	1.069	1.026	1.114	0.002
LMWH (OR)	1	0	2.325	0.602	14.906	1.145	3.505	10.223	3.141	33.272	<0.001

Abbreviations: Cat., category; CI, confidence interval; Est., estimated; LMWH, low-molecular-weight heparin; OR, odds ratio.

The baseline odds (estimated for a 64-year-old female with RDW-SD 45.78 and K 4.10 mmol/L, under no LMWH treatment) were 0.009, suggesting very high pro-survival tendency (9 deaths per 1000 individuals). These odds would be modulated (Figure 3) by the following effects: K (by 98% per each 1 mmol/L increase), male sex (by 2.798-fold), age (by 6.9% per each 1-year increase), RDW-SD (by 87.7% per every 15% increase) and administration of LMWH (by 10.223-fold).

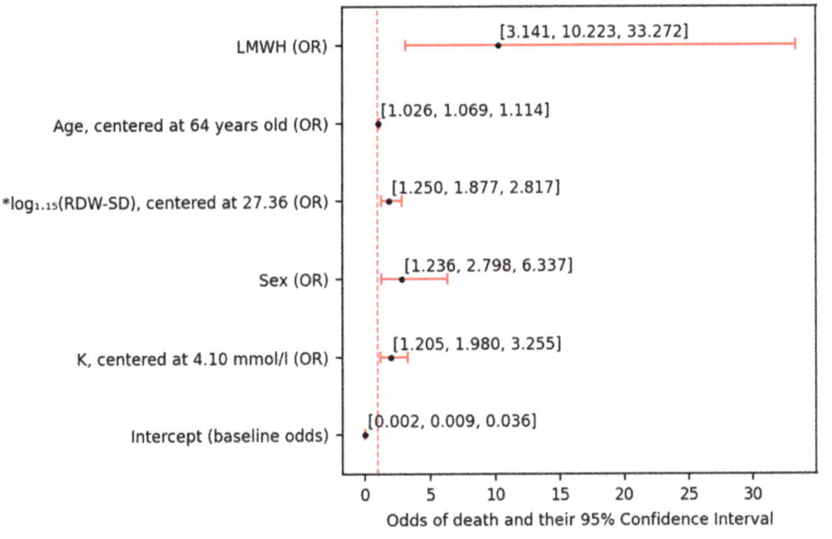

Figure 3. Multi-effect odds ratios (ORs) of death associated with the model derived through iteration (stepwise elimination). The baseline odds represent the odds of death among individuals with the following characteristics: female, neither low-molecular-weight heparin (LMWH), insulin nor remdesivir treatment, 45.78 RDW-SD, 4.10 mmol/L K, aged 64 years old. The ORs show the fold change in baseline odds ratios (ORs) associated with each effect (variable). Significant findings ($p < 0.05$) were marked with '*'.

The baseline odds of death were established for designated representatives. This allows for the simultaneous application of all variables in the model to calculate the odds ratio for death concerning specific characteristics (LMW, age, RDW-SD, sex, potassium centered at 4.10 mmol/L) relative to the baseline person. For a 64-year-old woman not taking LMWH, with an RDW-SD value of 45.78 fL, every increase in potassium by 1 mmol/L from the baseline value of 4.10 mmol/L increased the odds of death by 98%. Additionally, for every one-year increase in age beyond 64 years without taking LMWH, RDW-SD at 45.78 fL, and potassium concentration at 4.10 mmol/L, there was a 6.9% increase in the odds of death.

The baseline odds (estimated for a 64-year-old female with RDW-SD 45.78 and K 4.10 mmol/L, under no LMWH treatment) was 0.009, suggesting very high pro-survival tendency (9 deaths per 1000 individuals). These odds would be modulated (Figure 3) by the following effects: K (by 98% per each 1 mmol/L increase), male sex (by 2.798-fold), age (by 6.9% per each 1-year increase), RDW-SD (by 87.7% per every 15% increase) and administration of LMWH (by 10.223-fold).

3.4. Significant Contrasts. Part 1: How Both LMWH and Remdesivir Modulated the Effect of Metformin Intake on the Odds of Death

According to the model, the modulation of the odds of death by metformin treatment were dependent on administration of both LMWH and remdesivir, although the baseline odds differed between different types of treatment (Figure 4). The stratum administered with LMWH and remdesivir but no metformin was the only one that showed a baseline ratio approximately equal to 1 ($p \approx 0.617$), indicating nearly identical odds of death and survival. The other strata (Figure 4) showed significantly higher baseline odds of survival compared to the odds of death.

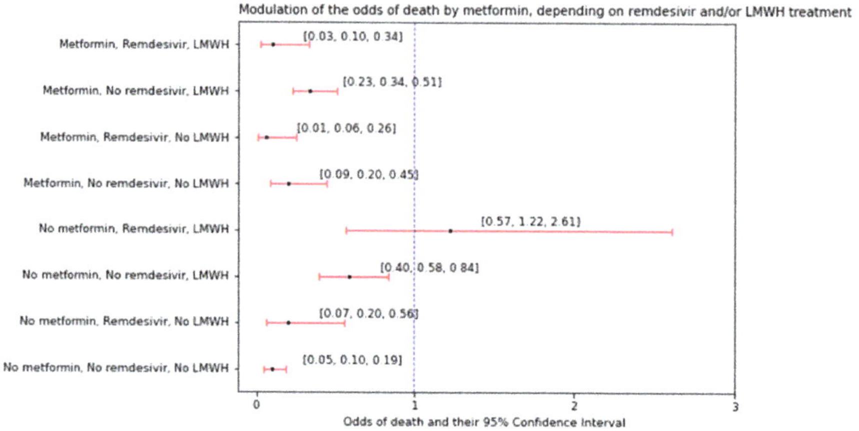

Figure 4. Estimated baseline odds of death depending on administration of metformin and/or remdesivir and/or low-molecular-weight heparin (LMWH).

Based on the estimations from the model among the stratum that did not undergo either remdesivir or LMWH treatment, individuals who were administered with metformin would show 2.10-fold higher odds of death compared to individuals who were not administered with metformin. This fold difference would be approximately 3.54-fold lower ($p \approx 0.036$) in the stratum administered with LMWH (in patients with or without remdesivir administration), or 6.93-fold lower ($p \approx 0.011$) in the stratum administered with remdesivir (in patients with or without LMWH administration). Interestingly, LMWH and remdesivir did not significantly affect each other in the way that they modulated the effect of metformin intake on the odds of death ($\beta = 0.069$, 95% CI: 0.004–1.32, $p \approx 0.076$). Based on the baseline odds of death for different patient characteristics, metformin intake was associated with higher odds of death under no treatment with LMWH and remdesivir, although it would promote survival if LMWH and/or remdesivir had been administered during hospitalization (Figure 4).

3.5. Significant Contrasts. Part 2: Insights into Aging. Inflammation and its Mutual Effect on How Insulin Affected the Odds of Death

Similar to the previous subsection, the interactions selected for further exploration were based on their significance upon applying the likelihood ratio (LR) test. To fully understand the interaction between age, hsCRP and insulin on the odds of death, one needs to assume that the baseline individual who would be referred to in this subsection was aged 64 with hsCRP equal to 48.88.

Interestingly, age- and inflammation-associated changes in the odds of death in the baseline individuals would depend on insulin administration (Table 3). Among patients not administered with insulin, every subsequent one-year increase in age or one-unit increase in hsCRP would cause, respectively, 0.6% or 6.1% increases in the odds of death ($p < 0.001$). Conversely, these age and inflammation-wise changes in odds of death were not observed among patients administered with insulin.

Table 3. Description of effects and their significant interactions in building a model to determine the modification of the impact of metformin intake on the likelihood of death in patients taking LMWH and/or remdesivir. (**A**) Reference group: no insulin administration, aged 64, with hsCRP 48.88. (**B**) Reference group: insulin administration, aged 64, with hsCRP 48.88.

A. Reference Group: No Insulin Administration, Aged 64, with hsCRP 48.88										
Effect/Interaction	**Description of the Analyzed Effect/Interaction**	**β**	**β SE**	**Wald Stat.**	**β −95% CI**	**β 95% CI**	**Est. Effect/ Interaction**	**Est. Effect/ Interaction −95% CI**	**Est. Effect/ Interaction 95% CI**	***p***
Intercept	Odds of death for a patient not administered with insulin, aged 64, with hsCRP 48.88 mg/L	−2.026	0.224	81.551	−2.465	−1.586	**0.1319**	0.0850	0.2047	**<0.001**
Insulin	Modulation of odds by insulin administration at age 64 and hsCRP 48.88 mg/L	1.152	0.355	10.554	0.457	1.847	**3.1647**	1.5793	6.3414	**0.001**
hsCRP (centered at 48.88)	Change in odds upon each subsequent 1-unit increase in hsCRP	0.006	0.001	17.667	0.003	0.009	**1.0061**	1.0033	1.0090	**<0.001**
Age (centered at 64)	Change in odds upon each subsequent 1-year increase in age	0.059	0.014	17.278	0.031	0.087	**1.0608**	1.0317	1.0907	**<0.001**
Insulin*hsCRP	Fold difference in how administration with insulin would change the odds of death, upon each subsequent 1-unit increase in hsCRP	−0.007	0.003	5.720	−0.012	−0.001	**0.9932**	0.9877	0.9988	**0.017**
Insulin*Age	Fold difference in how administration with insulin would change the odds of death, upon each subsequent 1-year increase in age	−0.056	0.023	5.706	−0.102	−0.010	**0.9457**	0.9034	0.9900	**0.017**
‡ hsCRP*Age	Fold change in how age and hsCRP modulated each other in changing the odds of death	−0.00009	0.00015	0.389	−0.00038	0.00020	0.9999	0.9996	1.0002	0.533
‡ Insulin*hsCRP*Age	Fold change in how hsCRP and hsCRP modulated the impact of each other on changing the impact of insulin on the odds of death	0.00040	0.00029	1.978	−0.00016	0.00096	1.0004	0.9998	1.0010	0.160
B. Reference Group: Insulin Administration, Aged 64, with hsCRP 48.88										
Effect/Interaction	**Description of the Analyzed Effect/Interaction**	**β**	**β SE**	**Wald Stat.**	**β −95% CI**	**β 95% CI**	**Est. Effect/ Interaction**	**Est. Effect/ Interaction −95% CI**	**Est. Effect/ Interaction 95% CI**	***p***
Intercept	Odds of death for a patient administered with insulin, aged 64, with hsCRP 48.88 mg/L	−0.874	0.275	10.119	−1.412	−0.335	**0.4174**	0.2437	0.7151	**0.001**
Insulin	Modulation of odds by the lack of insulin administration, at age 64 and hsCRP 48.88 mg/L	−1.152	0.355	10.554	−1.847	−0.457	**0.3160**	0.1577	0.6332	**0.001**
hsCRP (centered at 48.88)	Change in odds upon each subsequent 1-unit increase in hsCRP	−0.001	0.002	0.079	−0.005	0.004	0.9993	0.9946	1.0041	0.779
Age (centered at 64)	Change in odds upon each subsequent 1-year increase in age	0.003	0.019	0.031	−0.033	0.040	1.0033	0.9675	1.0404	0.861
Insulin*hsCRP	Fold difference in how the lack of administration with insulin would change the odds of death, upon each subsequent 1-unit increase in hsCRP	0.007	0.003	5.720	0.001	0.012	**1.0068**	1.0012	1.0124	**0.017**
Insulin*Age	Fold difference in how the lack of administration with insulin would change the odds of death, upon each subsequent 1-year increase in age	0.056	0.023	5.706	0.010	0.102	**1.0574**	1.0101	1.1069	**0.017**
‡ hsCRP*Age	Fold change in how age and hsCRP modulated each other in changing the odds of death	0.00031	0.00024	1.605	−0.00017	0.00079	1.0003	0.9998	1.0008	0.205
‡ Insulin*hsCRP*Age	Fold change in how hsCRP and hsCRP modulated the impact of each other on changing the impact of insulin on the odds of death	−0.00040	0.00029	1.978	−0.00096	0.00016	0.9996	0.9990	1.0002	0.160

'X*Y' terms denote interactions between variables (effects). ‡ denotes interactions that were explored upon the addition of both of them to the model. *p*-values lower than 0.05 and their corresponding ORs are marked **in bold**. Abbreviations: CI, confidence interval; hsCRP, high-sensitivity C-reactive protein; SE, standard error.

Let us further assume that the baseline individuals were not administered with insulin. Based on the model (Table 3), this stratum would show approximately 3.16-fold higher odds of death if insulin were administered ($p \approx 0.001$). This occurrence stemmed from different baseline odds of death depending on insulin administration (0.4174 if administered vs. 0.1319 if not). However, as both age and hsCRP modulated these odds only in individuals not administered with insulin (Figure 5A,B), there are age and hsCRP-related characteristics (Figure 5D,F) that would not only render the odds in this group higher than the 0.4174 (the baseline odds for patients administered with insulin), but also make death more probable than survival (odds > 1) among this sole group (e.g., not administered with insulin), as shown in Figure 5C,E.

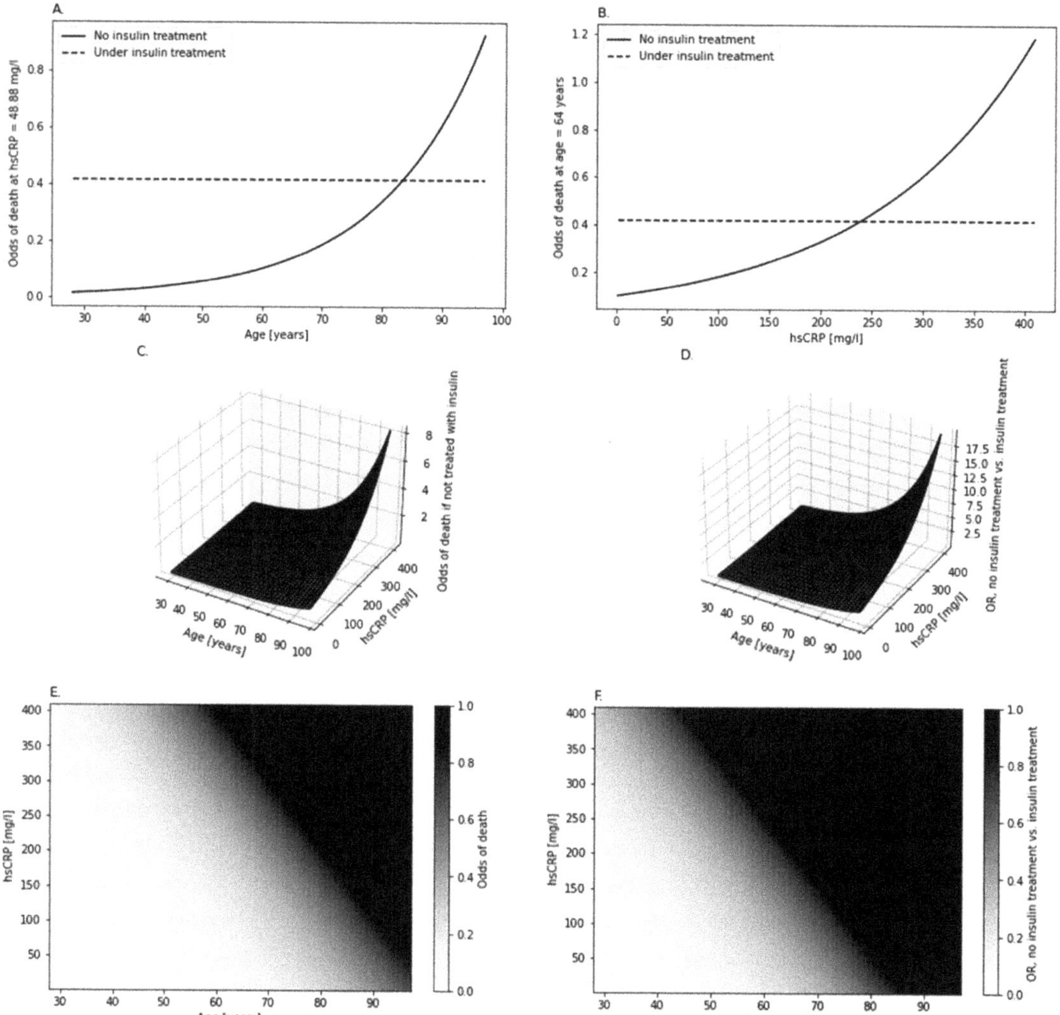

Figure 5. The three-way modulation of the odds of death by insulin, age and inflammation (high-sensitivity CRP—hsCRP). Plots (**A**,**B**) show how age (**A**) or hsCRP (**B**) change the odds of death depending on the administration of insulin. Plot (**C**) shows how age and hsCRP, together, change the odds of death among individuals not administered with insulin. Plot (**D**) presents the not administered/administered (with insulin) OR depending on both age and hsCRP. Plots (**E**,**F**) are

heatmaps created from plots (**C**,**D**), showing when the probability of death is higher than the probability of survival (odds > 1 shown in black plot (**E**)) or when the individuals not administered with insulin are of the higher odds of death compared to individuals who were administered with insulin (OR > 1 shown in black, plot (**F**)).

3.6. Significant Contrasts. Part 3: The Association between Death and LMWH Treatment Differed Depending on Age

The baseline individual referred to in this subsection was assumed to be 64 years old (Table 4). According to the model, such a patient would most probably survive (odds < 1), posing odds of death approximately 0.131 under no LMWH treatment or approximately 0.286 if LMWH was administered (OR $\approx$ 0.456, $p \approx 0.022$). As age, per se, would significantly alter the odds of death only among individuals administered with LMWH (5.5% increase of the odds with each one-year increase in age), the administered/not administered OR of death would be increasing by 6.1% with every one-year age increase above 64 years old ($p \approx 0.019$), as shown in Figure 6.

Table 4. Insights from a model aimed to assess the modulation of the association of LMWH treatment with the odds of death among COVID-19-positive diabetic patients by age.

A. Reference Group: No LMWH Administration, Aged 64										
Effect/Interaction	**Description of the Analyzed Effect/Interaction**	**β**	**β SE**	**Wald Stat.**	**β −95% CI**	**β 95% CI**	**Est. Effect/ Interaction**	**Est. Effect/ Interaction −95% CI**	**Est. Effect/ Interaction 95% CI**	***p***
Intercept	Odds of death for a patient not administered with LMWH, aged 64	−2.036	0.293	48.338	−2.610	−1.462	0.131	0.074	0.232	**<0.001**
LMWH	Modulation of odds by LMWH administration, at age 64	0.785	0.343	5.235	0.113	1.457	2.192	1.119	4.295	**0.022**
Age (centered at 64)	Change in odds upon each subsequent 1-year increase in age	−0.006	0.022	0.073	−0.048	0.037	0.994	0.953	1.037	0.788
LMWH*Age	Fold difference in how administration with LMWH would change the odds of death, upon each subsequent 1-year increase in age	0.059	0.025	5.472	0.010	0.109	1.061	1.010	1.115	**0.019**
B. Reference Group: LMWH Administration, Aged 64										
Effect/Interaction	**Description of the Analyzed Effect/Interaction**	**β**	**β SE**	**Wald Stat.**	**β −95% CI**	**β 95% CI**	**Est. Effect/ Interaction**	**Est. Effect/ Interaction −95% CI**	**Est. Effect/ Interaction 95% CI**	***p***
Intercept	Odds of death for a patient administered with LMWH, aged 64	−1.251	0.179	49.031	−1.602	−0.901	0.286	0.202	0.406	**<0.001**
LMWH	Modulation of odds by the lack of LMWH administration, at age 64	−0.785	0.343	5.235	−1.457	−0.113	0.456	0.233	0.894	**0.022**
Age (centered at 64)	Change in odds upon each subsequent 1-year increase in age	0.053	0.013	16.461	0.028	0.079	1.055	1.028	1.083	**<0.001**
LMWH*Age	Fold difference in how the lack of administration with LMWH would change the odds of death, upon each subsequent 1-year increase in age	−0.059	0.025	5.472	−0.109	−0.010	0.942	0.897	0.990	**0.019**

'X*Y' terms denote interactions between variables (effects). Values of the 'Age' variable were centered at 60 years of age. p-values lower than 0.05 are marked **in bold**. Abbreviations: CI, confidence interval; SE, standard error; LMWH, low-molecular-weight heparin.

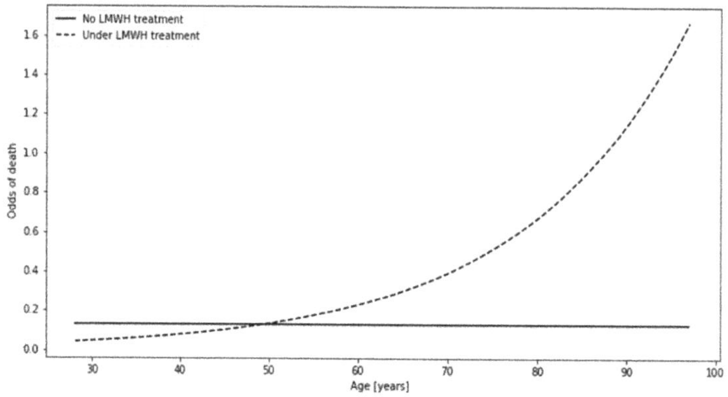

Figure 6. The relationship between the odds of death and the patient's age depending on the administration of low-molecular-weight heparin (LMWH).

4. Discussion

COVID-19, as many other inflammation-driving diseases/syndromes, induces the excessive production of inflammatory cytokines ('cytokine storm') leading to activation of CD4- and CD8-positive lymphocytes. This dysregulation leads to development of various aforementioned comorbidities, often leading to increased mortality [4,21]. In this study, non-survivors were characterized by male sex; higher age; the following traits upon their admission: $SpO_2 \leq 94\%$, undergoing oxygen therapy (in many cases due to the severity of the disease) and hemorrhage; and the following traits associated with their medical history: heart failure, heart infarction and chronic kidney disease. These findings were in line with the literature, which links higher mortality in patients suffering from COVID-19 and T2DM with male sex [22] heart failure, chronic kidney disease [23], hyperglycemia (poor diabetic control) [24], lower oxygen saturation [25] or heart infarction in the past [26]. Another study lists cardiovascular diseases (such as coronary artery disease) and stroke as other death-promoting factors [27]. Moreover, one of the aforementioned studies [21] also showed that death during hospitalization was more frequent among the patients who had developed the following during the hospitalization: hypovolemic shock, cardiogenic shock, heart infarction, sepsis, chronic obstructive pulmonary disease (COPD) or other inflammatory pulmonary syndromes [22]. However, to our knowledge, the literature does not sufficiently cover the topic of risk modeling in these patients (COVID-19 and T2DM), as it focuses on analyzing the effects of different factors on mortality with use of the models. Albeit the models correct the estimated values (odds, risk etc.) for characteristics such as sex, age and comorbidity, they do not utilize nor enable exploring the interactions between these factors, let alone exploring the interactions between the drugs administered during the hospitalization. An example of such a study carried out on the COVID-19- and T2DM-positive stratum [28] showed that COPD increased the odds of death. However, this effect was not further explored. In this situation, one would be left to their own interpretation, not knowing whether the COPD-associated increase in mortality would be further modulated by any comorbidity, requiring the use of a different set of patient characteristics depending on these comorbidities. Explorative interaction analysis could prove an answer to this question, possibly revealing the population strata that does not show an association between COPD and higher mortality. This and similar musings led to the conceptualization of our preliminary study [29–32].

The aim of this study was dichotomic. Univariate analysis and multivariate AI-assisted extraction of the key factors associated with the odds of death in the COVID-19- and T2DM-positive patient stratum acted as a prelude to exploring whether the pro-fatal effect of antidiabetic and anti-viral drugs administered during hospitalization was affected by any patient-specific characteristic upon admission.

Nearly all of the available parameters were associated with the odds of death based on univariate (not adjusted by any other variables) logistic regression analysis. The analysis revealed that older age and male sex (unsurprisingly) were positive factors for estimating mortality odds. Having an oxygen saturation under the physiological values (95%–100%), likewise, was positively associated with a fatal outcome. LMWH and acetylsalicylic acid were iatrogenic factors promoting in-hospital death. Moreover, among the laboratory parameters, hsCRP, K, creatinine, urea and RDW-SD were positive indicators of higher odds of death. While it is logical that the inflammation- and diuresis- related parameters would be associated with higher severity of the disease [29–31], the anisocytosis parameter (RDW-SD) may not be a first-pick candidate for a poor outcome predictor. In clinical practice, RDW is a predictor of outcome in critically ill and septic patients (an increase in RDW is caused by an increase in the number of old red blood cells, which have a lower volume). Several meta-analyses have demonstrated the association between RDW and the risk of mortality in patients with COVID-19 [33] and proved the important role of RDW in predicting prognosis [34]. RDW-SD has also been shown to be a strong independent predictor of infection severity and death in COVID-19 patients: an RDW-SD $\leq$ 43 showed no risk of death, while RDW-SD > 47 indicated severe disease and a high risk of mortality [35]. If the RDW-SD value would fall in the range of 43 < RDW-SD $\leq$ 47, the course of the disease would be severe, but the risk of death was low. Therefore, it seems likely that determining the value of RDW may prove important in undertaking early intervention to reduce mortality in COVID-19 patients, especially in the case of limited resources. However, so far, the role of RDW has not been previously demonstrated in patients with COVID-19 and type 2 diabetes. Therefore, univariate logistic regression analysis showed that age, male sex and RDW-SD are positive factors in estimating the odds of death. Moreover, RDW-SD is a strong independent predictor of infection severity and death in COVID-19 patients. An RDW-SD value > 47 indicated severe disease and a high risk of death.

It should be emphasized that during the first (univariate) step of our analysis, insulin and metformin administration were revealed to be insignificant in terms of mortality odds modulation. While this does not necessarily mean that insulin and metformin play no role in such predictions (as will be shown later in the discussion), it could be rightfully pointed out that insulin and metformin could not be used, on their own, in the process of estimating the risk of death in these patients.

In the next step of the analysis (deriving a multivariate model, Figure 3), the factors that were used in the previous step were all included in the initial pool of candidates for predictors of death. Subsequently, they were discarded one by one in a stepwise manner based on how much information they brought to the classifying (death/survival) model. As the pool of rejected factors began to increase, all of these variables were re-checked whether they should be again included in the model classifying mortality status. The multivariate model derived in the process enables estimation of the odds of death based on five factors: LMWH treatment, age, RDW-SD, sex and K. Calculating the odds of death of a patient admitted to the ward could be performed by multiplying the baseline odds (denoted by the intercept) based on the aforementioned characteristics. The value of the intercept and OR associated with sex show that survival would be the most frequent outcome (odds << 1) in a typical patient (described in the figure description) suffering from both COVID-19 and diabetes, regardless of sex (women: odds = 0.009, men: odds = $0.009 \cdot 2.798 \approx 0.025$). Had two patients of the same outcome been compared, each one-year gap between them would render the older patient 6.9% (odds = 1.069) more likely to die during the hospitalization. Each increase in potassium (by 1 mmol/L) and RDW-SD (by 15%) would, likewise promote death (by 98% and 87.7%, respectively). The association of these factors with death may be explained with cellular damage due to oxidative stress caused by inflammation. While, in this state, K would be simply liberated from the cells, the RDW-SD increase would be associated with the increase in anisocytosis in the state of constant/transient anemia—not only caused by their lysis per se but also correlated with kidney damage due to the lack of erythropoietin secretion. An over 10-fold increase in the odds of death upon

LMWH treatment does not indicate that LMWH promotes death—it should rather hint that the decision of its administration was made in case of patients of higher disease severity emerging from possible increase of D-dimers, which account for the increased fibrinolysis. The mentioned D-dimers have been posed as mortality predictors in COVID-19 patients [36]. Moreover, increase plasmatic concentration of D-dimers among T2DM patients was shown to be associated with increased risk of cardiovascular disease events, regardless of conventional risk factors or the treatment-wise factors [36]. However, to our knowledge, D-dimers have not been proven (due to not having been studied) to pose as direct predictors of death in patients with T2DM nor patients with both T2DM and COVID-19. The last observation, already used while analyzing the baseline odds, is that men were of markedly higher odds of dying (in this model, OR = 2.798). While, as mentioned before, the odds in both sexes would be favoring survival in typical patients (64-year-old, 45.78% RDW-SD, 4.10 mmol/L K, no LMWH treatment), this sex-related difference would, epidemiologically, play an important role among the patients of higher age and disease severity. While this risk assessment model needs to undergo validation and comparison to different models in future studies to be taken more seriously, one is certain that the multivariate models, likewise to univariate, provide a hint that the administration of insulin and metformin is not a factor informative enough to be used in risk assessment of the entire COVID-19- and T2DM-positive population. Potential possibilities stemming from this information were revealed upon the last part of the analysis. The developed multivariate model allowed for the estimation of the chance of death based on LMWH treatment, age, RDW-SD, gender and K. Each increase in the patient's age by one year increased the chance of death by 6.9%, each increase in potassium concentration by 1 mmol/L increased the chance of death by 98% and an increase in RDW-SD by 15% increased the chance of death by 87%, which was caused by cell damage by oxidative stress. LMWH was used in patients with advanced COVID-19, in whom an increase in D-dimer levels (increased fibrinolysis) was observed. The 10-fold increase in the risk of death after LMWH treatment was not due to the treatment itself, but to the stage of advancement of COVID-19. The association of gender with a higher risk of death concerned older patients with advanced disease. There was no gender effect observed for younger patients, aged 64.

The last part of the analysis explored the interactions between the variables (factors) in terms of changing the odds of death. What makes these interactions different to the convention used in the previous part of the study is that they explore whether any pair of factors (patient characteristics) has a multiplicative effect on the modulation of the odds of death by the third factor—a drug used during the hospitalization. LMWH and remdesivir were independent on each other in how they modulated the effect of metformin on the odds of death. Conversely, age and hsCRP interacted with each other, having a multiplicative effect on the difference in the odds of mortality between individuals who took insulin vs. the ones who did not. In the first observed interaction, remdesivir and LMWH treatments showed different patterns in affecting the odds of death, between patients administered with metformin and those under no such treatment. Upon analyzing the odds of death (N deaths/N survivals, Figure 4) it could be observed that the odds of death were different upon administration of remdesivir and LMWH, depending on whether the patient was under treatment with metformin. While metformin-administered patients showed an increasing pattern in the odds of death (LMWH and remdesivir > LMWH only > remdesivir only > neither LMWH nor remdesivir), such a pattern was not observed among the patients under no metformin treatment. One may argue about the novelty of this observation due to the fact that the treatment with remdesivir and LMWH blatantly shows the severity of the disease, thus implicating higher odds of death. However, to our knowledge, our study is the first one to show that this rationale was not universal for all of the COVID-19 T2DM patients. To gather more precise information on the odds of in-hospital death, before risk modeling, the entire population may need to be stratified in regards to metformin treatment and, perhaps, treatment with other antidiabetic agents as well. Another observation from this study was that metformin intake was associated with higher odds of death (0.20 vs. 0.10, Figure 4) compared to no intake among patients under no LMWH and remdesivir treatment. There is no possible way to discuss this matter referring to the literature since other studies did not report the odds of death in the same context as our study (three-way interaction). First and foremost, it is stated that metformin has both in vivo and in vitro effects on *SARS-CoV-2*, letting one assume there might be possibly different outcomes (and sets of its predictors) depending on metformin treatment [32]. Some studies on COVID-19 patients indicate lower likelihood of death upon metformin treatment [37–39]. However, DeFronzo et al. reported a lack of this association, but observed a markedly lower likelihood of heart failure among patients administered with metformin [38,40–42]. Analyzing interactions with inhibitors of dipeptydylpeptidase 4 (DPP-4i) may be a good choice for future analyses similar to ours, since this agent appears to have both direct and indirect effects on *SARS-CoV-2* infection. DPP-4i, being a gliptin [41] drug representative, owing to its anti-inflammatory action, could be hypothesized to indirectly (through lowering the CRP concentration) affect the severity of COVID-19 [38]. Another hypothesized indirect action of DPP-4i is combating the 'cytokine storm' through inhibiting the activation of TLR4 in the lung alveoli [5]. As *SARS-CoV-2* binds with these receptors, DPP-4i could help combat the pulmonary 'cytokine storm', leading to a decrease in lung injuries and collateral damage to other organs that could induce the state of multi-organ failure over the duration of COVID-19 [11,43]. Moreover, DPP-4i acts as a receptor for the *SARS-CoV-2* [13]; likewise, the drug binds with *MERS-CoV* [44]. This occurrence could have been associated with the observation of a lower concentration of soluble (in serum/plasma) DPP-4i among the diabetic COVID-19 patients [45]. So far, the idea behind using DPP-4i as a predictor of death/severity of the disease in the mentioned population could not be taken for granted due to the inconsistencies in the literature [46–49]. Likewise, remdesivir treatment had positive effects on the clinical improvement associated with the reduced risk of severe acute respiratory distress syndrome in need of intubation but it seemed not to affect mortality among COVID-19 patients [50]. In the presented publication, the analysis of interactions between variables (factors) in terms of the change in the probability of death showed that LMWH and remdesivir independently modulated the effect of metformin on the risk of death, while age and hsCRP interacted in their effect on the difference in the risk of death between people taking insulin and those not taking it. Metformin increased the risk of death the most in the group of people taking both LMWH and remdesivir. This observation was not demonstrated in the same group of people who did not take metformin. Additionally, age and hsCRP modulated the chance of death only in people who did not receive insulin.

However, DPP-4i could take part in interactions on which the information is scarce. Significant interaction of insulin with hsCRP and age hinted at different modulation of the odds of death by insulin, depending on these two other variables. This occurrence was due to fact that age and hsCRP did not significantly change the odds of death among patients administered with insulin (Table 3, Figure 5A,B), while the patients not administered with it showed a positive association between these odds and either hsCRP or age (Table 3, Figure 5A–C). This insulin-related difference between patients deepened the difference in odds between them when given more advanced age and/or higher hsCRP (Figure 5D,F). However, there is no universal answer to whether any of these groups would be more prone to showing a fatal outcome—it all is a matter of age and hsCRP (Figure 5F). Moreover, upon reaching a specific threshold of age and hsCRP, the odds would become of favor of death (e.g., more patients would die compared to the count of survivors) among the patients not administered with insulin. This interaction is not as complex as it could be, since age and hsCRP, although both simultaneously affecting the odds of death, had an isolated effect on it—hsCRP and age did not modulate the effect of each other on the odds ('hsCRP*Age' in Table 3) regardless of administration with insulin ('Insulin*hsCRP*Age' in Table 3). The cause of such a phenomenon, not discussed or mentioned in other studies, remains a mystery until validated and further analyzed on a bigger population, with possibly more factors brought into the model. A study [12] showed insulin treatment to be positively associated with the likelihood of death. However, the said study did not explore the possible effect of age on the insulin–mortality association. Perhaps a future model could employ both insulin–age and metformin–remdesivir–LMWH interactions. Hopefully, new research would investigate this matter on bigger retrospective data and/or a diabetic population not suffering from COVID-19 (assuming no COVID-19 outbreak in the future).

The third interaction was featured in this manuscript since it is associated with LMWH treatment, which is featured in both the multivariate model (Figure 3) and the aforementioned interaction (Figure 4). If one was to divide patients in the context of LMWH administration, the individuals under no such treatment would show constant odds of death equal to 0.202 regardless of age, meaning that the number of deceased patients would constitute about 1/5 of the survivors. Patients under LMWH treatment showed an increase in the odds with age, reaching the threshold which favors death at the age of approximately 85 years (odds > 1, thus N deaths > N survivors).

Before concluding the findings, study limitations need to be introduced. The first limitation comes from the rather low sample size (Figure 1). It should be emphasized that the data of all hospitalized T2DM patients from the Temporary COVID Hospital were employed for carrying out this study. Thus, we assumed the data to be randomly collected (in spite of the sample size), since all patients participated in the process. However, low sample size restricted us to study only up to two-way interactions and forming three-way interactions to be analyzed so as to avoid redundancy. Moreover, all of the observed interactions were not added to the multivariate model (Figure 3), having in mind that such a model would be highly prone to overfitting, thus would be biased with an increased false discovery rate. The sample size for such a model would need to be more than 1000 individuals (50–100 for every variable/interaction in the model), which exceeded the possibilities of our cooperation with this one hospital. The lack of comorbidities (seen in Table 1) in the initial set of variables was intentional so as to remove factors that could be so strongly associated with mortality that they would render other factors too weak to be spotted upon being analyzed in a population sample of such size. This choice was made upon assessing the comorbidity-associated frequencies and their statistics in regards to mortality (Table 1). Moreover, some patient features that could have had an impact on the observed were not registered upon creating this database in the times of COVID-19 onset. These features include BMI, diabetes duration, glycemic control, overall frailty, the stage of T2DM, and the severity of COVID-19. Since the decision on treatment with LMWH and remdesivir was made upon the admission of the study participants, there was no need for adjusting the models based on length of treatment with these agents. Our future study plans to gather the information from the patients regarding whether the treatment strategy for them changed after ending the hospitalization in the Temporary COVID-19 Hospital. Moreover, information on the post-hospitalization mortality in these individuals will be based on analyzing the national registry. Lastly, some may argue that the study shows neither goodness-of-fit metrics nor the classification quality of the model. While showing these properties of the model would be vital in a study that strived to determine the best death likelihood assessment model, our study focused on analyzing the models and interactions related to treatment. We explored the factors that may not even modulate the odds of risk per se, without their interactions with other patient characteristics (in this study: age, hsCRP and treatment with remdesivir or LMWH). Having these drawbacks in mind, we would like to encourage the readers to view this study as preliminary.

The insights from this study unfold to be rather peculiar, bringing some skepticism in the case of analyzing mortality risk with models based solely on logistic regression or (presumably) other regression methods. This study hints at possible caveats that could be encountered by simply using multivariate models without previously investigating whether the patterns of mortality changes associated with the predictors were affected by treatment. In this study, although insulin and/or metformin were not informative enough to be included in the multivariate assessment of the likelihood of death, the information about their administration revealed a contrast in how remdesivir and LMWH (in the case of metformin) compared to hsCRP and age (in the case of insulin) affected the odds of death in hospitalized T2DM patients suffering from COVID-19. Moreover, the association of LMWH treatment (one of the predictors in the multivariate model) with death was shown to be dependent on age. These observations not only show an importance of taking treatment into account when assessing death likelihood in the specific COVID-19 T2DM population, but hopefully may prove as grounds for future research into mortality modeling among T2DM patients. Although society has liberated itself from the grasp of the COVID-19 pandemic, the deleterious impact of the *SARS-CoV-2* infection may come with time in the form of newly studied post-COVID syndrome, leading to a sheer increase in the frequency of various comorbidities. If this time were to come, the analysis of interactions stemming from varying intakes of drugs may pose as a key to successful risk assessment, possibly saving thousands of lives and broadening our knowledge of other threats yet to come. In the further part of this research, we plan to analyze the mortality of patients included in the presented study in the second follow-up (after two years). We will also examine levels of early markers of kidney damage, neurological disorders and intravascular damage in patients who have had symptomatic COVID-19.

5. Conclusions

In a multivariate model, along with other multivariate-adjusted significant features (LMWH treatment, age, sex, K concentration), RDW-SD was associated with mortality among the patients suffering from COVID-19 and type 2 diabetes. For every 15% increase in RDW-SD, the odds of death increased by 87.7%.

Stratification by insulin administration revealed that age and hsCRP increased the odds of death exclusively among the patients who were not administered with insulin. Metformin intake was positively associated with death among those of low age and low hsCRP. Upon increase in both age and/or hsCRP above the threshold (mapped in Figure 5F), metformin intake started to be negatively associated with death. The impact of this effect kept rising with age and hsCRP.

Administration of remdesivir and/or LMWH changed the association between metformin and the odds of death from positive (if neither remdesivir nor LMWH were administered) to negative (if any of these drugs was administered). Moreover, remdesivir and LMWH had an additive effect on the magnitude of the pro-survival impact of metformin intake among the patients.

The association between LMWH administration and the odds of death changed from negative to positive with the increase in age.

The above findings ought to be taken with a pinch of salt until they have been validated with more sophisticated models (with these and other interactions), in a bigger population sample. Future research will, likewise, need to test these associations in a diabetic population not suffering from COVID-19.

Although metformin and insulin may not, per se, act as universal indicators of death in diabetic patients with COVID-19, their role could vary within the higher personalization of the risk assessment model (through adding and exploring their interactions with various patient characteristics). Such a practice, when utilized in large models, could provide a definite answer, cutting down the discussion of whether these agents are associated with death, when facing corroborating results from the literature. This conclusion applies regardless of whether the diabetic patients would be suffering from COVID-19 or not, since the studies into metformin and insulin in context of mortality lack the exploration of their interactions.

Author Contributions: Conceptualization, Ł.L., A.B.-S. and K.M.; methodology, M.M.; software, Ł.L.; validation, M.T. and P.L.; formal analysis, Ł.L.; investigation, M.R., A.M.-W., D.B.-C., E.K., J.S. and A.D.; resources, J.A.-M.; data curation, K.K.; writing—Ł.L., A.B.-S. and Ł.L., writing—review and editing, K.M.; visualization, Ł.L. and A.B.-S.; supervision, K.M. and E.A.J.; project administration, K.M. and E.A.J. All authors have read and agreed to the published version of the manuscript.

Funding: This research received no external funding.

Institutional Review Board Statement: The study was conducted in accordance with the Declaration of Helsinki, and approved Bioethical Committee and Ethics Committee of the Medical University in Wroclaw, Poland (No: KB-666/2019, 7 October 2019).

Informed Consent Statement: Informed consent was obtained from all subjects involved in the study.

Data Availability Statement: Access to the data is possible after sending an inquiry to the corresponding author by e-mail.

Acknowledgments: The authors thank researchers from the Faculty of Medicine, Wroclaw Medical University—Barbara Adamik, Krzysztof Kaliszewski, Katarzyna Kiliś-Pstrusińska, Michał Pomorski and Marcin Protasiewicz for their help in creating the database.

Conflicts of Interest: The authors declare no conflicts of interest.

Appendix A

Table A1. Results from the univariate analysis of the associations of the selected effects (variables) on the odds of death among COVID-19 patients suffering from type 2 diabetes.

Effect	Analyzed Cat.	Reference Cat.	OR	OR −95% CI	OR 95% CI	p
$SpO_2 \leq 94$ on room air	Yes	No	1.982	1.006	3.906	0.048
Sex	Male	Female	1.771	1.126	2.785	0.013
Insulin	Yes	No	1.364	0.832	2.236	0.219
Metformin	Yes	No	0.716	0.459	1.115	0.139
LMWH	Yes	No	3.506	1.972	6.234	<0.001
Acetylsalicylic acid	Yes	No	1.703	1.076	2.696	0.023
Convalescent plasma	Yes	No	1.618	0.878	2.981	0.123
Remdesivir	Yes	No	1.209	0.659	2.216	0.540
Age	-	-	1.038	1.017	1.060	<0.001
hsCRP	-	-	1.004	1.002	1.006	0.001
Na	-	-	1.026	0.988	1.066	0.184
K	-	-	1.886	1.399	2.543	<0.001
$\log_{1.15}$(RDW-SD)	-	-	1.538	1.235	1.915	<0.001
$\log_2$(Creatinine)	-	-	1.537	1.197	1.974	0.001
$\log_2$(Urea)	-	-	1.877	1.444	2.439	<0.001

Abbreviations: CI, confidence interval; OR, odds ratio. The visualization of this table (without the p-values) is given in Figure 2.

Table A2. The process of derivation of the multivariate model through stepwise elimination (cut-off $p = 0.05$).

Step	Effect	Wald Statistic	Wald Test p	Score Statistic	Score Test p	Effect Status
1	$SpO_2 \leq 94$ on room air	0.280	0.597			In the model
	Sex	5.731	0.017			In the model
	Insulin	0.550	0.458			In the model
	Metformin	<0.001	0.986			Excluded in this step
	LMWH	15.447	<0.001			In the model
	Acetylsalicylic acid	0.609	0.435			In the model
	Convalescent plasma	0.153	0.695			In the model
	Remdesivir	0.188	0.665			In the model
	Age	9.492	0.002			In the model
	hsCRP	1.822	0.177			In the model
	K	4.818	0.028			In the model
	$\log_2$(RDW-SD)	8.273	0.004			In the model
	$\log_2$(Creatinine)	0.426	0.514			In the model
2	$SpO_2 \leq 94$ on room air	0.282	0.596			In the model
	Sex	5.816	0.016			In the model
	Insulin	0.556	0.456			In the model
	$\log_2$(Creatinine)	0.433	0.511			In the model
	LMWH	15.510	<0.001			In the model
	Acetylsalicylic acid	0.610	0.435			In the model
	Convalescent plasma	0.154	0.695			Excluded in this step
	Remdesivir	0.188	0.664			In the model
	Age	9.684	0.002			In the model
	hsCRP	1.859	0.173			In the model
	K	4.817	0.028			In the model
	$\log_2$(RDW-SD)	8.299	0.004			In the model
	Metformin			0.000	0.986	Excluded in the previous step(s)
3	$SpO_2 \leq 94$ on room air	0.242	0.623			Excluded in this step
	Sex	5.731	0.017			In the model
	Insulin	0.483	0.487			In the model
	$\log_2$(Creatinine)	0.375	0.540			In the model
	LMWH	15.773	<0.001			In the model
	Acetylsalicylic acid	0.545	0.460			In the model
	$\log_2$(RDW-SD)	8.199	0.004			In the model
	Remdesivir	0.248	0.618			In the model
	Age	9.718	0.002			In the model
	hsCRP	1.924	0.165			In the model
	K	5.701	0.017			In the model

Table A2. *Cont.*

Step	Effect	Wald Statistic	Wald Test *p*	Score Statistic	Score Test *p*	Effect Status
3	Convalescent plasma			0.154	0.695	Excluded in the previous step(s)
	Metformin			0.001	0.981	Excluded in the previous step(s)
4	K	5.537	0.019			In the model
	Sex	5.628	0.018			In the model
	Insulin	0.602	0.438			In the model
	log_2(Creatinine)	0.314	0.575			In the model
	LMWH	15.516	<0.001			In the model
	Acetylsalicylic acid	0.464	0.496			In the model
	log_2(RDW-SD)	8.024	0.005			In the model
	Remdesivir	0.230	0.631			Excluded in this step
	Age	9.803	0.002			In the model
	hsCRP	1.686	0.194			In the model
	$SpO_2 \leq 94$ on room air			0.242	0.622	Excluded in the previous step(s)
	Convalescent plasma			0.113	0.736	Excluded in the previous step(s)
	Metformin			0.002	0.961	Excluded in the previous step(s)
5	K	5.740	0.017			In the model
	Sex	5.535	0.019			In the model
	Insulin	0.668	0.414			In the model
	log_2(Creatinine)	0.299	0.584			Excluded in this step
	LMWH	15.916	<0.001			In the model
	Acetylsalicylic acid	0.566	0.452			In the model
	log_2(RDW-SD)	7.903	0.005			In the model
	hsCRP	1.750	0.186			In the model
	Age	9.697	0.002			In the model
	Remdesivir			0.231	0.631	Excluded in the previous step(s)
	$SpO_2 \leq 94$ on room air			0.225	0.635	Excluded in the previous step(s)
	Convalescent plasma			0.167	0.683	Excluded in the previous step(s)
	Metformin			0.003	0.957	Excluded in the previous step(s)

Table A2. *Cont.*

Step	Effect	Wald Statistic	Wald Test *p*	Score Statistic	Score Test *p*	Effect Status
6	K	7.608	0.006			In the model
	Sex	6.115	0.013			In the model
	Insulin	0.745	0.388			In the model
	Age	10.004	0.002			In the model
	LMWH	15.954	<0.001			In the model
	Acetylsalicylic acid	0.513	0.474			Excluded in this step
	log_2(RDW-SD)	8.569	0.003			In the model
	hsCRP	1.815	0.178			In the model
	log_2(Creatinine)			0.300	0.584	Excluded in the previous step(s)
	Remdesivir			0.215	0.643	Excluded in the previous step(s)
	$SpO_2 \leq 94$ on room air			0.170	0.680	Excluded in the previous step(s)
	Convalescent plasma			0.114	0.736	Excluded in the previous step(s)
	Metformin			0.001	0.972	Excluded in the previous step(s)
7	K	7.387	0.007			In the model
	Sex	5.872	0.015			In the model
	Insulin	0.459	0.498			Excluded in this step
	Age	9.772	0.002			In the model
	LMWH	15.713	<0.001			In the model
	hsCRP	1.937	0.164			In the model
	log_2(RDW-SD)	8.993	0.003			In the model
	Acetylsalicylic acid			0.515	0.473	Excluded in the previous step(s)
	log_2(Creatinine)			0.244	0.621	Excluded in the previous step(s)
	Remdesivir			0.315	0.575	Excluded in the previous step(s)
	$SpO_2 \leq 94$ on room air			0.104	0.747	Excluded in the previous step(s)
	Convalescent plasma			0.080	0.777	Excluded in the previous step(s)
	Metformin			0.007	0.934	Excluded in the previous step(s)
8	K	8.559	0.003			In the model
	Sex	5.788	0.016			In the model
	log_2(RDW-SD)	8.793	0.003			In the model
	Age	9.999	0.002			In the model
	LMWH	15.825	<0.001			In the model
	hsCRP	2.036	0.154			Excluded in this step

Table A2. *Cont.*

Step	Effect	Wald Statistic	Wald Test *p*	Score Statistic	Score Test *p*	Effect Status
8	Insulin			0.461	0.497	Excluded in the previous step(s)
	Acetylsalicylic acid			0.235	0.628	Excluded in the previous step(s)
	log_2(Creatinine)			0.317	0.573	Excluded in the previous step(s)
	Remdesivir			0.347	0.556	Excluded in the previous step(s)
	$SpO_2 \leq 94$ on room air			0.184	0.668	Excluded in the previous step(s)
	Convalescent plasma			0.031	0.859	Excluded in the previous step(s)
	Metformin			0.024	0.878	Excluded in the previous step(s)
9	K	7.739	0.005			In the model
	Sex	6.134	0.013			In the model
	log_2(RDW-SD)	9.450	0.002			In the model
	Age	9.779	0.002			In the model
	LMWH	16.552	<0.001			In the model
	hsCRP			2.070	0.150	Excluded in the previous step(s)
	Insulin			0.556	0.456	Excluded in the previous step(s)
	Acetylsalicylic acid			0.288	0.592	Excluded in the previous step(s)
	log_2(Creatinine)			0.385	0.535	Excluded in the previous step(s)
	Remdesivir			0.442	0.506	Excluded in the previous step(s)
	$SpO_2 \leq 94$ on room air			0.001	0.970	Excluded in the previous step(s)
	Convalescent plasma			0.095	0.758	Excluded in the previous step(s)
	Metformin			0.171	0.679	Excluded in the previous step(s)

The Wald test was utilized in assessing the value of the factors to be included in the model. The score test (Lagrange multiplier test) was used to check if, at any step, the previously excluded factors should be re-included into the current model. The final model is described in Table 2 and visualized in Figure 3.

Table A3. A list of all possible second-degree (two-way) interactions composed of the selected variables (effects, featured in Tables A1 and A2, inter alia) in context of their significance (compared to the naïve model—LR type 1 test) in modulating the odds of death among COVID-19-positive individuals suffering from type 2 diabetes.

Effect 1	Effect 2	χ^2	*p* (LR Test)
Metformin	Remdesivir	10.257	**0.0014**
LMWH	Metformin	5.6121	**0.0178**
hsCRP	Insulin	5.3447	**0.0208**
LMWH	Age	5.2361	**0.0221**
Age	Insulin	4.368	**0.0366**
K	Remdesivir	3.9539	**0.0468**
$\log_2$(Creatinine)	Insulin	3.8179	0.0507
LMWH	Insulin	3.743	0.053
Convalescent plasma	Metformin	3.7268	0.0535
K	$SpO_2 \leq 94$ on room air	3.7061	0.0542
hsCRP	$SpO_2 \leq 94$ on room air	3.037	0.0814
log2(RDW-SD)	Age	2.9078	0.0882
Metformin	Insulin	2.796	0.0945
Sex	Remdesivir	2.7621	0.0965
$\log_2$(Creatinine)	Metformin	2.7294	0.0985
LMWH	$\log_2$(Creatinine)	2.7034	0.1001
$\log_2$(Urea)	Remdesivir	2.6518	0.1034
K	hsCRP	2.3899	0.1221
LMWH	K	2.1219	0.1452
Acetylsalicylic acid	Metformin	2.0447	0.1527
hsCRP	Metformin	2.0331	0.1539
K	$\log_2$(Urea)	1.9158	0.1663
$\log_2$(RDW-SD)	hsCRP	1.9001	0.1681
K	Metformin	1.5692	0.2103
$\log_2$(RDW-SD)	$SpO_2 \leq 94$ on room air	1.5311	0.2159
LMWH	Remdesivir	1.5194	0.2177
Age	Metformin	1.4653	0.2261
Acetylsalicylic acid	Insulin	1.4478	0.2289
K	Acetylsalicylic acid	1.4253	0.2325
$\log_2$(Urea)	$\log_2$(RDW-SD)	1.3581	0.2439
$\log_2$(RDW-SD)	Metformin	1.1828	0.2768
LMWH	Acetylsalicylic acid	1.1417	0.2853
$\log_2$(Creatinine)	Remdesivir	1.1405	0.2856
$\log_2$(Urea)	Metformin	0.9777	0.3228
$\log_2$(RDW-SD)	Sex	0.9316	0.3344
Age	Convalescent plasma	0.9268	0.3357
LMWH	$SpO_2 \leq 94$ on room air	0.8762	0.3493

Table A3. *Cont.*

Effect 1	Effect 2	χ^2	*p* (LR Test)
hsCRP	Convalescent plasma	0.8687	0.3513
hsCRP	Remdesivir	0.8583	0.3542
Acetylsalicylic acid	Remdesivir	0.8463	0.3576
Sex	Acetylsalicylic acid	0.8111	0.3678
LMWH	hsCRP	0.7506	0.3863
$SpO_2 \leq 94$ on room air	Remdesivir	0.7191	0.3964
log_2(Urea)	Insulin	0.6931	0.4051
K	log_2(Creatinine)	0.6634	0.4153
Convalescent plasma	Remdesivir	0.5695	0.4504
log_2(Creatinine)	Convalescent plasma	0.5348	0.4646
Sex	Metformin	0.5297	0.4668
Age	hsCRP	0.5284	0.4673
log_2(Creatinine)	Sex	0.5032	0.4781
log_2(Creatinine)	Acetylsalicylic acid	0.4948	0.4818
Convalescent plasma	Insulin	0.4787	0.489
LMWH	Sex	0.3969	0.5287
K	log_2(RDW-SD)	0.367	0.5446
K	Insulin	0.3392	0.5603
log_2(Creatinine)	hsCRP	0.2903	0.59
Age	$SpO_2 \leq 94$ on room air	0.2817	0.5956
log_2(RDW-SD)	Acetylsalicylic acid	0.258	0.6115
Insulin	Remdesivir	0.2404	0.6239
log_2(Urea)	$SpO_2 \leq 94$ on room air	0.2237	0.6362
Age	Acetylsalicylic acid	0.2162	0.6419
LMWH	log_2(Urea)	0.2161	0.642
$SpO_2 \leq 94$ on room air	Insulin	0.2128	0.6446
Age	Sex	0.2001	0.6547
Sex	$SpO_2 \leq 94$ on room air	0.1967	0.6574
Age	log_2(Creatinine)	0.1935	0.66
LMWH	Convalescent plasma	0.1814	0.6702
log_2(Creatinine)	$SpO_2 \leq 94$ on room air	0.1459	0.7025
hsCRP	Sex	0.1422	0.7061
log_2(Urea)	log_2(Creatinine)	0.1385	0.7098
log_2(RDW-SD)	Insulin	0.1155	0.734
$SpO_2 \leq 94$ on room air	Convalescent plasma	0.1132	0.7365
$SpO_2 \leq 94$ on room air	Metformin	0.09	0.7642
log_2(Urea)	hsCRP	0.0846	0.7711
K	Convalescent plasma	0.0605	0.8058
Acetylsalicylic acid	Convalescent plasma	0.0507	0.8218
Acetylsalicylic acid	$SpO_2 \leq 94$ on room air	0.0459	0.8303

Table A3. *Cont.*

Effect 1	Effect 2	χ^2	*p* (LR Test)
Age	Remdesivir	0.0427	0.8363
$\log_2$(RDW-SD)	Convalescent plasma	0.0339	0.8538
hsCRP	Acetylsalicylic acid	0.0254	0.8733
K	Sex	0.0216	0.8831
$\log_2$(RDW-SD)	$\log_2$(Creatinine)	0.0209	0.8851
$\log_2$(Urea)	Acetylsalicylic acid	0.0186	0.8914
$\log_2$(RDW-SD)	Remdesivir	0.015	0.9026
K	Age	0.0086	0.9262
$\log_2$(Urea)	Sex	0.0066	0.935
Sex	Convalescent plasma	0.0041	0.9488
$\log_2$(Urea)	Age	0.0023	0.9621
Sex	Insulin	0.0019	0.9654
LMWH	$\log_2$(RDW-SD)	0.0016	0.9678
$\log_2$(Urea)	Convalescent plasma	0.0009	0.9767

Significant findings ($p < 0.05$) are marked **in bold**.

References

1. COVID-19 Cases | WHO COVID-19 Dashboard. Available online: https://data.who.int/dashboards/covid19/cases?n=c (accessed on 10 January 2024).
2. Raman, B.; Bluemke, D.A.; Lüscher, T.F.; Neubauer, S. Long COVID: Post-Acute Sequelae of COVID-19 with a Cardiovascular Focus. *Eur. Heart J.* **2022**, *43*, 1157–1172. [CrossRef] [PubMed]
3. Singh, A.K.; Khunti, K. COVID-19 and Diabetes. *Annu. Rev. Med.* **2022**, *73*, 129–147. [CrossRef]
4. Steenblock, C.; Hassanein, M.; Khan, E.G.; Yaman, M.; Kamel, M.; Barbir, M.; Lorke, D.E.; Rock, J.A.; Everett, D.; Bejtullah, S.; et al. Diabetes and COVID-19: Short- and Long-Term Consequences. *Horm. Metab. Res.* **2022**, *54*, 503–509. [CrossRef] [PubMed]
5. Nag, S.; Mandal, S.; Mukherjee, O.; Mukherjee, S.; Kundu, R. DPP-4 Inhibitors as a Savior for COVID-19 Patients with Diabetes. *Future Virol.* **2023**, *18*, 321–333. [CrossRef] [PubMed]
6. Singh, A.K.; Gillies, C.L.; Singh, R.; Singh, A.; Chudasama, Y.; Coles, B.; Seidu, S.; Zaccardi, F.; Davies, M.J.; Khunti, K. Prevalence of Co-morbidities and Their Association with Mortality in Patients with COVID-19: A Systematic Review and Meta-analysis. *Diabetes Obes. Metab.* **2020**, *22*, 1915–1924. [CrossRef] [PubMed]
7. Barron, E.; Bakhai, C.; Kar, P.; Weaver, A.; Bradley, D.; Ismail, H.; Knighton, P.; Holman, N.; Khunti, K.; Sattar, N.; et al. Associations of Type 1 and Type 2 Diabetes with COVID-19-Related Mortality in England: A Whole-Population Study. *Lancet Diabetes Endocrinol.* **2020**, *8*, 813–822. [CrossRef]
8. Bode, B.; Garrett, V.; Messler, J.; McFarland, R.; Crowe, J.; Booth, R.; Klonoff, D.C. Glycemic Characteristics and Clinical Outcomes of COVID-19 Patients Hospitalized in the United States. *J. Diabetes Sci. Technol.* **2020**, *14*, 813–821. [CrossRef]
9. Tittel, S.R.; Rosenbauer, J.; Kamrath, C.; Ziegler, J.; Reschke, F.; Hammersen, J.; Mönkemöller, K.; Pappa, A.; Kapellen, T.; Holl, R.W. Did the COVID-19 Lockdown Affect the Incidence of Pediatric Type 1 Diabetes in Germany? *Diabetes Care* **2020**, *43*, e172–e173. [CrossRef]
10. Holman, N.; Knighton, P.; Kar, P.; O'Keefe, J.; Curley, M.; Weaver, A.; Barron, E.; Bakhai, C.; Khunti, K.; Wareham, N.J.; et al. Risk Factors for COVID-19-Related Mortality in People with Type 1 and Type 2 Diabetes in England: A Population-Based Cohort Study. *Lancet Diabetes Endocrinol.* **2020**, *8*, 823–833. [CrossRef]
11. Alshnbari, A.; Idris, I. Can Sodium-Glucose Co-Transporter-2 (SGLT-2) Inhibitor Reduce the Risk of Adverse Complications Due to COVID-19?—Targeting Hyperinflammation. *Curr. Med. Res. Opin.* **2022**, *38*, 357–364. [CrossRef]
12. Varghese, E.; Samuel, S.M.; Liskova, A.; Kubatka, P.; Büsselberg, D. Diabetes and Coronavirus (*SARS-CoV-2*): Molecular Mechanism of Metformin Intervention and the Scientific Basis of Drug Repurposing. *PLoS Pathog.* **2021**, *17*, e1009634. [CrossRef] [PubMed]
13. Li, Y.; Zhang, Z.; Yang, L.; Lian, X.; Xie, Y.; Li, S.; Xin, S.; Cao, P.; Lu, J. The *MERS-CoV* Receptor DPP4 as a Candidate Binding Target of the *SARS-CoV-2* Spike. *iScience* **2020**, *23*, 101160. [CrossRef] [PubMed]
14. Zelniker, T.A.; Wiviott, S.D.; Raz, I.; Im, K.; Goodrich, E.L.; Bonaca, M.P.; Mosenzon, O.; Kato, E.T.; Cahn, A.; Furtado, R.H.M.; et al. SGLT2 Inhibitors for Primary and Secondary Prevention of Cardiovascular and Renal Outcomes in Type 2 Diabetes: A Systematic Review and Meta-Analysis of Cardiovascular Outcome Trials. *Lancet* **2019**, *393*, 31–39. [CrossRef] [PubMed]

15. Carino, A.; Moraca, F.; Fiorillo, B.; Marchianò, S.; Sepe, V.; Biagioli, M.; Finamore, C.; Bozza, S.; Francisci, D.; Distrutti, E.; et al. Hijacking *SARS-CoV-2*/ACE2 Receptor Interaction by Natural and Semi-Synthetic Steroidal Agents Acting on Functional Pockets on the Receptor Binding Domain. *Front. Chem.* **2020**, *8*, 572885. [CrossRef] [PubMed]
16. Baggen, J.; Jacquemyn, M.; Persoons, L.; Vanstreels, E.; Pye, V.E.; Wrobel, A.G.; Calvaresi, V.; Martin, S.R.; Roustan, C.; Cronin, N.B.; et al. TMEM106B Is a Receptor Mediating ACE2-Independent *SARS-CoV-2* Cell Entry. *Cell* **2023**, *186*, 3427–3442.e22. [CrossRef] [PubMed]
17. Wang, K.; Chen, W.; Zhang, Z.; Deng, Y.; Lian, J.-Q.; Du, P.; Wei, D.; Zhang, Y.; Sun, X.-X.; Gong, L.; et al. CD147-Spike Protein Is a Novel Route for *SARS-CoV-2* Infection to Host Cells. *Signal Transduct. Target. Ther.* **2020**, *5*, 283. [CrossRef] [PubMed]
18. Masre, S.F.; Jufri, N.F.; Ibrahim, F.W.; Abdul Raub, S.H. Classical and Alternative Receptors for *SARS-CoV-2* Therapeutic Strategy. *Rev. Med. Virol.* **2021**, *31*, 1–9. [CrossRef] [PubMed]
19. Clinical Management of Severe Acute Respiratory Infection When Novel Coronavirus (nCoV) Infection Is Suspected: Interim Guidance, 12 January 2020. Available online: https://iris.who.int/handle/10665/332299 (accessed on 5 January 2024).
20. Levey, A.S.; Coresh, J.; Greene, T.; Stevens, L.A.; Zhang, Y.; Hendriksen, S.; Kusek, J.W.; Van Lente, F. Using Standardized Serum Creatinine Values in the Modification of Diet in Renal Disease Study Equation for Estimating Glomerular Filtration Rate. *Ann. Intern. Med.* **2006**, *145*, 247–254. [CrossRef]
21. Alwani, M.; Yassin, A.; Al-Zoubi, R.M.; Aboumarzouk, O.M.; Nettleship, J.; Kelly, D.; AL-Qudimat, A.R.; Shabsigh, R. Sex-based Differences in Severity and Mortality in COVID-19. *Rev. Med. Virol.* **2021**, *31*, e2223. [CrossRef]
22. Muniyappa, R.; Gubbi, S. COVID-19 Pandemic, Coronaviruses, and Diabetes Mellitus. *Am. J. Physiol. Endocrinol. Metab.* **2020**, *318*, E736–E741. [CrossRef]
23. Rajpal, A.; Rahimi, L.; Ismail-Beigi, F. Factors Leading to High Morbidity and Mortality of COVID-19 in Patients with Type 2 Diabetes. *J. Diabetes* **2020**, *12*, 895–908. [CrossRef]
24. Norouzi, M.; Norouzi, S.; Ruggiero, A.; Khan, M.S.; Myers, S.; Kavanagh, K.; Vemuri, R. Type-2 Diabetes as a Risk Factor for Severe COVID-19 Infection. *Microorganisms* **2021**, *9*, 1211. [CrossRef]
25. Solerte, S.B.; D'Addio, F.; Trevisan, R.; Lovati, E.; Rossi, A.; Pastore, I.; Dell'Acqua, M.; Ippolito, E.; Scaranna, C.; Bellante, R.; et al. Sitagliptin Treatment at the Time of Hospitalization Was Associated With Reduced Mortality in Patients With Type 2 Diabetes and COVID-19: A Multicenter, Case-Control, Retrospective, Observational Study. *Diabetes Care* **2020**, *43*, 2999–3006. [CrossRef]
26. Pitt, B.; Agarwal, R.; Anker, S.D.; Ruilope, L.M.; Rossing, P.; Ahlers, C.; Brinker, M.; Joseph, A.; Lambelet, M.; Lawatscheck, R.; et al. Association of Finerenone Use With Reduction in Treatment-Emergent Pneumonia and COVID-19 Adverse Events Among Patients With Type 2 Diabetes and Chronic Kidney Disease. *JAMA Netw. Open* **2022**, *5*, e2236123. [CrossRef]
27. Jung, H.S.; Choi, J.W. Association between COVID-19 and Incidence of Cardiovascular Disease and All-Cause Mortality among Patients with Diabetes. *Front. Endocrinol.* **2023**, *14*, 1–8. [CrossRef] [PubMed]
28. Gazzaz, Z.J. Diabetes and COVID-19. *Open Life Sci.* **2021**, *16*, 297–302. [CrossRef] [PubMed]
29. Li, J.; Huang, D.Q.; Zou, B.; Yang, H.; Hui, W.Z.; Rui, F.; Yee, N.T.S.; Liu, C.; Nerurkar, S.N.; Kai, J.C.Y.; et al. Epidemiology of COVID-19: A Systematic Review and Meta-analysis of Clinical Characteristics, Risk Factors, and Outcomes. *J. Med. Virol.* **2021**, *93*, 1449–1458. [CrossRef] [PubMed]
30. Liu, S.; Zhang, L.; Weng, H.; Yang, F.; Jin, H.; Fan, F.; Zheng, X.; Yang, H.; Li, H.; Zhang, Y.; et al. Association Between Average Plasma Potassium Levels and 30-Day Mortality During Hospitalization in Patients with COVID-19 in Wuhan, China. *Int. J. Med. Sci.* **2021**, *18*, 736–743. [CrossRef] [PubMed]
31. Mahroum, N.; Alghory, A.; Kiyak, Z.; Alwani, A.; Seida, R.; Alrais, M.; Shoenfeld, Y. Ferritin—From Iron, through Inflammation and Autoimmunity, to COVID-19. *J. Autoimmun.* **2022**, *126*, 102778. [CrossRef] [PubMed]
32. McCarthy, M.W. Metformin as a Potential Treatment for COVID-19. *Expert. Opin. Pharmacother.* **2023**, *24*, 1199–1203. [CrossRef] [PubMed]
33. Gama, S. RDW Shows Prognostic Potential in Hospitalized Patients with COVID-19. *J. Med. Virol.* **2022**, *94*, 3498–3500. [CrossRef] [PubMed]
34. Soni, M.; Gopalakrishnan, R. Significance of RDW in Predicting Mortality in COVID-19—An Analysis of 622 Cases. *Int. J. Lab. Hematol.* **2021**, *43*, O221–O223. [CrossRef] [PubMed]
35. Pouladzadeh, M.; Safdarian, M.; Choghakabodi, P.M.; Amini, F.; Sokooti, A. Validation of Red Cell Distribution Width as a COVID-19 Severity Screening Tool. *Future Sci. OA* **2021**, *7*, FSO712. [CrossRef]
36. Soni, M.; Gopalakrishnan, R.; Vaishya, R.; Prabu, P. D-Dimer Level Is a Useful Predictor for Mortality in Patients with COVID-19: Analysis of 483 Cases. *Diabetes Metab. Syndr. Clin. Res. Rev.* **2020**, *14*, 2245–2249. [CrossRef]
37. Bramante, C.T.; Ingraham, N.E.; Murray, T.A.; Marmor, S.; Hovertsen, S.; Gronski, J.; McNeil, C.; Feng, R.; Guzman, G.; Abdelwahab, N.; et al. Metformin and Risk of Mortality in Patients Hospitalised with COVID-19: A Retrospective Cohort Analysis. *Lancet Healthy Longev.* **2021**, *2*, e34–e41. [CrossRef] [PubMed]
38. Kim, M.K.; Jeon, J.-H.; Kim, S.-W.; Moon, J.S.; Cho, N.H.; Han, E.; You, J.H.; Lee, J.Y.; Hyun, M.; Park, J.S.; et al. The Clinical Characteristics and Outcomes of Patients with Moderate-to-Severe Coronavirus Disease 2019 Infection and Diabetes in Daegu, South Korea. *Diabetes Metab. J.* **2020**, *44*, 602. [CrossRef] [PubMed]
39. Chen, Y.; Yang, D.; Cheng, B.; Chen, J.; Peng, A.; Yang, C.; Liu, C.; Xiong, M.; Deng, A.; Zhang, Y.; et al. Clinical Characteristics and Outcomes of Patients With Diabetes and COVID-19 in Association With Glucose-Lowering Medication. *Diabetes Care* **2020**, *43*, 1399–1407. [CrossRef] [PubMed]

40. DeFronzo, R.; Fleming, G.A.; Chen, K.; Bicsak, T.A. Metformin-Associated Lactic Acidosis: Current Perspectives on Causes and Risk. *Metabolism* **2016**, *65*, 20–29. [CrossRef]
41. Bugliani, M.; Syed, F.; Paula, F.M.M.; Omar, B.A.; Suleiman, M.; Mossuto, S.; Grano, F.; Cardarelli, F.; Boggi, U.; Vistoli, F.; et al. DPP-4 Is Expressed in Human Pancreatic Beta Cells and Its Direct Inhibition Improves Beta Cell Function and Survival in Type 2 Diabetes. *Mol. Cell Endocrinol.* **2018**, *473*, 186–193. [CrossRef]
42. Ali, N. Elevated Level of C-reactive Protein May Be an Early Marker to Predict Risk for Severity of COVID-19. *J. Med. Virol.* **2020**, *92*, 2409–2411. [CrossRef]
43. Choudhury, A.; Mukherjee, S. In Silico Studies on the Comparative Characterization of the Interactions of *SARS-CoV-2* Spike Glycoprotein with ACE-2 Receptor Homologs and Human TLRs. *J. Med. Virol.* **2020**, *92*, 2105–2113. [CrossRef] [PubMed]
44. Vankadari, N.; Wilce, J.A. Emerging COVID-19 Coronavirus: Glycan Shield and Structure Prediction of Spike Glycoprotein and Its Interaction with Human CD26. *Emerg. Microbes Infect.* **2020**, *9*, 601–604. [CrossRef] [PubMed]
45. Schlicht, K.; Rohmann, N.; Geisler, C.; Hollstein, T.; Knappe, C.; Hartmann, K.; Schwarz, J.; Tran, F.; Schunk, D.; Junker, R.; et al. Circulating Levels of Soluble Dipeptidylpeptidase-4 Are Reduced in Human Subjects Hospitalized for Severe COVID-19 Infections. *Int. J. Obes.* **2020**, *44*, 2335–2338. [CrossRef] [PubMed]
46. Rakhmat, I.I.; Kusmala, Y.Y.; Handayani, D.R.; Juliastuti, H.; Nawangsih, E.N.; Wibowo, A.; Lim, M.A.; Pranata, R. Dipeptidyl Peptidase-4 (DPP-4) Inhibitor and Mortality in Coronavirus Disease 2019 (COVID-19)—A Systematic Review, Meta-Analysis, and Meta-Regression. *Diabetes Metab. Syndr. Clin. Res. Rev.* **2021**, *15*, 777–782. [CrossRef] [PubMed]
47. Bonora, B.M.; Avogaro, A.; Fadini, G.P. Disentangling Conflicting Evidence on DPP-4 Inhibitors and Outcomes of COVID-19: Narrative Review and Meta-Analysis. *J. Endocrinol. Investig.* **2021**, *44*, 1379–1386. [CrossRef]
48. Wargny, M.; Potier, L.; Gourdy, P.; Pichelin, M.; Amadou, C.; Benhamou, P.-Y.; Bonnet, J.-B.; Bordier, L.; Bourron, O.; Chaumeil, C.; et al. Predictors of Hospital Discharge and Mortality in Patients with Diabetes and COVID-19: Updated Results from the Nationwide CORONADO Study. *Diabetologia* **2021**, *64*, 778–794. [CrossRef] [PubMed]
49. Strollo, R.; Maddaloni, E.; Dauriz, M.; Pedone, C.; Buzzetti, R.; Pozzilli, P. Use of DPP4 Inhibitors in Italy Does Not Correlate with Diabetes Prevalence among COVID-19 Deaths. *Diabetes Res. Clin. Pract.* **2021**, *171*, 108444. [CrossRef]
50. Attena, E.; Caturano, A.; Annunziata, A.; Maraolo, A.E.; De Rosa, A.; Fusco, F.M.; Halasz, G.; Dall'Ospedale, V.; Conte, M.; Parisi, V.; et al. Remdesivir treatment and clinical outcome in non-severe hospitalized COVID-19 patients: A propensity score matching multicenter Italian hospital experience. *Eur. J. Clin. Pharmacol.* **2023**, *79*, 967–974. [CrossRef]

biomedicines

MDPI

Article

In Association with Other Risk Factors, Smoking Is the Main Predictor for Lower Transcutaneous Oxygen Pressure in Type 2 Diabetes

Tomislav Bulum [1,2,*], Neva Brkljačić [1], Angelika Tičinović Ivančić [3], Maja Čavlović [1], Ingrid Prkačin [2,4] and Martina Tomić [1]

1 Vuk Vrhovac University Clinic for Diabetes, Endocrinology and Metabolic Diseases, Merkur University Hospital, 10000 Zagreb, Croatia
2 School of Medicine, University of Zagreb, 10000 Zagreb, Croatia
3 Zagreb Country Public Health Institute, 10430 Samobor, Croatia
4 Department of Internal Medicine, Merkur University Hospital, 10000 Zagreb, Croatia
* Correspondence: tomobulum@gmail.com

Abstract: Type 2 diabetes mellitus (T2DM) significantly increases the risk of peripheral artery disease (PAD), and diabetes is the leading cause of nontraumatic amputations. This study investigated the risk factors for transcutaneous oxygen pressure (TcPO2) in T2DM, a noninvasive method to quantify skin oxygenation and the underlying microvascular circulation. The study included 119 T2DM patients (91 male/28 female). TcPO2 measurements were conducted with the Tina TCM4 Series transcutaneous monitor (Radiometer, Copenhagen, Sweden) and skin electrodes. Patients with TcPO2 < 40 mmHg were younger ($p = 0.001$), had significantly higher systolic blood pressure (SBP) ($p = 0.023$), glycated hemoglobin (HbA_1c) ($p = 0.013$), fasting plasma glucose (fPG) ($p = 0.038$), total cholesterol ($p = 0.006$), LDL cholesterol ($p = 0.004$), and had more frequent smoking habits ($p = 0.001$) than those with TcPO2 $\geq$ 40 mmHg. The main predictors for the TcPO2 value ($R^2 = 0.211$) obtained via stepwise regression analysis were age, smoking, SBP, HbA_1c, fPG, and total and LDL cholesterol. Among all the listed predictors, smoking, HbA_1c, and LDL cholesterol were found to be the most significant, with negative parameter estimates of −3.051310 ($p = 0.0007$), −2.032018 ($p = 0.0003$), and −2.560353 ($p = 0.0046$). The results of our study suggest that in association with other risk factors, smoking is the main predictor for lower TcPO2 in T2DM.

Keywords: smoking; type 2 diabetes; atherosclerosis; peripheral artery disease; transcutaneous oxygen pressure

1. Introduction

Diabetes is a chronic disease with harmful chronic complications that is still the leading cause of blindness in the adult working population, nontraumatic amputations, and chronic kidney disease. Peripheral artery disease (PAD), caused by atherosclerosis and aggravated with several risk factors, affects the lower extremities and increases the risk of cardiovascular disease and death [1–5]. Compared to non-diabetic individuals, diabetes is associated with a two- to fourfold higher risk of PAD, while the presence of diabetes worsens outcomes in patients with PAD [6–9]. The worst diabetes complication is diabetic foot developed because of diabetic neuropathy and/or PAD [10].

Patients with type 2 diabetes mellitus (T2DM) usually have metabolic syndrome with a set of metabolic disturbances, like obesity, dyslipidemia, hypertension, and arterial stiffness, that increase the risk of cardiovascular disease and the risk of PAD [11–14]. It should be noted that PAD in diabetic patients is different at biological and clinical levels, and the effects of good glycemic control on the regression of microvascular disease are not reflected in macrovascular disease in the short term. There is a bidirectional relationship between T2DM and PAD; one disease may play an underlying role in the pathophysiology of the other and vice versa [15–17]. The ankle–brachial pressure index (ABI) is a noninvasive method to detect the presence and severity of PAD widely used in clinical practice [18,19]. However, in patients with diabetes, ABI has limited reliability in the diagnosis of PAD because of medial artery calcification, and the toe–brachial index (TBI) is more often estimated than ABI [20]. These two methods have limitations when examining the microcirculation in patients with PAD. A transcutaneous oxygen pressure (TcPO2) measurement provides information about the supply and delivery of oxygen to the underlying microvascular circulation by recording the partial pressure of oxygen at the skin surface. It can be considered a metabolic test, while ABI and TBI are hemodynamic tests [21,22].

ABI and TBI, as the most widely used noninvasive methods to detect the presence and severity of PAD in clinical practice, have limitations when examining microcirculation. Since diabetes is strongly associated with both macrovascular and microvascular complications, this study aimed to investigate the risk factors for lower $TcPO_2$ in T2DM, a metabolic test that provides information about microvascular circulation.

2. Materials and Methods

2.1. Study Design and Ethics Statement

This study was cross-sectional and conducted at the Department of Diabetes and Endocrinology and the Department of Cardiology. It included 119 patients with T2DM, referred by a diabetologist/neurologist/vascular surgeon due to suspicion of PAD. PAD has been diagnosed using the color Doppler ultrasound of the superficial femoral and other more distal arteries of both legs. A normal spectral arterial waveform was triphasic, while biphasic and monophasic waveforms of one or several arteries were considered PAD [23]. In those with PAD, ABI and TcPO2 measurements were performed. Patients with an ABI ≤ 1.3 were included in the study. The study was approved by the Hospital's Ethics Committee (protocol number 04/38-299, approval date: 7 August 2019). All T2DM patients, before any study procedures, received oral and written information about the study protocol and finally signed the written informed consent.

2.2. Demographic Data and Clinical Characteristics

Age at the time of the study, gender, and diabetes duration were basic demographic data of patients included in the study. Weight in kilograms (kg) and height in centimeters (cm) were measured to calculate body mass index (BMI) by dividing weight by the square of height in meters (kg/m^2). The waist circumference (WC) and hip circumference were measured with a tailor meter on standard places on bare skin to calculate the waist-to-hip ratio (WHR). A digital sphygmomanometer was used to measure systolic blood pressure (SBP) and diastolic blood pressure (DBP) in a sitting position after the period of a 10 min rest and expressed in mmHg. A smoker was defined as a person who had a history of smoking a minimum of 100 cigarettes during life with current smoking on some days or every day.

2.3. Markers of Glycemic Control and Lipid Metabolism

Fasting plasma glucose (fPG), serum lipids (total cholesterol, triglycerides, low-density lipoprotein (LDL) cholesterol, and high-density lipoprotein (HDL) cholesterol), and hemoglobin A_1c were measured in the morning after an overnight fast. Postprandial plasma glucose (ppPG) was measured two hours after a meal. Glycated hemoglobin (HbA_1c) was measured using an automated turbidimetric inhibition immunoassay (HbA_1c Gen 3, Cobas Integra 400 Plus, Roche Diagnostic, Basel, Switzerland) and expressed in % according to the National Glycohemoglobin Standardization Program (NGSP). This method is traceable to the International Federation of Clinical Chemistry and Laboratory Medicine (IFCC) reference system. Standard enzymatic methods were used to determine serum lipids, fPG, and ppPG on an automated analyzer (Beckman Coulter AU680, Beckman Coulter, Inc., Brea, CA, USA).

2.4. Transcutaneous Oxygen Pressure Measurement

The sensor/electrode of the Tina TCM4 series transcutaneous monitor (Radiometer, Copenhagen, Sweden) was put on the skin, where it heated the underlying tissue to create local hyperemia (making the arteries dilate), intensify the blood perfusion, and increase the oxygen pressure. Electrodes were heated up to 45 °C and transmitted a temperature of about 43 °C on the skin, improving oxygenation of the capillary blood. The sensor received an electric current corresponding to the oxygen concentration in the capillary blood. The oxygen diffused according to pressure from the capillary blood via the vascular epidermis to the electrode placed on the skin surface. After application, the sensor required a 10 to 15 min warm period and needed calibration every four to eight hours. A site reading involved an average of 35 min. Sensors were placed over a homogeneous capillary bed without hair, skin defects, ulcers, and prominent veins. Electrodes were not placed over a bone, on previous operation sites, in scar tissue, or in severe edema because they may have given unreliable results. Patients were advised to avoid prior smoking or caffeine use. During the monitoring, patients were in the supine position.

2.5. Ankle–Brachial Index

To calculate the ABI, measurements of the SBP in the brachial, posterior tibial, and dorsalis pedis arteries were conducted. The ABI represents higher resting SBP at the ankle divided by the higher systolic brachial pressure. A handheld 5 or 10 mHz Doppler instrument (Sonotrax Pro ultrasonic pocket Doppler, Edan, San Diego, CA, USA) was used to note the systolic pressures. A standard blood pressure cuff was placed immediately above the ankle to obtain the most precise pressure measurements. During the ABI measurement, patients were in the supine position. Normal ABI values are between 0.9 and 1.4. Values < 0.9 are indicative of peripheral atherosclerosis, while values over 1.4 are indicative of vascular calcification.

2.6. Statistical Analysis

Statistical analysis was conducted, and the graphs were created using the statistical package Statistica™ 14.0.1 (TIBCO Software Inc., Palo Alto, CA, USA). In all analyses, a *p*-value of less than 0.05 was considered statistically significant. After testing the normality of data distribution with the Kolmogorov–Smirnov test, normally distributed continuous variables were expressed as mean ± SD and non-normally distributed variables as the median with range. All categorical variables were expressed as numbers and percentages. Differences between the two groups were for continuous data examined using parametric (*t*-test) or non-parametric tests (Mann–Whitney), depending on the data distribution, and for categorical data testing, the chi-squared test was used. The Spearman rank correlation test was used to evaluate the relationship between the studied variables. Differences in TcPO2 between the groups according to the smoking habit (no, yes) and HbA_1c value (<8.0%, ≥8.0%) and their interactions were tested using the two-way analysis of variance (ANOVA). Stepwise regression was used to detect the main predictors of TcPO2.

3. Results

This study included 119 T2DM patients (91 male/28 female) with a mean age of 68.5 ± 7.8 years and a mean diabetes duration of 19.7 ± 9 years. All included patients had PAD. According to the Fontaine classification [23], 34 were asymptomatic (stage I), 43 had intermittent claudication after more than 200 m of pain-free walking (stage IIa), 22 had intermittent claudication after less than 200 m of walking (stage IIb), 1 had stage III (ischemic rest pain), and 19 had stage IV (18 neuropathic ischemic ulcers and 1 gangrene). Asymptomatic patients were declared those who did not have typical pain symptoms in the leg muscles provoked by the effort that passes at rest but had a pathological color

Doppler ultrasound finding regardless of the finding of ABI. ABI's median (min–max) in those patients was 0.81 (0.34–1.25). Furthermore, all our included patients had some stage of diabetic neuropathy, i.e., 12 had stage 1 (intermittent numbness and pain), 99 had stage 2 (persistent numbness and pain), and 8 had stage 3 (debilitating pain). Their mean/median values of TcPO2, basic characteristics, all analyzed risk factors, and ABI are shown in Table 1.

Table 1. Transcutaneous oxygen pressure, basic characteristics, risk factors, and ankle–brachial index of all type 2 diabetic patients (n = 119) included in the study.

	All Patients Included in the Study (n = 119)
TcPO2 (mmHg)	40.85 ± 13.97
Smoking (no/yes) (%)	50.4/49.6
BMI (kg/m^2)	29.39 ± 4.88
WC (cm)	106.2 ± 12.5
WHR	0.99 ± 0.07
SBP (mmHg)	140 (90–235)
DBP (mmHg)	80 (41–115)
HbA$_1$c (%)	7.90 ± 1.62
fPG (mmol/L)	8.16 ± 2.72
ppPG (mmol/L)	10.78 ± 3.54
Total cholesterol (mmol/L)	4.5 (2.5–9.2)
HDL cholesterol (mmol/L)	1.2 (0.4–2.3)
LDL cholesterol (mmol/L)	2.4 (0.3–4.9)
Triglycerides (mmol/L)	1.6 (0.6–9.5)
ABI	0.8 (0.3–1.3)

Legend: values are means ± SD, percentages, or median (min–max). BMI indicates body mass index; WC, waist circumference; WHR, waist-to-hip ratio; SBP, systolic blood pressure; DBP, diastolic blood pressure; HbA$_1$c, glycated hemoglobin; fPG, fasting plasma glucose; ppPG, postprandial plasma glucose; HDL, high-density lipoprotein cholesterol; LDL, low-density lipoprotein cholesterol; ABI, ankle–brachial index.

Regarding the TcPO2 value, patients were split into two groups: group 1 (TcPO2 ≥ 40 mmHg; n = 66) and group 2 (TcPO2 < 40 mmHg; n = 53) (Table 2). The two TcPO2 groups did not significantly differ in gender, diabetes duration, anthropometric parameters, BMI, WC and WHR, DBP, ppPG, HDL cholesterol, and triglycerides ($p > 0.05$). However, patients with TcPO2 < 40 mmHg were younger ($p = 0.001$) and had more frequent smoking habits ($p = 0.001$) than those with TcPO2 ≥ 40 mmHg. Furthermore, those with lower TcPO2 had significantly higher SBP ($p = 0.023$), HbA$_1$c ($p = 0.013$), fPG ($p = 0.038$), total cholesterol ($p = 0.006$), and LDL cholesterol ($p = 0.004$), while they had a significantly lower ABI ($p < 0.001$) than those with higher TcPO2.

Table 2. Transcutaneous oxygen pressure, risk factors, and ankle–brachial index of type 2 diabetic patients (n = 119) divided into two groups according to the transcutaneous oxygen pressure.

	TcPO2 ≥ 40 (n = 66)	TcPO2 < 40 (n = 53)	t^a χ^b Z^c	p
TcPO2 (mmHg)	50.34 ± 8.85	29.12 ± 9.49	17.767 [a]	<0.001
Age (years)	70.00 ± 7.45	66.75 ± 7.89	3.248 [a]	0.001
Smoking (no/yes) (%)	59.5/40.5	38.7/61.3	10.201 [b]	0.001
SBP (mmHg)	140 (90–230)	148 (100–235)	−2.267 [c]	0.023
HbA$_1$c (%)	7.67 ± 1.58	8.20 ± 1.64	−2.517 [a]	0.013
fPG (mmol/L)	7.85 ± 2.14	8.58 ± 3.25	−2.082 [a]	0.038
Total cholesterol (mmol/L)	4.3 (2.5–9.1)	4.8 (2.9–9.2)	−2.722 [c]	0.006

Table 2. *Cont.*

	TcPO2 ≥ 40 (n = 66)	TcPO2 < 40 (n = 53)	t^a χ^b Z^c	p
LDL cholesterol (mmol/L)	2.2 (0.3–4.7)	2.6 (1.2–4.9)	−2.848 ^{c}	0.004
ABI	0.8 (0.5–1.2)	0.7 (0.3–1.3)	3.539 ^{c}	<0.001

Legend: values are means ± SD, percentages, or medians (min–max). t^a represents t-test, χ^b represents chi-square test, Z^c represents Mann–Whitney test, p represents comparison between patients with different level of TcPO2. SBP indicates systolic blood pressure; HbA_1c, glycated hemoglobin; LDL, low-density lipoprotein cholesterol; ABI, ankle–brachial index.

The correlation between TcPO2 and smoking and their relation to other risk factors and ABI are shown in Table 3. A significant negative correlation was found between the TcPO2 value and smoking (R = −0.242166, p = 0.000167) (Figure 1A). TcPO2 correlated significantly positively with age (R = 0.217315, p = 0.000757) while negatively with SBP (R = −0.200125, p = 0.001962) (Figure 1B), HbA_1c (R = −0.218749, p = 0.000696) (Figure 1C), fPG (R = −0.153979, p = 0.017687), total cholesterol (R = −0.223532, p = 0.000526) (Figure 1D), and LDL cholesterol (R = −0.220646, p = 0.000624) (Figure 1E). In contrast, smoking related significantly negatively to age (R = −0.320846, p = 0.000000) and gender (m/f; R = −0.233076, p = 0.000287) but significantly positively to HbA_1c (R = 0.294675, p = 0.000004) and ppPG (R = 0.137999, p = 0.033343) (Table 3). ABI was associated significantly positively with TcPO2 (R = 0.286434, p = 0.000039), while no significant correlation was observed between ABI and smoking (Table 3).

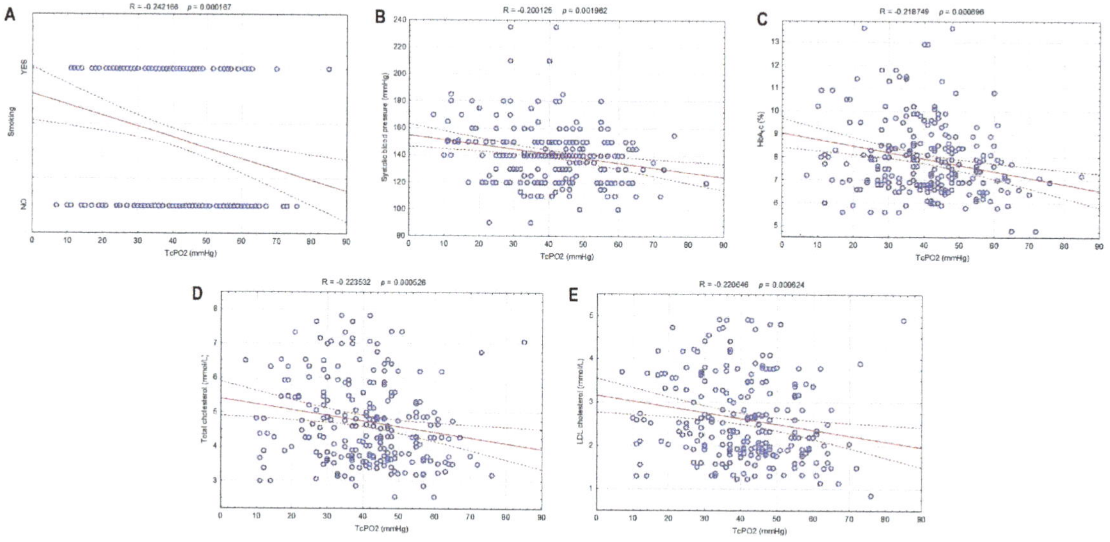

Figure 1. Correlations between transcutaneous oxygen pressure and smoking (**A**), systolic blood pressure (**B**), hemoglobin A_1c (**C**), total cholesterol (**D**), and LDL cholesterol (**E**) in type 2 diabetic patients included in the study.

Figure 2 presents the correlation of ABI and TcPO2 within different stages of the Fontaine scale. The most significant association was observed in stages 1 (R = 0.501668, p = 0.000151) (Figure 2A) and 2 (R = 0.219206, p = 0.018070) (Figure 2B); in stage 3 (Figure 2C), there was a small number of patients to analyze, while in stage 4 (R = −0.038659, p = 0.839275) (Figure 2D), no significant relation between ABI and TcPO2 was observed.

Table 3. Correlations between transcutaneous oxygen pressure, smoking, the other risk factors, and ankle–brachial index in type 2 diabetic patients included in the study.

	TcPO2	Smoking
Smoking	−0.242 **	1.000
Age	0.217 **	−0.321 **
Gender (m/f)	−0.067	−0.233 **
SBP	−0.200 *	0.011
HbA_1c	−0.219 **	0.295 **
fPG	−0.154 *	0.051
ppPG	−0.032	0.138 *
Total cholesterol	−0.224 **	0.096
LDL cholesterol	−0.129 *	0.059
ABI	0.286 **	−0.006

Legend: values are Spearman R-values. ** represents $p < 0.001$, * $p < 0.05$. SBP indicates systolic blood pressure; HbA_1c, glycated hemoglobin; fPG, fasting plasma glucose; ppPG, postprandial plasma glucose; HDL, high-density lipoprotein cholesterol; LDL, low-density lipoprotein cholesterol; ABI, ankle–brachial index.

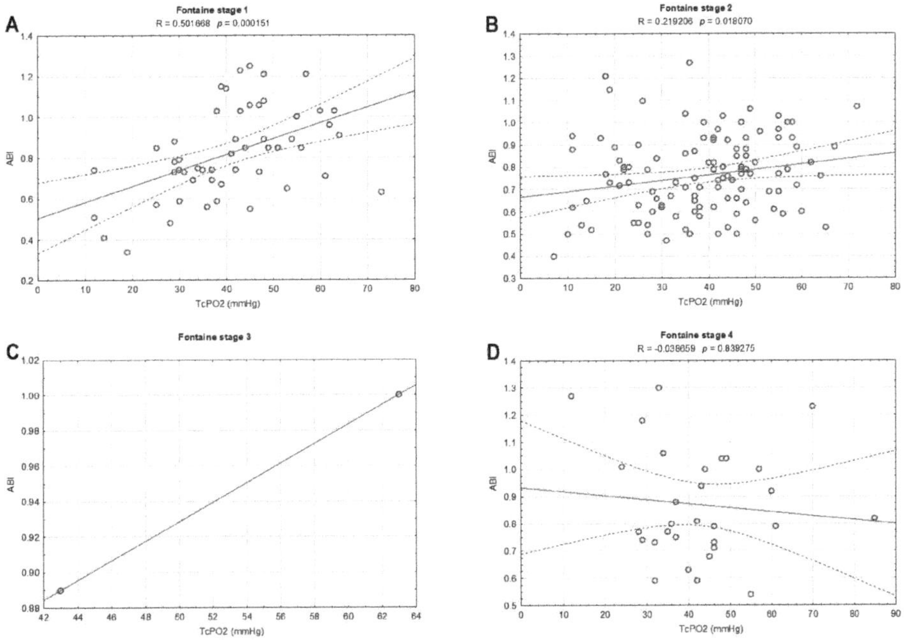

Figure 2. Correlations between the ankle–brachial index and transcutaneous oxygen pressure within different stages of the Fontaine scale: stage 1 (**A**), stage 2 (**B**), stage 3 (**C**), and stage 4 (**D**).

With a special emphasis on the two essential risk factors, smoking and HbA_1c, Table 4 presents the differences in TcPO2 of T2DM divided into two groups according to their smoking habit (no, yes) and the level of HbA_1c (<8.0%, ≥8.0%) tested via ANOVA with two main factors and their interaction. The statistically significant differences in TcPO2 were found according to the smoking habit ($p = 0.016$) and the level of HbA_1c ($p = 0.002$), though the difference in TcPO2 observed according to the interaction between the groups of smoking and HbA_1c was not significant ($p = 0.419$). The differences in TcPO2 found via ANOVA with two main factors and their interaction are graphically shown in Figure 3.

Table 4. Results of two-way ANOVA for the differences between transcutaneous oxygen pressure according to the smoking habit, hemoglobin A_1c, and their interaction.

	TcPO2		
	df	**F**	***p***
Smoking	1	5.932	0.016
HbA_1c gr.	1	9.394	0.002
Smoking and HbA_1c gr.	1	0.656	0.419

Legend: TcPO2 indicates transcutaneous oxygen pressure; HbA_1c, glycated hemoglobin.

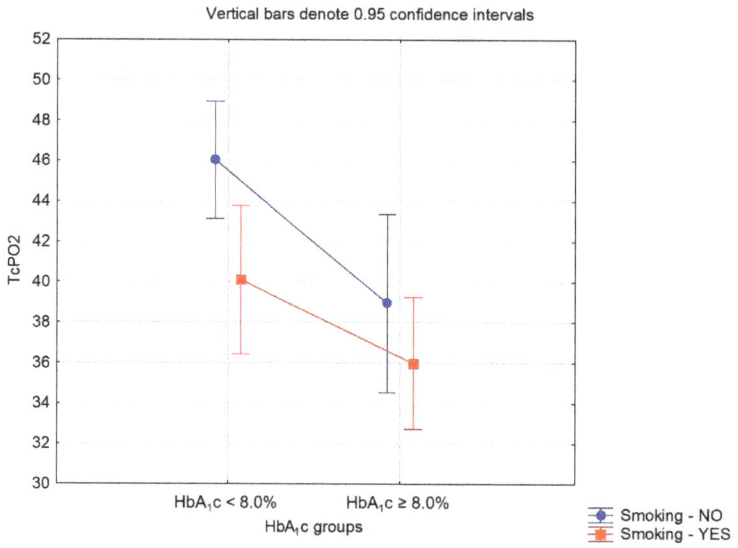

Figure 3. Differences in transcutaneous oxygen pressure (TcPO2) according to the smoking habit and glycated hemoglobin (HbA_1c) value.

The main predictors for the TcPO2 value ($R^2 = 0.211$) obtained via stepwise regression analysis were age, smoking, SBP, HbA_1c, fPG, and total and LDL cholesterol (Table 5). Among all the listed predictors, smoking, HbA_1c, and LDL cholesterol were found to be the most significant, with negative parameter estimates of −3.051310 ($p = 0.0007$), −2.032018 ($p = 0.0003$), and −2.560353 ($p = 0.0046$) influencing the TcPO2 value relative to a one-unit change of each and representing the negatively significant impact of the correlation between smoking and well-known risk factors on the reduction in TcPO2 value.

Table 5. Results of stepwise regression analysis for the transcutaneous oxygen pressure as a dependent variable.

Variable	Estimate	Standard Error	F	*p*	Adjusted R^2	R^2
Age	0.355	13.716	9.65	0.0021	0.0353	
Smoking	−3.051	13.656	11.83	0.0007	0.0439	
SBP	−0.145	13.645	12.21	0.0006	0.0454	
HbA_1c	−2.032	13.598	13.93	0.0003	0.0519	0.211
fPG	−1.109	13.665	11.46	0.0008	0.0424	
Total cholesterol	−1.959	13.771	7.71	0.0059	0.0277	
LDL cholesterol	−2.560	13.757	8.19	0.0046	0.0296	

Legend: TcPO2 indicates transcutaneous oxygen pressure; SBP, systolic blood pressure; HbA1c, glycated hemoglobin; fPG, fasting plasma glucose; LDL, low-density lipoprotein cholesterol.

4. Discussion

The results of our study suggest that the main predictors for the lower TcPO2 value in T2DM obtained via stepwise regression analysis are age, smoking, SBP, HbA_1c, fPG, total and LDL cholesterol. Among all the listed predictors, smoking, HbA_1c, and LDL cholesterol were found to be the most significant. In contrast, no significant correlation was observed between ABI and smoking. TcPO2 is a metabolic test that measures oxygen pressure at the skin surface, while ABI and TBI, the preferred noninvasive indicators of PAD, have limitations when examining microcirculation in patients with PAD [21–25]. Diabetes mellitus facilitates the progression of medial artery calcification, which increases the values of systolic pressure at the ankle, and thus, T2DM patients diagnosed with PAD via a Doppler ultrasound might have a falsely normal ABI [24]. TcPO2 measurement should be conducted to assess the ischemia grade in those with arterial calcification where ABI and TBI are unreliable, in those without clinical symptoms like claudication and rest pain, and in those with diabetic foot complications [26–28]. This is following our results where no significant relation between ABI and TcPO2 was observed in stage 4 of the Fontaine classification (in our case, 18 patients with neuropathic ischemic ulcers and 1 with gangrene).

The mean age of T2DM patients in our study was 68.5 ± 7.8 years. It is well known that the prevalence of PAD increases with higher age. The prevalence of PAD in those over 50 years is up to 29% [29]. However, most elderly patients with PAD are asymptomatic because they walk slowly and cannot induce symptoms of PAD, such as rest pain and claudication [30,31]. Considering this, in older patients with T2DM and suspected PAD, TcPO2 might be a better diagnostic option in the assessment of PAD. In our study, older age was associated with better TCO2, which can be explained by the fact that older patients smoked less often and therefore had better TcPO2 results. The median blood pressure in our cohort was 140/80 mmHg, and SBP was slightly increased according to the latest diabetes guidelines [32]. A study that included over 4 million people between 30 and 90 years suggests that a 20 mmHg higher than the recommended SBP is associated with a 63% higher risk of PAD independent of sex or smoking status [33]. In addition, isolated systolic hypertension is the most prevalent form of hypertension in the population with PAD [34]. On the contrary, only those with lower DBP (<70 mm Hg) had a higher risk of PAD events in the lower extremities [35]. Intensive blood pressure control is effective and safe in patients with PAD [36]. Hypertension induces thickness of the smooth muscle cell layer of the media, fibrosis, remodeling of large arteries, and arterial stiffness, contributing to PAD [37–39].

In our study, HbA_1c and fPG were significant predictors for the TcPO2 value. Advanced glycation end-products (AGE), promoted by hyperglycemia, accumulate in patients and may accelerate the progression of microvascular complications in diabetes [40]. In contrast, the relationship between hyperglycemia and the atherosclerosis of large arteries appears weaker [41]. AGE activates the expression of adhesion molecules on the surface and promotes the adhesion and entrance of monocytes/macrophages into the subendothelial space. AGE also modifies extracellular matrix molecules involved in developing atherosclerotic lesions [42]. Hyperglycemia also promotes proinflammatory responses via the activation of protein kinase C-beta and aldose reductase [43]. Hyperglycemia induces oxidative stress with superoxide overproduction in endothelial cells that activates several significant pathways involved in the pathogenesis of micro- and macrovascular complications of diabetes [44]. Finally, increased glucose uptake by vascular cells activates protein kinase C, an essential protein kinase mediating the cellular signaling pathway, and has several pro-atherogenic effects [45,46]. In ischemic conditions, hyperglycemia per se increases the susceptibility to limb necrosis [47].

Diabetic dyslipidemia is a known risk factor for PAD, and in T2DM nitrated lipoproteins, modified lipoproteins produced by the nitration of the tyrosyl residues of apolipoproteins by myeloperoxidase are also linked with cardiovascular disease [12]. The relationship between the level of LDL cholesterol, notably small dense LDL cholesterol, and the risk of atherosclerosis in T2DM is one of the most studied connections. In our study, total and LDL cholesterol were significant predictors for the TcPO2 value. In T2DM and insulin resistance, there is a predominance of small dense subclasses of LDL cholesterol that undergo several modifications, making them more atherogenic [48]. Small dense LDL cholesterol is associated with poor outcomes after vascular angioplasty in patients with PAD. Since our study included overweight T2DM, we can assume there was a predominance of small dense LDL particles in our patients [49,50]. In patients with type 1 diabetes with similar total and LDL cholesterol levels, as in our study, higher serum lipid levels were associated with lower TcPO2 [51].

The results of our study indicate that, in association with other risk factors, smoking is the main predictor for lower TcPO2 in T2DM. Smoking influences the distribution and composition of serum lipids, increases the total cholesterol content, promotes longer circulation of LDL in plasma and uptake in vessels, and accelerates the formation of plaques [52–54]. Cigarette smoke may induce the dysfunction of endothelial cells via decreased endothelial nitric oxide synthase activity and smooth muscle cells via several mechanisms [55,56]. Cigarette smoke directly damages cellular and sub-cellular structures via reactive oxygen and nitrogen species and the resulting oxidative stress [57]. Smoking causes vascular wall contraction by activating Rho kinase, promoting monocyte adhesion to endothelial cells and entering monocytes and macrophages into endothelium [58,59]. Nicotine from cigarette smoke causes migration, proliferation, apoptosis, phenotypic changes, and the contraction of smooth muscle cells in the arterial wall [60]. Smoking has a direct effect on the TcPO2 value because smoking increases carboxyhemoglobin and reduces oxyhemoglobin, therefore decreasing the TcPO2 value as well. However, a study that included 129 patients with PAD found that only the presence of diabetes adversely affected TcPO2 and clinical disease severity but not smoking [61]. Croatia has one of the highest smoking rates in Europe despite various anti-smoking campaigns. According to 2020 study data, the prevalence of smoking in Croatia was 36%, the third-highest tobacco prevalence in Europe [62].

Some limitations of the present study should be addressed. First, the cross-sectional design of our study limited the ability to infer a causal relation between TcPO2 and risk for the progression of PAD. Second, our study was a single hospital-based study; therefore, selection bias is likely. Third, this cohort had little racial/ethnic diversity, and our data would be primarily relevant to a white European population. Fourth, in patients with diabetes, TBI is more often estimated than ABI. Finally, a major limitation of the study is that smoking is recorded as a dichotomous variable, whereas it should be treated as a continuous one, given its effects vary significantly with the dosage consumed.

5. Conclusions

Our results suggest that, in association with other risk factors, smoking is the main predictor for lower TcPO2 in T2DM. No significant correlation was observed between ABI and smoking, and no significant relation between ABI and TcPO2 was observed in patients in the worst stage of the Fontaine classification, indicating that the TcPO2 measurement might be the preferable option to assess the ischemia grade in those with diabetic foot complications. In our everyday clinical practice, besides the optimal control of systemic risk factors, we need to be much more aware of the harmful effects of smoking, and patients with T2DM and PAD should be strongly advised to stop smoking.

Author Contributions: Conceptualization, T.B., M.T. and N.B.; data curation, M.T.; formal analysis, T.B. and M.T.; methodology, T.B., M.T. and N.B., project administration, T.B. and M.T.; resources, T.B.; supervision, N.B. and T.B.; writing—original draft, T.B. and M.T.; writing—review and editing, T.B., N.B., M.T., A.T.I., I.P. and M.Č. All authors have read and agreed to the published version of the manuscript.

Funding: This research received no specific grant from public, commercial, or not-for-profit funding agencies.

Institutional Review Board Statement: The study was conducted following the Declaration of Helsinki and approved by the Hospital's Ethics Committee (Merkur University Hospital, protocol number 04/38-299, approval date: 7 August 2019).

Informed Consent Statement: Informed consent was obtained from all subjects included in the study.

Data Availability Statement: The data presented in this study are available on a specific request from the corresponding author.

Conflicts of Interest: All authors declare no competing interests.

References

1. Saeedi, P.; Petersohn, I.; Salpea, P.; Malanda, B.; Karuranga, S.; Unwin, N.; Colagiuri, S.; Guariguata, L.; Motala, A.A.; Ogurtsova, K.; et al. IDF Diabetes Atlas Committee. Global and regional diabetes prevalence estimates for 2019 and projections for 2030 and 2045: Results from the International Diabetes Federation Diabetes Atlas, 9th edition. *Diabetes Res. Clin. Pract.* **2019**, *157*, 107843. [CrossRef] [PubMed]
2. Aronson, D.; Rayfield, E.J. How hyperglycemia promotes atherosclerosis: Molecular mechanisms. *Cardiovasc. Diabetol.* **2002**, *1*, 1. [CrossRef]
3. Nishikawa, T.; Edelstein, D.; Du, X.L.; Yamagishi, S.; Matsumura, T.; Kaneda, Y.; Yorek, M.A.; Beebe, D.; Oates, P.J.; Hammes, H.P.; et al. Normalizing mitochondrial superoxide production blocks three pathways of hyperglycemic damage. *Nature* **2000**, *404*, 787–790. [CrossRef]
4. American Diabetes Association. Peripheral arterial disease in people with diabetes. *Diabetes Care* **2003**, *26*, 3333–3341. [CrossRef]
5. Creager, M.A.; White, C.J.; Hiatt, W.R.; Criqui, M.H.; Josephs, S.C.; Alberts, M.J.; Pearce, W.H.; Gray, B.H.; Rocha-Singh, K.J. Atherosclerotic peripheral vascular disease symposium II: Executive summary. *Circulation* **2008**, *118*, 2811–2825. [CrossRef]
6. Marso, S.P.; Hiatt, W.R. Peripheral arterial disease in patients with diabetes. *J. Am. Coll. Cardiol.* **2006**, *47*, 921–929. [CrossRef]
7. Mukherjee, D. Peripheral and cerebrovascular atherosclerotic disease in diabetes mellitus. *Best Pract. Res. Clin. Endocrinol. Metab.* **2009**, *23*, 335–345. [CrossRef] [PubMed]
8. Fadini, G.P.; Spinetti, G.; Santopaolo, M.; Madeddu, P. Impaired regeneration contributes to poor outcomes in diabetic peripheral artery disease. *Arterioscler. Thromb. Vasc. Biol.* **2020**, *40*, 34–44. [CrossRef]
9. Fitridge, R.; Pena, G.; Mills, J.L. The patient presenting with chronic limb-threatening ischaemia. Does diabetes influence presentation, limb outcomes and survival? *Diabetes Metab. Res. Rev.* **2020**, *36* (Suppl. S1), e3242. [CrossRef]
10. Bandyk, D.F. The diabetic foot: Pathophysiology, evaluation, and treatment. *Semin. Vasc. Surg.* **2018**, *31*, 43–48. [CrossRef]
11. Regufe, V.; Pinto, C.; Perez, P. Metabolic syndrome in type 2 diabetic patients: A review of current evidence. *Porto Biomed. J.* **2020**, *6*, e101. [CrossRef]
12. Jakubiak, G.K.; Cie'slar, G.; Stanek, A. Nitrotyrosine, Nitrated Lipoproteins, and Cardiovascular Dysfunction in Patients with Type 2 Diabetes: What Do We Know and What Remains to Be Explained? *Antioxidants* **2022**, *11*, 856. [CrossRef]
13. Stanek, A.; Grygiel-Górniak, B.; Brożyna-Tkaczyk, K.; Myśliński, W.; Cholewka, A.; Zolghadri, S. The Influence of Dietary Interventions on Arterial Stiffness in Overweight and Obese Subjects. *Nutrients* **2023**, *15*, 1440. [CrossRef]
14. Bello-Chavolla, O.Y.; Antonio-Villa, N.E.; Vargas-Vázquez, A.; Martagón, A.J.; Mehta, R.; Arellano-Campos, O.; Gómez-Velasco, D.V.; Almeda-Valdés, P.; Cruz-Bautista, I.; Melgarejo-Hernandez, M.A.; et al. Prediction of incident hypertension and arterial stiffness using the non–insulin-based metabolic score for insulin resistance (METS-IR) index. *J. Clin. Hypertens.* **2019**, *21*, 1063–1070. [CrossRef]
15. Achim, A.; Stanek, A.; Homorodean, C.; Spinu, M.; Onea, H.L.; Lazăr, L.; Marc, M.; Ruzsa, Z.; Olinic, D.M. Approaches to Peripheral Artery Disease in Diabetes: Are There Any Differences? *Int. J. Environ. Res. Public Health* **2022**, *19*, 9801. [CrossRef]
16. Wilcox, T.; Newman, J.D.; Maldonado, T.S.; Rockman, C.; Berger, J.S. Peripheral vascular disease risk in diabetic individuals without coronary heart disease. *Atherosclerosis* **2018**, *275*, 419–425. [CrossRef] [PubMed]
17. Jakubiak, G.K.; Pawlas, N.; Cieślar, G.; Stanek, A. Chronic Lower Extremity Ischemia and Its Association with the Frailty Syndrome in Patients with Diabetes. *Int. J. Environ. Res. Public Health* **2020**, *17*, 9339. [CrossRef] [PubMed]
18. Aboyans, V.; Ricco, J.B.; Bartelink, M.E.L.; Björck, M.; Brodmann, M.; Cohnert, T.; Collet, J.P.; Czerny, M.; De Carlo, M.; Debus, S.; et al. 2017 ESC Guidelines on the Diagnosis and Treatment of Peripheral Arterial Diseases, in collaboration with the European Society for Vascular Surgery (ESVS): Document covering atherosclerotic disease of extracranial carotid and vertebral, mesenteric, renal, upper and lower extremity arteriesEndorsed by: The European Stroke Organization (ESO)The Task Force for the Diagnosis and Treatment of Peripheral Arterial Diseases of the European Society of Cardiology (ESC) and of the European Society for Vascular Surgery (ESVS). *Eur. Heart J.* **2018**, *39*, 763–816. [CrossRef] [PubMed]
19. Casey, S.; Lanting, S.; Oldmeadow, C.; Chuter, V. The reliability of the ankle brachial index: A systematic review. *J. Foot Ankle Res.* **2019**, *12*, 39. [CrossRef] [PubMed]
20. Chang, C.-W.; Sung, Y.-W.; Huang, Y.-T.; Chung, Y.-C.; Lee, M.-Y. Better Detection of Peripheral Arterial Disease with Toe-Brachial Index Compared to Ankle-Brachial Index among Taiwanese Patients with Diabetic Kidney Disease. *J. Clin. Med.* **2023**, *12*, 7393. [CrossRef] [PubMed]

21. Leenstra, B.; Wijnand, J.; Verhoeven, B.; Koning, O.; Teraa, M.; Verhaar, M.C.; de Borst, G.J. Applicability of Transcutaneous Oxygen Tension Measurement in the Assessment of Chronic Limb-Threatening Ischemia. *Angiology* **2020**, *71*, 208–216. [CrossRef]
22. Leenstra, B.; de Kleijn, R.; Kuppens, G.; Verhoeven, B.A.N.; Hinnen, J.W.; de Borst, G.J. Photo-Optical Transcutaneous Oxygen Tension Measurement Is of Added Value to Predict Diabetic Foot Ulcer Healing: An Observational Study. *J. Clin. Med.* **2020**, *9*, 3291. [CrossRef]
23. Nasra, K.; Osher, M. Sonography Vascular Peripheral Arterial Assessment, Protocols, and Interpretation. In *StatPearls [Internet]*; StatPearls Publishing: Treasure Island, FL, USA, 2023. Available online: https://www.ncbi.nlm.nih.gov/books/NBK570577/ (accessed on 30 January 2024).
24. Kim, T.I.; Guzman, R.J. Medial artery calcification in peripheral artery disease. *Front. Cardiovasc. Med.* **2023**, *10*, 1093355. [CrossRef]
25. Fontaine, R.; Kim, M.; Kieny, R. Surgical treatment of peripheral circulation disorders. *Helv. Chir. Acta* **1954**, *21*, 499–533. (In German) [PubMed]
26. López-Moral, M.; García-Madrid, M.; Molines-Barroso, R.J.; García-Álvarez, Y.; Tardáguila-García, A.; Lázaro-Martínez, J.L. Analyses of transcutaneous oxygen pressure values stratified for foot angiosomes to predict diabetic foot ulcer healing. *J. Tissue Viability* **2023**, *32*, 480–486. [CrossRef] [PubMed]
27. Ren, B.; Li, B.; Pan, T.; Zhao, E.; Ju, S.; Li, X.; Li, X.; Zhu, Y.; Cai, Y.; Huang, L.; et al. Risk factors for at-risk foot and peripheral artery disease among the population with diabetes: A multicommunity-based cross-sectional study. *Diabetes Res. Clin. Pract.* **2023**, *203*, 110869. [CrossRef] [PubMed]
28. Catella, J.; Long, A.; Mazzolai, L. What Is Currently the Role of TcPO2 in the Choice of the Amputation Level of Lower Limbs? A Comprehensive Review. *J. Clin. Med.* **2021**, *10*, 1413. [CrossRef] [PubMed]
29. Thiruvoipati, T.; Kielhorn, C.E.; Armstrong, E.J. Peripheral artery disease in patients with diabetes: Epidemiology, mechanisms, and outcomes. *World J. Diabetes* **2015**, *6*, 961–969. [CrossRef] [PubMed]
30. Aronow, W.S. Peripheral arterial disease in the elderly. *Clin. Interv. Aging* **2007**, *2*, 645–654. [CrossRef]
31. Aronow, W.S.; Ahn, C.; Gutstein, H. Prevalence and incidence of cardiovascular disease in 1160 older men and 2464 older women in a long-term health care facility. *J. Gerontol. A Biol. Sci. Med. Sci.* **2002**, *57*, M45–M46. [CrossRef] [PubMed]
32. American Diabetes Association Professional Practice Committee. Cardiovascular disease and risk management: Standards of care in diabetes-2024. *Diabetes Care* **2024**, *47* (Suppl. S1), S179–S218. [CrossRef]
33. Emdin, C.A.; Anderson, S.G.; Callender, T.; Conrad, N.; Salimi-Khorshidi, G.; Mohseni, H.; Woodward, M.; Rahimi, K. Usual blood pressure, peripheral arterial disease, and vascular risk: Cohort study of 4.2 million adults. *BMJ* **2015**, *351*, h4865. [CrossRef]
34. Safar, M.E.; Priollet, P.; Luizy, F.; Mourad, J.-J.; Cacoub, P.; Levesque, H.; Benelbaz, J.; Michon, P.; Herrmann, M.-A.; Blacher, J. Peripheral arterial disease and isolated systolic hypertension: The ATTEST study. *J. Hum. Hypertens.* **2009**, *23*, 182–187. [CrossRef] [PubMed]
35. Itoga, N.K.; Tawfik, D.S.; Lee, C.K.; Maruyama, S.; Leeper, N.J.; Chang, T.I. Association of Blood Pressure Measurements with Peripheral Artery Disease Events. *Circulation* **2018**, *138*, 1805–1814. [CrossRef] [PubMed]
36. Frary, J.M.C.; Pareek, M.; Byrne, C.; Vaduganathan, M.; Biering-Sørensen, T.; Rujic, D.; Kragholm, K.H.; Olesen, T.B.; Olsen, M.H.; Bhatt, D.L. Intensive blood pressure control appears to be effective and safe in patients with peripheral artery disease: The Systolic Blood Pressure Intervention Trial. *Eur. Heart J. Cardiovasc. Pharmacother.* **2021**, *7*, e38–e40. [CrossRef] [PubMed]
37. Shimizu, Y. Progression of Carotid Intima-Media Thickness Partly Indicates the Prevention of Hypertension among Older Individuals in the General Population. *Life* **2023**, *13*, 1588. [CrossRef]
38. Rubio-Guerra, A.F.; Garro-Almendaro, A.K.; Lozano-Nuevo, J.L.; Arana-Pazos, K.C.; Duran-Salgado, M.B.; Morales-López, H. Prehypertension is associated with peripheral arterial disease and low ankle-brachial index. *Indian Heart J.* **2018**, *70*, 502–505. [CrossRef]
39. Omboni, S.; Posokhov, I.N.; Rogoza, A.N. Relationships between 24-h blood pressure variability and 24-h central arterial pressure, pulse wave velocity and augmentation index in hypertensive patients. *Hypertens. Res.* **2017**, *40*, 385–391. [CrossRef]
40. Poznyak, A.; Grechko, A.V.; Poggio, P.; Myasoedova, V.A.; Alfieri, V.; Orekhov, A.N. The Diabetes Mellitus–Atherosclerosis Connection: The Role of Lipid and Glucose Metabolism and Chronic Inflammation. *Int. J. Mol. Sci.* **2020**, *21*, 1835. [CrossRef]
41. Bornfeldt, K.E. Does Elevated Glucose Promote Atherosclerosis? Pros and Cons. *Circ. Res.* **2016**, *119*, 190–193. [CrossRef]
42. Katakami, N. Mechanism of Development of Atherosclerosis and Cardiovascular Disease in Diabetes Mellitus. *J. Atheroscler. Thromb.* **2018**, *25*, 27–39. [CrossRef]
43. Tabit, C.E.; Shenouda, S.M.; Holbrook, M.; Fetterman, J.L.; Kiani, S.; Frame, A.A.; Kluge, M.A.; Held, A.; Dohadwala, M.M.; Gokce, N.; et al. Protein kinase C-β contributes to impaired endothelial insulin signaling in humans with diabetes mellitus. *Circulation* **2013**, *127*, 86–95. [CrossRef]
44. Giacco, F.; Brownlee, M. Oxidative stress and diabetic complications. *Circ. Res.* **2010**, *107*, 1058–1070. [CrossRef]
45. Newton, A.C. Regulation of the ABC kinases by phosphorylation: Protein kinase C as a paradigm. *Biochem. J.* **2008**, *88*, 1341–1378. [CrossRef] [PubMed]
46. Zeadin, M.G.; Petlura, C.I.; Werstuck, G.H. Molecular mechanisms linking diabetes to the accelerated development of atherosclerosis. *Can. J. Diabetes* **2013**, *37*, 345–350. [CrossRef] [PubMed]
47. Lévigne, D.; Tobalem, M.; Modarressi, A.; Pittet-Cuénod, B. Hyperglycemia Increases Susceptibility to Ischemic Necrosis. *BioMed Res. Int.* **2013**, *2013*, 490964. [CrossRef] [PubMed]

48. Ivanova, E.A.; Myasoedova, V.A.; Melnichenko, A.A.; Grechko, A.V.; Orekhov, A.N. Small dense low-density lipoprotein as biomarker for atherosclerotic diseases. *Oxidative Med. Cell. Longev.* **2017**, *2017*, 1273042. [CrossRef]
49. Klop, B.; Elte, J.W.F.; Cabezas, M.C. Dyslipidemia in obesity: Mechanisms and potential targets. *Nutrients* **2013**, *5*, 1218–1240. [CrossRef]
50. Jacomella, V.; Gerber, P.A.; Mosimann, K.; Husmann, M.; Thalhammer, C.; Wilkinson, I.; Berneis, K.; Amann-Vesti, B.R. Small Dense Low Density Lipoprotein Particles Are Associated with Poor Outcome after Angioplasty in Peripheral Artery Disease. *PLoS ONE* **2014**, *9*, e108813. [CrossRef]
51. Neubauer-Geryk, J.; Wielicka, M.; Kozera, G.M.; Brandt-Varma, A.; Wołoszyn-Durkiewicz, A.; Myśliwiec, M.; Bieniaszewski, L. Skin oxygenation impairment is associated with increased total cholesterol level in children with short-lasting type 1 diabetes mellitus. *Adv. Dermatol. Allergol.* **2021**, *38*, 615–621. [CrossRef]
52. Wang, W.; Zhao, T.; Geng, K.; Yuan, G.; Chen, Y.; Xu, Y. Smoking and the Pathophysiology of Peripheral Artery Disease. *Front. Cardiovasc. Med.* **2021**, *8*, 704106. [CrossRef]
53. Lietz, M.; Berges, A.; Lebrun, S.; Meurrens, K.; Steffen, Y.; Stolle, K.; Schueller, J.; Boue, S.; Vuillaume, G.; Vanscheeuwijck, P.; et al. Cigarette-smoke-induced atherogenic lipid profiles in plasma and vascular tissue of apolipoprotein E-deficient mice are attenuated by smoking cessation. *Atherosclerosis* **2013**, *229*, 86–93. [CrossRef]
54. Ma, B.; Chen, Y.; Wang, X.; Zhang, R.; Niu, S.; Ni, L.; Di, X.; Han, Q.; Liu, C. Cigarette smoke exposure impairs lipid metabolism by decreasing low-density lipoprotein receptor expression in hepatocytes. *Lipids Health Dis.* **2020**, *19*, 88. [CrossRef]
55. Siasos, G.; Tsigkou, V.; Kokkou, E.; Oikonomou, E.; Vavuranakis, M.; Vlachopoulos, C.; Verveniotis, A.; Limperi, M.; Genimata, V.; Papavassiliou, A.G.; et al. Smoking and atherosclerosis: Mechanisms of disease and new therapeutic approaches. *Curr. Med. Chem.* **2014**, *21*, 3936–3948. [CrossRef]
56. Donato, A.J.; Morgan, R.G.; Walker, A.E.; Lesniewski, L.A. Cellular and molecular biology of aging endothelial cells. *J. Mol. Cell. Cardiol.* **2015**, *89*, 122–135. [CrossRef]
57. Caliri, A.W.; Tommasi, S.; Besaratinia, A. Relationships among smoking, oxidative stress, inflammation, macromolecular damage, and cancer. *Mutat. Res. Rev. Mutat. Res.* **2021**, *787*, 108365. [CrossRef]
58. Higashi, Y. Smoking cessation and vascular endothelial function. *Hypertens. Res.* **2023**, *46*, 2670–2678. [CrossRef] [PubMed]
59. Wang, C.; Petriello, M.C.; Zhu, B.; Hennig, B. PCB 126 induces monocyte/macrophage polarization and inflammation through AhR and NF-κB pathways. *Toxicol. Appl. Pharmacol.* **2019**, *367*, 71–81. [CrossRef] [PubMed]
60. Duong-Quy, S.; Dao, P.; Hua-Huy, T.; Guilluy, C.; Pacaud, P.; Dinh-Xuan, A.T. Increased Rho-kinase expression and activity and pulmonary endothelial dysfunction in smokers with normal lung function. *Eur. Respir. J.* **2011**, *37*, 349–355. [CrossRef] [PubMed]
61. Rooke, T.W.; Osmundson, P.J. The influence of age, sex, smoking, and diabetes on lower limb transcutaneous oxygen tension in patients with arterial occlusive disease. *Arch. Intern. Med.* **1990**, *150*, 129–132. [CrossRef] [PubMed]
62. European Commission. Special Eurobarometer 429: Attitudes of Europeans towards Tobacco and Electronic Cigarettes. 2020. Available online: https://health.ec.europa.eu/tobacco/overview_en#documents (accessed on 17 January 2023).

biomedicines

MDPI

Article

Hyperglycaemia and Its Prognostic Value in Patients with COVID-19 Admitted to the Hospital in Lithuania

Lina Zabuliene [1], Ieva Kubiliute [2], Mykolas Urbonas [3], Ligita Jancoriene [2], Jurgita Urboniene [4] and Ioannis Ilias [5,*]

1 Institute of Clinical Medicine, Faculty of Medicine, Vilnius University, 03101 Vilnius, Lithuania; lina.zabuliene@mf.vu.lt

2 Clinic of Infectious Diseases and Dermatovenerology, Institute of Clinical Medicine, Faculty of Medicine, Vilnius University, 08661 Vilnius, Lithuania; ieva.kubiliute@santa.lt (I.K.); ligita.jancoriene@mf.vu.lt (L.J.)

3 Faculty of Medicine, Vilnius University, 03101 Vilnius, Lithuania

4 Center of Infectious Diseases, Vilnius University Hospital Santaros Klinikos, 08661 Vilnius, Lithuania; jurgita.urboniene@santa.lt

5 Department of Endocrinology, Diabetes and Metabolism, Elena Venizelou Hospital, 11521 Athens, Greece

* Correspondence: iiliasmd@yahoo.com

Abstract: Background and objectives: Increased blood glucose levels atadmission are frequently observed in COVID-19 patients, even in those without pre-existing diabetes. Hyperglycaemia is associated with an increased incidence of severe COVID-19 infection. The aim of this study was to evaluate the association between hyperglycaemia at admission with the need for invasive mechanical ventilation (IMV) and in-hospital mortality in patients without diabetes who were hospitalized for COVID-19 infection. Materials and methods: This retrospective observational study was conducted at Vilnius University Hospital Santaros Clinics, Lithuania with adult patients who tested positive for severe acute respiratory syndrome coronavirus 2 SARS-CoV-2 and were hospitalized between March 2020 and May 2021. Depersonalized data were retrieved from electronic medical records. Based on blood glucose levels on the day of admission, patients without diabetes were divided into 4 groups: patients with hypoglycaemia (blood glucose below 4.0 mmol/L), patients with normoglycaemia (blood glucose between ≥4.0 mmol/L and <6.1 mmol/L), patients with mild hyperglycaemia (blood glucose between ≥6.1 mmol/L and <7.8 mmol/L), and patients with intermittent hyperglycaemia (blood glucose levels ≥7.8 mmol/L and <11.1 mmol/L). A multivariable binary logistic regression model was created to determine the association between hyperglycaemia and the need for IMV. Survival analysis was performed to assess the effect of hyperglycaemia on outcome within 30 days of hospitalization. Results: Among 1945 patients without diabetes at admission, 1078 (55.4%) had normal glucose levels, 651 (33.5%) had mild hyperglycaemia, 196 (10.1%) had intermittent hyperglycaemia, and 20 (1.0%) had hypoglycaemia. The oddsratio (OR) for IMV in patients with intermittent hyperglycaemia was 4.82 (95% CI 2.70–8.61, $p < 0.001$), and the OR was 2.00 (95% CI 1.21–3.31, $p = 0.007$) in those with mild hyperglycaemia compared to patients presenting normal glucose levels. The hazardratio (HR) for 30-day in-hospital mortality in patients with mild hyperglycaemia was 1.62 (95% CI 1.10–2.39, $p = 0.015$), while the HR was 3.04 (95% CI 2.01–4.60, $p < 0.001$) in patients with intermittent hyperglycaemia compared to those with normoglycaemia at admission. Conclusions: In COVID-19 patients without pre-existing diabetes, the presence of hyperglycaemia at admission is indicative of COVID-19-induced alterations in glucose metabolism and stress hyperglycaemia. Hyperglycaemia at admission in COVID-19 patients without diabetes is associated with an increased risk of invasive mechanical ventilation and in-hospital mortality. This finding highlights the importance for clinicians to carefully consider and select optimal support and treatment strategies for these patients. Further studies on the long-term consequences of hyperglycaemia in this specific population are warranted.

Keywords: coronavirus; SARS-CoV-2; COVID-19; glucose on admission; hyperglycaemia; in-hospital mortality

1. Introduction

Since the beginning of the severe acute respiratory syndrome coronavirus 2 (SARS-CoV-2) pandemic, diabetes mellitus has emerged as one of the most common comorbidities predisposing to coronavirus disease 2019 (COVID-19) and an important risk factor for hospitalization and mortality [1–3]. People with diabetes face a compromised immune system, making them more susceptible to severe outcomes of COVID-19. Diabetes is known for causing a pro-inflammatory syndrome, so patients with diabetes are more vulnerable to increased production of cytokines, which consequently lead to the deterioration of COVID-19 due to the development of acute respiratory distress syndrome and shock. Moreover, the hyperactivation of the coagulation cascade in COVID-19, particularly in the presence of pre-existing pro-thrombotic hypercoagulability associated with diabetes, intensifies the risk of severe thromboembolic complications [3]. Increased glucose levels at admission are frequently observed in COVID-19 patients, even in those without a history of diabetes.

Stress hyperglycaemia is a common condition in patients with any acute illness when the interaction of various cytokines and stress hormones leads to a state of insulin resistance and increased glucose production [4]. Inflammatory cytokines, such as interleukin-1 (IL-1), interleukin-6 (IL-6), and tumour necrosis factor-α (TNF-α), suppress insulin release and induce insulin resistance, and elevated levels of IL-6 promote hyperglycaemia by releasing glucose from hepatic glycogen reserves. Cortisol, catecholamines, glucagon, and growth hormone decrease insulin release by amplifying the activity of pancreatic alpha cells. Catecholamines further limit insulin binding, and, together with growth hormone, prevent insulin activation by suppressing tyrosine kinase activity. Moreover, catecholamines and glucocorticoids restrict glucose uptake in peripheral skeletal muscles through modulation of the glucose transporter type 4 [4].

Recent studies reported that stress hyperglycaemia increases the risk of mortality in critically ill patients [5] and patients with myocardial infarction [6] and stroke [7]. A single-centre study involving 1000 patients admitted to the intensive care unit found that in patients without diabetes, the risk of death increased by 20% for each 1 mmol/l increase in acute glycaemia [5]. Another study with 660 patients experiencing ST elevation myocardial infarction and treated with primary percutaneous coronary intervention showed significantly higher rates of mortality, cardiogenic shock, contrast-induced nephropathy, and the no-reflow phenomenon in the stress hyperglycaemia patient group [6]. A large study involving 8622 patients revealed that stress hyperglycaemia independently predicted severe neurological deficit within 1 year in patients with acute ischemic stroke, regardless of diabetes status. This association with mortality at 1 year is more pronounced in people without diagnosed or underlying diabetes [7]. In New Zealand, a study involving 739,152 ICU patients without a pre-existing diabetes diagnosis demonstrated a clear dose-response relationship between hyperglycaemia and hospital mortality, as well as an extended duration of hospital stay [8].

The appearance of hyperglycaemia in COVID-19 patients without diabetes likely indicates increased systemic stress as well. Furthermore, recent evidence from experimental studies suggests that SARS-CoV-2 infects human pancreatic β-cells and leads to morphological, transcriptional, and functional changes [9].

Hyperglycaemia is associated with a higher incidence of a severe course of COVID-19 infection, including the need for oxygen therapy [10,11], invasive mechanical ventilation (IMV) [10,11], and admission to the intensive care unit (ICU) [10–12] and has been found to be a predictor of in-hospital mortality in COVID-19 patients [12–15].

While extensive research has been conducted on the impact of hyperglycaemia in patients with diabetes and COVID-19, there remains a noticeable gap in our understanding of hyperglycaemia's role in individuals without pre-existing diabetes. The aim of this study was to evaluate the association between hyperglycaemia at admission with the need for IMV and in-hospital mortality in patients without diabetes who were hospitalized for COVID-19 infection. By addressing this research gap, our study aims to contribute valuable insights that can inform clinical strategies and interventions tailored to patients without pre-existing diabetes, ultimately enhancing our ability to optimize care and improve outcomes in this specific population.

2. Materials and Methods

A single centre, retrospective observational cohort study was conducted at Vilnius University Hospital Santaros Klinikos (VUH SK), Vilnius, Lithuania [16].

2.1. Participants

Adult patients (18 years of age and older) who were hospitalized at VUH SK between March 2020 and May 2021 for confirmed COVID-19 infection and treated in the standard care unit, high dependency unit, or intensive care unit (ICU) were included in the study. The infection was verified based on a positive SARS-CoV-2 reverse transcriptase polymerase chain reaction result or a rapid antigen test conducted on a nasopharyngeal sample for symptomatic patients within 5 days from the onset of COVID-19 symptoms [16]. A total of 2561 hospitalized patients with COVID-19, who had their blood glucose tested during their hospital stay, were included in the analysis. Out of the 2561 patients hospitalized with COVID-19, 2054 had no pre-existing diabetes or a blood glucose concentration meeting the criteria for newly diagnosed diabetes during the hospital stay (Figure 1).

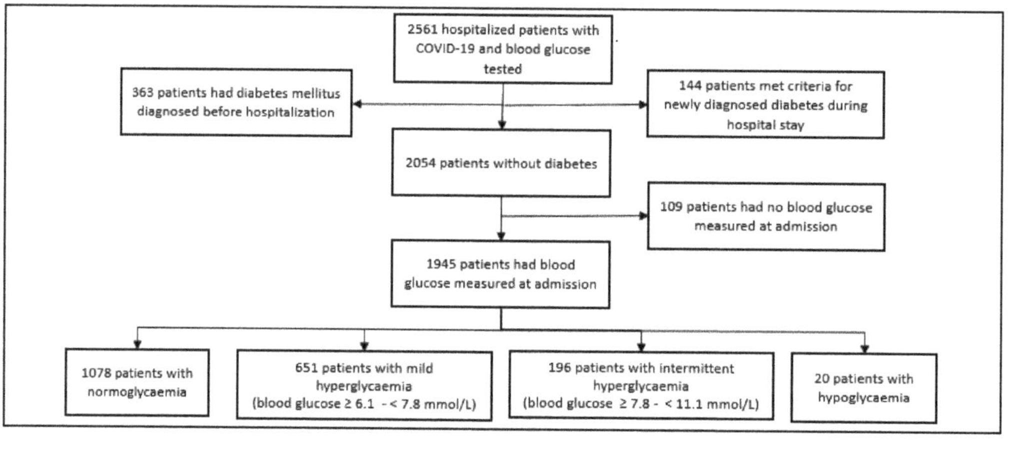

Figure 1. Distribution of patients hospitalized with COVID-19 infection.

2.2. Data Collection and Variables

Depersonalized data were retrieved from the electronic medical records (EMR) of VUH SK and provided by the informatics and development centre in accordance with hospital-approved procedures [16].

Demographic variables included gender and age. Data on comorbidities included arterial hypertension (AH), coronary artery disease (CAD), congestive heart failure (CHF), diabetes mellitus, obesity, chronic obstructive pulmonary disease (COPD), chronic kidney disease (CKD), and previous stroke. Comorbidity data were extracted using the relevant codes from the International Statistical Classification of Diseases and Related Health Problems, Tenth Revision, Australian Modification (ICD-10-AM). AH was defined by the presence of comorbidities with ICD-10-AM codes I10, I11.0, and I11.9; CAD by the presence of comorbidities with ICD-10-AM codes I20.0, I20.2, I20.8, and I20.9; CHF by the presence of comorbidities with ICD-10-AM codes I50.0, I50.1, and I50.9; diabetes by the presence of comorbidities with ICD-10-AM codes E10 and E11; obesity by the presence of comorbidities with ICD-10-AM codes E66, E66.0, E66.2, E66.8, and E66.9; COPD by the presence of comorbidities with ICD-10-AM codes J44.0, J44.1, J44.8, and J44.9; CKD by the presence of comorbidities with ICD-10-AM codes N18.1, N18.2, N18.3, N18.4, N18.5, and N18.9; and previous stroke by the presence of comorbidities with ICD-10-AM code I69.If the condition was not documented in the patient's EMR during hospitalization for COVID-19 infection, the patient was classified as not having that condition. Information regarding the utilization of antibiotics, systemic steroids, antivirals, IMV, length of hospital stay, and in-hospital mortality data was also extracted from depersonalized EMR.

Data from initial laboratory tests, including complete blood count, creatinine, urea, sodium, estimated glomerular filtration rate (eGFR), potassium, alanine aminotransferase (ALT), aspartate aminotransferase (AST), lactate dehydrogenase (LDH), C-reactive protein (CRP), ferritin, interleukin 6 (IL-6), D-dimer, and troponin I, were also retrieved and evaluated.The neutrophil-to-lymphocyte ratio (NLR) and AST to ALT ratio was calculated.

Data from blood glucose measurements conducted during hospitalization were obtained. Patients who had a blood glucose level of 11.1 mmol/L or higher during hospitalization were classified as having newly diagnosed diabetes mellitus. Based on the blood glucose level on the day of admission (if multiple blood glucose tests were performed within the first 24 h after admission, the mean glucose value was considered), patients without diabetes were divided into the following 4 groups: patients with hypoglycaemia were defined as those with blood glucose levels at admission below 4.0 mmol/L, patients with normoglycaemia had blood glucose levels at admission between ≥4.0 mmol/L and <6.1 mmol/L, patients with mild hyperglycaemia had blood glucose levels at admission was between ≥6.1 mmol/L and <7.8 mmol/L, and patients with intermittent hyperglycaemia had blood glucose levels atadmission between ≥7.8 mmol/L and <11.1 mmol/L.

Data from 2561 COVID-19 patients were analysed.

2.3. Main Outcome

The main outcome of the study was to evaluate the relationship between glycemia on admission in patients without diabetes and the severity of COVID-19 outcomes, including the need for mechanical ventilation and 30-day in-hospital mortality.

2.4. Statistical Analysis

Continuous and categorical variables were presented as medians (interquartile range [IQR]) and numbers (percentages, %), respectively. The Mann–Whitney U test was used to compare continuous variables, and the χ^2 test was used to compare categorical variables. A multivariable binary logistic regression model was created to determine association of glucose levels and the need for IMV. The model included the need for IMV as the dependent variable, and age, gender, comorbidities which proportions statistically significantly differed between groups as predictors. We conducted survival analysis to assess the effects of glucose level on outcome within 30 days of hospitalization. We created a Cox proportional hazards regression model with in-hospital mortality as the dependent variable and age, gender, comorbidities with proportions that statistically significantly differed between groups, systemic steroids use, and treatment with remdesivir as predictors and plotted curves for survival stratified by glucose level. A two-sided *p*-value less than 0.05 was considered statistically significant. Analysis was performed using IBM Statistical Package for the Social Sciences software version 20.0 (IBM SPSS Statistics for Windows, Version 20.0, 2018, Armonk, NY, USA: IBM Corp.), and Microsoft Excel (Microsoft Corporation, 2018, Microsoft Excel, Available at: https://office.microsoft.com/excel, accessed on 18 December 2023) was used to produce figures.

3. Results

Among 2561 hospitalized adults, 55.1% were men. The median age was 60 years (IQR 49–70). Patients' demographic, clinical characteristics, and initial laboratory parameters are presented in Table 1.

Table 1. Demographic, clinical, and initial laboratory characteristics of patients hospitalized with COVID-19 infection.

Demographic and Clinical Characteristic (2561 Patients)	N (%)	Laboratory Characteristics	N	Median (IQR)
Age, years, median (IQR)	60 (49–70)	Haemoglobin, g/L	2561	138 (124–149)
Male	1412 (55.1)	WBC, $\times 10^9$/L	2561	6.48 (4.84–9.03)
Female	1149 (44.9)	Neutrophils, $\times 10^9$/L	2561	4.76 (3.30–7.13)
Any concommitant condition	1252 (48.9)	Lymphocytes, $\times 10^9$/L	2561	1 (0.70–1.40)
Arterial hypertension	983 (38.4)	NLR	2558	4.70 (2.86–8.05)
Coronary artery disease	90 (3.5)	Platelets, $\times 10^9$/L	2561	198 (153–258)
Congestive heart failure	198 (7.7)	Glucose, mmol/L	2561	6.12 (5.43–7.28)
Diabetes mellitus	363 (14.2)	Creatinine, µmol/L	2557	82 (67–105)
Obesity	123 (4.8)	Urea, mmol/L	2371	5.73 (4.12–8.74)
COPD	42 (1.6)	eGFR, mL/min/1.73 m^2	2513	83 (58.95–96)
Chronic kidney disease	205 (8.0)	Sodium, mmol/L	2551	140 (137–143)
Previous stroke	32 (1.2)	Potassium, mmol/L	2551	4.20 (3.90–4.60)
Invasive mechanical ventilation	192 (7.5)	ALT, U/L	2500	31.42 (19.65–52)
Antibiotics use	1863 (72.7)	AST, U/L	2485	36 (26–57)
Antivirals (remdesivir)	808 (31.6)	AST to ALT ratio	2483	1.17 (0.87–1.67)
Systemic steroids	1630 (63.6)	LDH, U/L	2302	303 (236–408.04)
In-hospital mortality	313 (12.2)	CRP, mg/L	2558	62.15 (22.78–124.88)
Length of hospital stay, days, median (IQR)	11 (7–16)	Ferritin, µg/L	2367	479.85 (236–1009.44)
		IL-6, ng/L	2254	29.60 (14.40–57.30)
		D-dimer, µg/L	2344	510 (305–985)
		Troponin I, ng/L	2122	10 (5–26)

ALT—alanine aminotransferase; AST—aspartate aminotransferase; COPD—chronic obstructive pulmonary disease, CRP—C-reactive protein; eGFR—estimated glomerular filtration rate; IL-6—interleukin 6; IQR—interquartile range; LDH—lactate dehydrogenase; N—number; NLR—neutrophil-to-lymphocyte ratio; WBC—white blood cell count.

Reference values: Haemoglobin: 128–160 g/L (for males), 117–145 g/L (for females); WBC: 4.0–9.8 $\times$ 10^9/L; neutrophils: 1.5–6.0 $\times$ 10^9/L; lymphocytes: 1.0–4.0 $\times$ 10^9/L; NLR—1–2; platelets: 140–450 $\times$ 10^9/L; glucose: 4.2–6.1 mmol/L; creatinine: 64–104 µmol/L (for males), 49–90 µmol/L (for females); urea: 2.5–7.5 mmol/L; sodium: 134–145 mmol/L; potassium: 3.8–5.3 mmol/L; ALT: $\leq$40 U/L; AST: $\leq$40 U/L; AST to ALT ratio: <1; LDH: 125–243 U/L; CRP: <5 mg/L; ferritin: 25–350 µg/L (for men), 13–232 µg/L (for women); IL-6: 0–7 ng/L; D-dimer: <250 µg/L; and troponin I: <19 ng/L.

Out of a total of 2561 patients, 363 (14.2%) had a pre-existing diagnosis of diabetes before hospitalization, and 144 (5.6%) met the diagnostic criteria for newly diagnosed diabetes during their hospital stay.

Glucose levels at admission were measured for 1945 patients without diabetes. Out of a total of 1945 patients without diabetes, 1078 (55.4%) had a normal glucose level at admission, 651 (33.5%) patients had mild hyperglycaemia at admission, and 196 (10.1%) patients had intermittent hyperglycaemia at admission. Additionally, 20 (1.0%) patients without diabetes had hypoglycaemia upon admission (Figure 1).

Patients with mild hyperglycaemia and intermittent hyperglycaemia were older compared to patients with normoglycaemia (Table 2).

Table 2. Demographic and clinical characteristics of COVID-19 patients without diabetes based on glycaemia levels on admission.

Demographic and Clinical Characteristic	Normoglycaemia N = 1078	Mild Hyperglycaemia, N = 651	Intermittent Hyperglycaemia, N = 196	p-Value [1]	p-Value [2]	p-Value [3]
Age in years, median (IQR)	55 (43–66)	60 (50–68)	67 (59–76)	<0.001	<0.001	<0.001
Male	604 (56.0%)	379 (58.2%)	108 (55.1%)	0.373	0.810	0.439
Female	474 (44.0%)	272 (41.8%)	88 (44.9%)	0.373	0.810	0.439
Any underlying condition	373 (34.6%)	307 (47.2%)	119 (60.7%)	<0.001	<0.001	0.001
Arterial hypertension	299 (27.7%)	246 (37.8%)	96 (49.0%)	<0.001	<0.001	0.005
Coronary artery disease	23 (2.1%)	19 (2.9%)	10 (5.1%)	0.304	0.016	0.141
Congestive heart failure	48 (4.5%)	38 (5.8%)	21 (10.7%)	0.200	<0.001	0.019
Obesity	24 (2.2%)	22 (3.4%)	12 (6.1%)	0.149	0.002	0.086
COPD	12 (1.1%)	10 (1.5%)	2 (1.0%)	0.447	1.000	0.743
Chronic kidney disease	58 (5.4%)	30 (4.6%)	18 (9.2%)	0.479	0.039	0.015
Previous stroke	8 (0.7%)	5 (0.8%)	5 (2.6%)	1.000	0.037	0.057
Invasive mechanical ventilation	29 (2.7%)	38 (5.8%)	29 (14.8%)	0.001	<0.001	<0.001
Antibiotics	763 (70.8%)	486 (74.7%)	141 (71.9%)	0.081	0.742	0.447
Antivirals (remdesivir)	326 (30.2%)	242 (37.2%)	64 (32.7%)	0.003	0.500	0.248
Systemic steroids	634 (58.8%)	465 (71.4%)	134 (68.4%)	<0.001	0.012	0.409
In-hospital mortality	57 (5.3%)	61 (9.4%)	44 (22.4%)	0.001	<0.001	<0.001
Length of hospital stay, days, median (IQR)	10 (7–14)	11 (8–16)	11.50 (7–16)	0.001	0.059	0.996

1—p value comparing patients with normoglycaemia vs. patients with mild hyperglycaemia. 2—p value comparing patients with normoglycaemia vs. patients with intermittent hyperglycaemia. 3—p value comparing patients with mild hyperglycaemia vs. patients with intermittent hyperglycaemia.

The prevalence of AH, CAD, CHF, obesity, CKD, and previous stroke was higher in patients with intermittent hyperglycaemia compared to patients with normoglycaemia. The prevalence of AH, CHF, and CKD was higher in patients with intermittent hyperglycaemia compared to patients with mild hyperglycaemia.

The higher proportion of patients with intermittent hyperglycaemia required IMV compared to patients with mild hyperglycaemia (14.8% vs. 5.8%, $p < 0.001$) and normoglycaemia (14.8% vs. 2.7%, $p < 0.001$).

A total of 1233 (64.1%) patients without diabetes received systemic steroids, with 1201 of them treated with dexamethasone for a course lasting 9 (IQR 6–10) days. A higher proportion of patients with mild hyperglycaemia (74.4% vs. 58.8%, $p < 0.001$) and intermittent hyperglycaemia (68.4% vs. 58.8%, $p = 0.012$) received systemic steroids compared to patients with normal glucose levels at admission.

A total of 632 (32.8%) patients without diabetes received remdesivir for a course lasting 5 (IQR 5–5) days. A higher proportion of patients with mild hyperglycaemia (37.2% vs. 30.2%, $p = 0.003$) received systemic steroids compared to patients with normal glucose levels at admission. However, there was no statistically significant difference between the mild and intermittent hyperglycaemia groups regarding the percentage of patients treated with remdesivir.

The highest in-hospital mortality rate was noted in patients with intermittent hyperglycaemia at admission reaching 22.4% compared to those with mild hyperglycaemia (9.4%) and normoglycaemia (5.3%) (Table 2).

Patients with intermittent hyperglycaemia on admission had higher levels of white blood cell (WBC) counts, neutrophil counts, NLR, platelet counts, creatinine, urea, ALT, AST, LDH, CRP, ferritin, IL-6, D-dimer, and troponin I compared to patients with normoglycaemia, whereas lymphocyte count, eGFR, potassium, and sodium concentration were significantly lower (Table 3).

Table 3. Initial laboratory characteristics of COVID-19 patients without diabetes based on glycaemia levels upon admission.

Laboratory Characteristics	Normoglycaemia		Mild Hyperglycaemia		Intermittent Hyperglycaemia		p-Value [1]	p-Value [2]	p-Value [3]
	n	Value, Median (IQR)	n	Value, Median (IQR)	n	Value, Median (IQR)			
Haemoglobin, g/L	1078	139 (125–150)	651	140 (127–151)	196	141 (124–151)	0.120	0.693	0.621
WBC, $\times10^9$/L	1078	5.87 (4.43–7.62)	651	6.54 (5.05–8.91)	196	8.22 (6.07–11.68)	<0.001	<0.001	<0.001
Neutrophils, $\times10^9$/L	1078	4.10 (2.90–5.80)	651	5 (3.60–7.16)	196	6.60 (4.50–9.90)	<0.001	<0.001	<0.001
Lymphocytes, $\times10^9$/L	1078	1.07 (0.80–1.46)	651	0.93 (0.66–1.26)	196	0.90 (0.60–1.33)	<0.001	<0.001	0.732
NLR	1076	3.73 (2.45–5.91)	650	5.20 (3.30–8.46)	196	7.47 (4.50–12.54)	<0.001	<0.001	<0.001
Platelets, $\times10^9$/L	1078	194 (151–254)	651	195 (153–253)	196	213.50 (168.25–277.75)	0.832	0.001	0.003
Glucose at admission, mmol/L	1078	5.46 (5.09–5.77)	651	6.60 (6.33–7.06)	196	8.70 (8.16–9.57)	<0.001	<0.001	<0.001
Creatinine, µmol/L	1075	78.2 (65–96)	651	81.01 (68–98.93)	196	87 (70.25–130.93)	0.015	<0.001	0.001
Urea, mmol/L	970	4.98 (3.71–6.68)	608	5.60 (4.10–7.82)	182	7.13 (4.88–14.15)	<0.001	<0.001	<0.001
eGFR	1052	88.95 (70–99.50)	638	83.60 (63.28–95.45)	194	68.05 (41–88.15)	<0.001	<0.001	<0.001
Sodium, mmol/L	1073	141 (138–143)	650	140 (137–143)	196	139 (136–142)	0.007	<0.001	0.012
Potassium, mmol/L	1073	4.20 (3.90–4.53)	650	4.10 (3.80–4.44)	196	4.10 (3.77–4.50)	<0.001	0.013	0.882
ALT, U/L	1059	30.11 (19–49)	633	35 (22–55.66)	190	38.50 (21–57)	<0.001	0.002	0.780
AST, U/L	1050	33.12 (24–50)	629	39 (29–60.15)	188	41 (28–76.75)	<0.001	<0.001	0.531
AST to ALT ratio	1050	1.13 (0.86–1.58)	628	1.13 (0.88–1.58)	188	1.25 (0.85–1.73)	0.806	0.123	0.178
LDH, U/L	993	282 (220–359)	592	318 (263–420.81)	165	362 (253.50–534)	<0.001	<0.001	0.024
CRP, mg/L	1077	48.65 (17.1–94.9)	650	68.21 (31.34–129.73)	196	100.05 (42.53–181.85)	<0.001	<0.001	0.001
Ferritin, µg/L	1007	409.33 (204.63–802.70)	612	568.50 (296.25–1223.25)	170	659.98 (294.24–1402.31)	<0.001	<0.001	0.288
IL-6, ng/L	958	26.15 (13.57–48.5)	581	32.40 (15.80–61.24)	161	36.90 (14.5–77.1)	<0.001	0.003	0.454
D-dimer, µg/L	990	420 (260– 726.25)	614	522.50 (320–926.25)	179	780 (365–1745)	<0.001	<0.001	<0.001
Troponin I, ng/L	899	7.97 (4–15)	561	10 (6–22)	161	20.20 (8.25–116)	<0.001	<0.001	<0.001

ALT—alanine aminotransferase; AST—aspartate aminotransferase; CRP—C-reactive protein; IL-6—interleukin 6; IQR—interquartile range; LDH—lactate dehydrogenase; NLR—neutrophil-to-lymphocyte ratio; WBC—white blood cell count. 1—p value comparing patients with normoglycaemia vs. patients with mild hyperglycaemia. 2—p value comparing patients with normoglycaemia vs. patients with intermittent hyperglycaemia. 3—p value comparing patients with mild hyperglycaemia vs. patients with intermittent hyperglycaemia.

Reference values: haemoglobin: 128–160 g/L (for males), 117–145 g/L (for females); WBC: 4.0–9.8 $\times$ 10^9/L; neutrophils: 1.5–6.0 $\times$ 10^9/L; lymphocytes: 1.0–4.0 $\times$ 10^9/L; NLR—1–2; platelets: 140–450 $\times$ 10^9/L; glucose: 4.2–6.1 mmol/L; creatinine: 64–104 µmol/L (for males), 49–90 µmol/L (for females); urea: 2.5–7.5 mmol/L; sodium: 134–145 mmol/L; potassium: 3.8–5.3 mmol/L; ALT: $\leq$40 U/L; AST: $\leq$40 U/L; AST to ALT ratio: <1; LDH: 125–243 ULl; CRP: <5 mg/L; ferritin: 25–350 µg/L (for men), 13–232 µg/L (for women); IL-6: 0–7 ng/L; D-dimer: <250 µg/L; and troponin I: <19 ng/L.

Patients with mild hyperglycaemia had higher levels of WBCs, neutrophil counts, NLR, creatinine, urea, ALT, AST, LDH, CRP, ferritin, IL-6, D-dimer, and troponin I compared to patients with normoglycaemia, whereas lymphocyte counts and eGFR, potassium, and sodium concentrations were significantly lower (Table 3).

Among patients with intermittent hyperglycaemia on admission, the odds ratio (OR) for IMV was 4.82 (95% CI 2.70–8.61, $p < 0.001$), while the OR was 2.00 (95% CI 1.21–3.31, $p = 0.007$) in those with mild hyperglycaemia compared to patients presenting normal glucose levels at admission. Other risk factors associated with the need for IMV were male gender, obesity, and CHF (Figure 2).

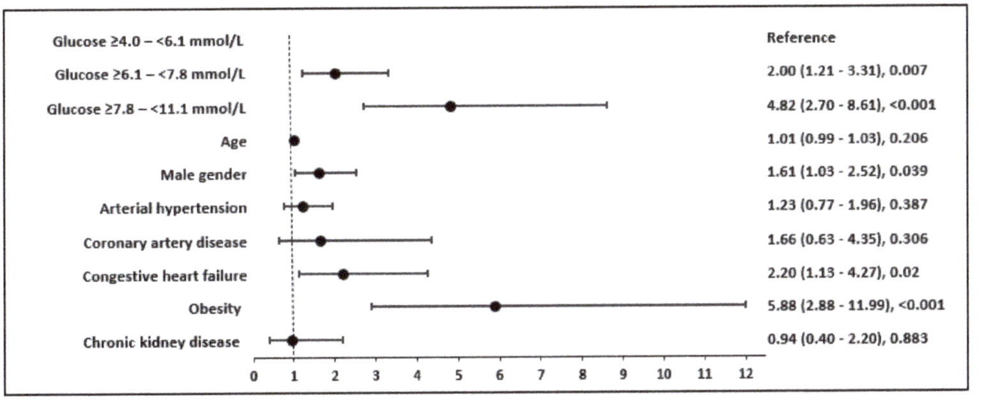

Figure 2. Risk factors and odds ratios (OR) associated with the need for invasive mechanical ventilation in COVID-19 patients without diabetes.

Cox regression analysis revealed that the hazard ratio (HR) for 30-day in-hospital mortality in patients with mild hyperglycaemia on admission was 1.62 (95% CI 1.10–2.39, $p = 0.015$), whilethe HR was 3.04 (95% CI 2.01–4.60, $p < 0.001$) in patients with intermittent hyperglycaemia compared to those with normoglycaemia (Figure 3).

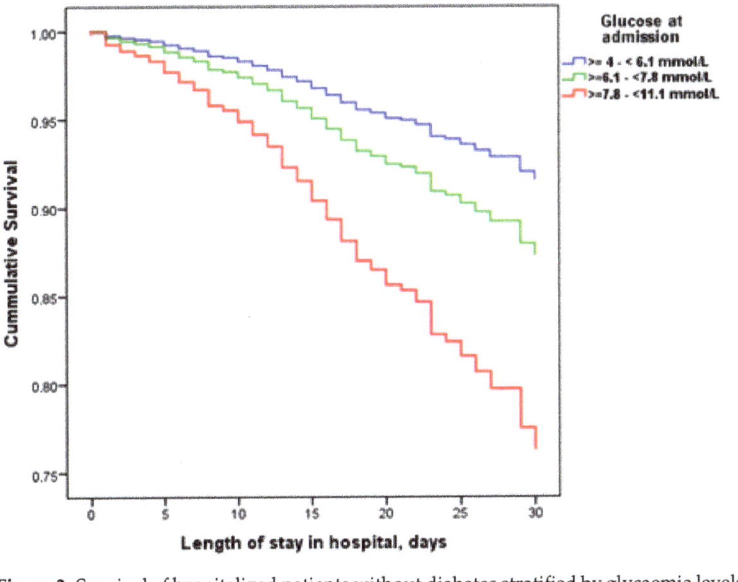

Figure 3. Survival of hospitalized patients without diabetes stratified by glycaemia levels atadmission.

Other risk factors associated with increased HR for 30 days in-hospital mortality were age, obesity, CHF, and previous stroke. Treatment with Remdesivir was associated with reduced HR (0.56 (95% CI 0.37–0.85, $p = 0.006$) for 30-day in-hospital mortality) (Table 4).

Table 4. Hazard ratios for 30-day in-hospital mortality.

Characteristic	In-Hospital Mortality	
	HR (95% CI)	p
Normoglycaemia	Reference	
Mild hyperglycaemia	1.62 (1.10–2.39)	0.015
Intermittent hyperglycaemia	3.04 (2.01–4.60)	<0.001
Age in years	1.06 (1.05–1.08)	<0.001
Male gender	1.07 (0.77–1.49)	0.689
Hypertension	0.94 (0.67–1.33)	0.729
Coronary artery disease	1.23 (0.69–2.18)	0.487
Congestive heart failure	1.97 (1.33–2.93)	0.001
Obesity	2.94 (1.56–5.57)	0.001
Previous stroke	3.86 (1.95–7.65)	<0.001
Chronic kidney disease	0.61 (0.36–1.04)	0.069
Antivirals (Remdesivir)	0.56 (0.37–0.85)	0.006
Systemic steroids	1.36 (0.94–1.99)	0.108

4. Discussion

Infection induces significant alterations in glucose metabolism. During infection, there is an upsurge in glucose production attributed to hepatic gluconeogenesis and glycogenolysis accompanied by reduced peripheral glucose uptake due to decreased blood flow in muscles (reversible insulin resistance) and increased anaerobic glycolysis due to hypoxia, resulting in elevated blood glucose levels, regardless of pre-existing diabetes status. Such a response is believed to be influenced by a combination of neurohumoral changes, activation of counterregulatory hormones (glucagon, epinephrine, cortisol, and growth hormone), excessive release of proinflammatory cytokines (IL-6, IL-1β, and tumour necrosis factor (TNF)-α), reactive oxygen species production, impaired immune cell function, and the release of lipid mediators [17–20].

Various viral infections, including cytomegalovirus, enteroviruses, Epstein-Barr virus, hepatitis B and C virus, human immunodeficiency virus, and influenza, use distinct mechanisms to promote hyperglycaemia and can directly affect glucose metabolism and insulin signaling pathways, leading to dysregulation of glucose homeostasis [21]. Recent findings have shed light on the interplay among viral factors, immune response, inflammation, pancreatic function, and the potential role of insulin resistance in driving the occurrence of hyperglycaemia during COVID-19 infection [21–25].

Our study demonstrated that 43.6% of patients without pre-existing diabetes hospitalized for COVID-19 infection had increased blood glucose levels atadmission. Data on the prevalence of hyperglycaemia in COVID-19 patients without diabetes varies and depends on the definition of hyperglycaemia and the population studied. Our study data are comparable to data from Montefusco et al., who reported that 46% of COVID-19 patients had hyperglycaemia, defined as blood glucose levels between 5.6 mmol/L and 11.1 mmol/L or two blood glucose measurements of >5.6 mmol/Land < 7.0 mmol/L [26]. Mamtani et al. reported that 20.6% of COVID-19 patients without pre-existing diabetes had blood glucose levels at admission $\geq$ 7.78 mmol/L [8]. Zhang et al. found that 20% of COVID-19 patients were in a state of impaired fasting glucose (defined as fasting blood glucose between $\geq$5.6 mmol/L and <7.0 mmol/L) [15].

The prognostic importance of hyperglycaemia on the outcomes of COVID-19 infection has been emphasized in multiple studies. Hyperglycaemia atadmission in patients without diabetes is associated with a higher incidence of a severe course of COVID-19 infection, need for IMV, admission to the ICU [10–12,24–30], and higher mortality [13,14,27,29,31,32].

Our study showed that a higher proportion of patients with intermittent hyperglycaemia at admission (14.8%) required IMV compared to patients with mild hyperglycaemia (5.8%) and patients with normoglycaemia (2.7%). The risk of IMV in patients with intermittent hyperglycaemia was 4.82-fold higher than in those with normoglycaemia. Iacobellis et al. noted that average blood glucose level at admission was the strongest independent predictor of bilateral pulmonary opacities suggestive of acute respiratory distress in the radiographic imaging of COVID-19 patients [27]. Fadine et al. reported that for every 2 mmol/L increase in glucose level at admission, the probability of severe COVID-19 increased by approximately15% independently from any other clinical-biochemical variables [28]. We determined that the HR for 30-day in-hospital mortality in patients with mild hyperglycaemia was 1.62, while the HR was 3.04in patients with intermittent hyperglycaemia compared to those with normoglycaemia. A meta-analysis including sixteen observational studies with 6386 COVID-19 patients demonstrated that the group of patients with hyperglycaemia at admission had an increased risk of mortality compared to the control group with euglycaemia (OR = 3.45, 95% CI 2.26–5.26) [30]. Morse et al. retrospectively showed that among patients without a pre-existing diabetes diagnosis, any hyperglycaemic value was associated with a substantial increase in the odds of mortality (OR = 3.07, 95% CI 2.79–3.37) compared to patients without hyperglycaemia [33].

The association between hyperglycaemia and increased mortality in COVID-19 patients is likely multifactorial, involving inflammation, immune dysfunction, vascular damage, and underlying comorbidities. Hyperglycaemia is known to contribute to a state of systemic inflammation, which can worsen the severity of infection and outcome in COVID-19 patients [34]. High blood glucose levels have been shown to impair the function of various immune cells, such as T cells and macrophages, thereby compromising the immune response against the virus [35]. Hyperglycaemia can contribute to endothelial dysfunction and arteriopathy, leading to complications such as thrombosis and impaired oxygen delivery, which can further exacerbate the severity of COVID-19 and increase the mortality risk [36]. Furthermore, individuals with newly developed hyperglycaemia during COVID-19 infection may be older and have underlying comorbidities, which can increase vulnerability and in-hospital mortality [34,37–39]. In our study, patients with mild or intermittent hyperglycaemia were older and had more comorbid conditions compared to patients with normoglycaemia. Furthermore, we observed elevated troponin I levels at admission in patients with intermittent hyperglycaemia.

The cytokine storm is a characteristic feature of COVID-19 infection and is strongly associated with disease severity and mortality [40]. The laboratory features of cytokine storms include haematological anomalies, such as leucocytosis or leukopenia, thrombocytopenia, and disseminated intravascular coagulation; high fibrinogen levels; elevated IL-6; and general markers of end-organ dysfunction [41]. We observed a significantly lower lymphocyte count, higher NLR, and higher IL-6 and CRP levels in patients with mild and intermittent hyperglycaemia, presuming that the inflammatory response is more pronounced in patients with increased glucose levels at admission. Our results are comparable to the findings of Coppelli et al., as we also observed a higher neutrophil count, lower lymphocyte count, and higher CRP in patients without known diabetes with hyperglycaemia (glucose level $\geq$ 7.78 mmol/L) at admission compared to patients with normoglycaemia [29].

Beyond the immediate impact on glucose metabolism, investigating the long-term consequences of COVID-19 infection and potential implications for metabolic health emerges as a crucial direction of exploration. Montefusco et al. highlighted the profound impact of COVID-19 on disrupting insulin signalling and beta cell function. They reported significant alterations in hormone profiles, both at basal levels and after stimulation testing, demonstrating elevated insulin, proinsulin, and C-peptide levels in patients who had recovered from COVID-19 compared to healthy controls [26]. In a recent meta-analysis that scrutinized the occurrence of new-onset diabetes and hyperglycaemia after COVID-19 infection in patients without pre-existing diabetes, the proportions of patients with new-onset diabetes was 3% and new-onset hyperglycaemia was 30%. Additionally, the meta-analysis found that new-onset diabetes and hyperglycaemia were 1.75 times higher in COVID-19 patients compared to non-COVID-19 patients [42]. Recommendations have been made for COVID-19 hyperglycaemic patients, emphasizing the need for follow-up at the first month and at intervals of 3–6 months during the first year post-discharge to discern whether hyperglycaemia is permanent or transient [43].

This study has several limitations. Comorbidities were identified based on ICD-10-AM coding, which may have resulted in some incomplete attributions. Additionally, information about fasting status on admission and glycated haemoglobin (HbA1c) was not available for all patients, potentially biasing the detection of pre-existing hyperglycaemia. Furthermore, the absence of data on body mass index limited our ability to accurately determine obesity in patients. Lastly, we were unable to control for the pre-admission use of glucocorticoids and other medications, which could have influenced our findings. An additional challenge relates to missing information on the duration of COVID-19 symptoms before hospital admission. While our research was conducted at the largest hospital in the capital of Lithuania, limiting the study to a single centre introduces the potential for selection bias and reduces the generalizability of our findings. The healthcare practices, patient demographics, and treatment protocols at this specific centre may not fully represent the broader population. An additional limitation of our retrospective study is the lack of information on the long-term consequences of hyperglycaemia in COVID-19 patients. As a retrospective analysis primarily focused on immediate outcomes during hospitalization, we did not have the opportunity to explore the extended effects of hyperglycaemia beyond the acute phase of the disease. Nonetheless, our study has several strengths, including the comprehensive clinical characterization of all patients who were hospitalized for COVID-19 infection over a period of more than one year in the largest university hospital in the country, as well as the evaluation of multiple laboratory parameters.

5. Conclusions

In COVID-19 patients without pre-existing diabetes, the presence of hyperglycaemia at admission is indicative of COVID-19-induced alterations in glucose metabolism and stress hyperglycaemia. Hyperglycaemia at admission in COVID-19 patients without diabetes is associated with an increased risk of invasive mechanical ventilation and in-hospital mortality. This finding highlights the importance for clinicians to carefully consider and select optimal support and treatment strategies for these patients. Further studies on the long-term consequences of hyperglycaemia in this specific population are warranted.

Author Contributions: L.Z., Conceptualization, Methodology, Writing—Original draft preparation, Supervision; I.K., Writing—Original draft preparation, Reviewing and Editing; M.U., Writing—Original draft preparation, Reviewing and Editing, Visualization; L.J., Data curation, Supervision; J.U., Data curation, Formal analysis, Writing—Reviewing and Editing, Visualization; I.I., Writing—Reviewing and Editing. All authors participated in manuscript writing and read and approved the final manuscript. All authors have read and agreed to the published version of the manuscript.

Funding: APC funded by the University of Vilnius.

Institutional Review Board Statement: Ethical review and approval were waived for this study due to the use of anonymized clinical data.

Informed Consent Statement: Waived for this study due to the use of anonymized clinical data.

Data Availability Statement: From Corresponding Author.

Conflicts of Interest: The authors declare no conflict of interest.

References

1. Roy, S.; Demmer, R.T. Impaired glucose regulation, SARS-CoV-2 infections and adverse COVID-19 outcomes. *Transl. Res.* **2022**, *241*, 52–69. [CrossRef] [PubMed]
2. Apicella, M.; Campopiano, M.C.; Mantuano, M.; Mazoni, L.; Coppelli, A.; Del Prato, S. COVID-19 in people with diabetes:Understanding the reasons for worse outcomes. *Lancet Diabetes Endocrinol.* **2020**, *8*, 782–792. [CrossRef] [PubMed]

3. Sharma, P.; Behl, T.; Sharma, N.; Singh, S.; Grewal, A.S.; Albarrati, A.; Albratty, M.; Meraya, A.M.; Bungau, S. COVID-19 and diabetes: Association intensify risk factors fo rmorbidity and mortality. *Biomed. Pharmacother.* **2022**, *151*, 113089. [CrossRef] [PubMed]
4. Vedantam, D.; Poman, D.S.; Motwani, L.; Asif, N.; Patel, A.; Anne, K.K. Stress-InducedHyperglycemia: Consequences and Management. *Cureus* **2022**, *14*, e26714. [PubMed]
5. Plummer, M.P.; Bellomo, R.; Cousins, C.E.; Annink, C.E.; Sundararajan, K.; Reddi, B.A.; Raj, J.P.; Chapman, M.J.; Horowitz, M.; Deane, A.M. Dysglycaemia in the critically ill and the interaction of chronic and acute glycaemia with mortality. *Intensive Care Med.* **2014**, *40*, 973–980. [CrossRef] [PubMed]
6. Khalfallah, M.; Abdelmageed, R.; Elgendy, E.; Hafez, Y.M. Incidence, predictors and outcomes of stress hyperglycemia in patients with ST elevation myocardial infarction undergoing primary percutaneous coronary intervention. *Diabetes Vasc. Dis. Res.* **2020**, *17*, 1479164119883983. [CrossRef]
7. Li, J.; Quan, K.; Wang, Y.; Zhao, X.; Li, Z.; Pan, Y.; Li, H.; Liu, L.; Wang, Y. Effect of Stress Hyperglycemiaon Neurological Deficit and Mortality in the Acute Ischemic Stroke People with and Without Diabetes. *Front. Neurol.* **2020**, *11*, 576895. [CrossRef]
8. Mamtani, M.; Kulkarni, H.; Bihari, S.; Prakash, S.; Chavan, S.; Huckson, S.; Pilcher, D. Degree of hyperglycemia independently associates with hospital mortality and length of stay in critically ill, nondiabetic patients: Results from the ANZICSCORE binational registry. *J. Crit. Care* **2020**, *55*, 149–156. [CrossRef]
9. Müller, J.A.; Groß, R.; Conzelmann, C.; Krüger, J.; Merle, U.; Steinhart, J.; Weil, T.; Koepke, L.; Bozzo, C.P.; Read, C.; et al. SARS-CoV-2 infects and replicates in cells of the human endocrine and exocrine pancreas. *Nat. Metab.* **2021**, *3*, 149–165. [CrossRef]
10. Matias, A.A.; Manique, I.; Sabino, T.; Rego, T.; Mihon, C.; Panarra, A.; Rizzo, M.; Silva-Nunes, J. Absolute Hyperglycemia versus Stress Hyperglycemia Ratio for the Prognosis of Hospitalized Patients with COVID-19 in the First Months of the Pandemic: A Retrospective Study. *Diabetes Ther.* **2022**, *14*, 335–346. [CrossRef]
11. Manique, I.; Abegão Matias, A.; Bouça, B.; Rego, T.; Cortez, L.; Sabino, T.; Panarra, A.; Rizzo, M.; Silva-Nunes, J. Does the Hyperglycemia Impact on COVID-19 Outcomes Depend upon the Presence of Diabetes? An Observational Study. *Metabolites* **2022**, *12*, 1116. [CrossRef]
12. Liu, S.P.; Zhang, Q.; Wang, W.; Zhang, M.; Liu, C.; Xiao, X.; Liu, Z.; Hu, W.-M.; Jin, P. Hyperglycemia is astrong predictor of poor prognosis in COVID-19. *Diabetes Res. Clin. Pract.* **2020**, *167*, 108338. [CrossRef]
13. Wang, S.; Ma, P.; Zhang, S.; Song, S.; Wang, Z.; Ma, Y.; Xu, J.; Wu, F.; Duan, L.; Yin, Z.; et al. Fasting blood glucose on admission is an independent predictor for 28-daymortality in patients with COVID-19 without previous diagnosis of diabetes: A multi-centre retrospective study. *Diabetologia* **2020**, *63*, 2102–2111. [CrossRef]
14. Mamtani, M.; Athavale, A.M.; Abraham, M.; Vernik, J.; Amarah, A.R.; Ruiz, J.P.; Joshi, A.J.; Itteera, M.; Zhukovski, S.D.; Madaiah, R.P.; et al. Association of hyperglycaemia with hospital mortality in nondiabetic COVID-19 patients: A cohort study. *Diabetes Metab.* **2021**, *47*, 101254. [CrossRef]
15. Zhang, J.; Kong, W.; Xia, P.; Xu, Y.; Li, L.; Li, Q.; Yang, L.; Wei, Q.; Wang, H.; Li, H.; et al. Impaired Fasting Glucose and Diabetes Are Related to Higher Risks of Complications and MortalityAmong Patients with Coronavirus Disease 2019. *Front. Endocrinol.* **2020**, *11*, 525. [CrossRef]
16. Kubiliute, I.; Vitkauskaite, M.; Urboniene, J.; Svetikas, L.; Zablockiene, B.; Jancoriene, L. Clinical characteristics and predictors for in-hospital mortality in adult COVID-19 patients: A retrospective single center cohort study in Vilnius, Lithuania. *PLoS ONE* **2023**, *18*, e0290656. [CrossRef]
17. McGuinness, O.P. Defective glucose homeostasis during infection. *Annu. Rev. Nutr.* **2005**, *25*, 9–35. [CrossRef]
18. Boonen, E.; Vanden Berghe, G. Endocrine responses to critical illness:Novel insights and therapeutic implications. *J. Clin. Endocrinol. Metab.* **2014**, *99*, 1569–1582. [CrossRef]
19. Gunst, J.; De Bruyn, A.; Vanden Berghe, G. Glucose control in the ICU. *Curr. Opin. Anaesthesiol.* **2019**, *32*, 156–162. [CrossRef]
20. Sasidharakurup, H.; Kumar, G.; Nair, B.; Diwakar, S. Mathematical Modeling of Severe Acute Respiratory Syndrome Coronavirus 2 Infection Network with Cytokine Storm, Oxidative Stress, Thrombosis, Insulin Resistance, and Nitric Oxide Pathways. *OMICS* **2021**, *25*, 770–781. [CrossRef] [PubMed]
21. Rajsfus, B.F.; Mohana-Borges, R.; Allonso, D. Diabetogenic viruses: Linking viruses to diabetes mellitus. *Heliyon* **2023**, *9*, e15021. [CrossRef]
22. Tsilingiris, D.; Dalamaga, M.; Liu, J. SARS-CoV-2 adipose tissue infection and hyperglycemia: A further step towards the understanding of severe COVID-19. *Metab. Open* **2022**, *13*, 100163. [CrossRef]
23. He, X.; Liu, C.; Peng, J.; Li, Z.; Li, F.; Wang, J.; Hu, A.; Peng, M.; Huang, K.; Fan, D.; et al. COVID-19 induces new-onset insulin resistance and lipid metabolic dysregulation via regulation of secreted metabolic factors. *Signal Transduct. Target. Ther.* **2021**, *6*, 427. [CrossRef]
24. Ilias, I.; Jahaj, E.; Kokkoris, S.; Zervakis, D.; Temperikidis, P.; Magira, E.; Pratikaki, M.; Vassiliou, A.G.; Routsi, C.; Kotanidou, A.; et al. Clinical Study of Hyperglycemia and SARS-CoV-2 Infection in Intensive Care Unit Patients. *In Vivo* **2020**, *34*, 3029–3032. [CrossRef]
25. Ilias, I.; Diamantopoulos, A.; Pratikaki, M.; Botoula, E.; Jahaj, E.; Athanasiou, N.; Pratikaki, M.; Vassiliou, A.G.; Routsi, C.; Kotanidou, A.; et al. Glycemia, Beta-Cell Function and Sensitivity to Insulin in Mildly to Critically Ill COVID-19 Patients. *Medicina* **2021**, *57*, 68. [CrossRef]

26. Montefusco, L.; Ben Nasr, M.; D'Addio, F.; Loretelli, C.; Rossi, A.; Pastore, I.; Daniele, G.; Abdelsalam, A.; Maestroni, A.; Dell'Acqua, M.; et al. Acute and long-term disruption of glycometabolic control after SARS-CoV-2 infection. *Nat. Metab.* **2021**, *3*, 774–785. [CrossRef]
27. Iacobellis, G.; Penaherrera, C.A.; Bermudez, L.E.; Bernal Mizrachi, E. Admission hyperglycemia and radiological findings of SARS-CoV2 in patients with and without diabetes. *Diabetes Res. Clin. Pract.* **2020**, *164*, 108185. [CrossRef]
28. Fadini, G.P.; Morieri, M.L.; Boscari, F.; Fioretto, P.; Maran, A.; Busetto, L.; Bonora, B.M.; Selmin, E.; Arcidiacono, G.; Pinelli, S.; et al. Newly-diagnosed diabetes and admission hyperglycemia predict COVID-19 severity by aggravating respiratory deterioration. *Diabetes Res. Clin. Pract.* **2020**, *168*, 108374. [CrossRef] [PubMed]
29. Coppelli, A.; Giannarelli, R.; Aragona, M.; Penno, G.; Falcone, M.; Tiseo, G.; Ghiadoni, L.; Barbieri, G.; Monzani, F.; Virdis, A.; et al. Hyperglycemia at Hospital Admission Is Associated with Severity of the Prognosis in Patients Hospitalized for COVID-19: The Pisa COVID-19 Study. *Diabetes Care* **2020**, *43*, 2345–2348. [CrossRef] [PubMed]
30. Yang, Y.; Cai, Z.; Zhang, J. Hyperglycemia at admission is astrong predictor of mortality and severe/critical complications in COVID-19 patients: Ameta-analysis. *Biosci. Rep.* **2021**, *41*, BSR20203584. [CrossRef] [PubMed]
31. Nateghi, S.; Gomari, M.M.; Roudsari, Y.J.; Foroughi, A.; Mansouri, F.; Shiva, A.; Nasrollahizadeh, A.; Nasiri, Z.; Faraji, N. Moderately hyperglycemia as an independent prognostic factor for the worse outcome of COVID-19. *Prim. Care Diabetes* **2022**, *16*, 361–364. [CrossRef] [PubMed]
32. Li, H.; Tian, S.; Chen, T.; Cui, Z.; Shi, N.; Zhong, X.; Qiu, K.; Zhang, J.; Zeng, T.; Chen, L.; et al. Newly diagnosed diabetes is associated with a higher risk of mortality than known diabetes in hospitalized patients with COVID-19. *Diabetes Obes. Metab.* **2020**, *22*, 1897–1906. [CrossRef]
33. Morse, J.; Gay, W.; Korwek, K.M.; McLean, L.E.; Poland, R.E.; Guy, J.; Sands, K.; Perlin, J.B. Hyperglycaemia increases mortality risk in non-diabetic patients with COVID-19 even more than in diabeticpatients. *Endocrinol. Diabetes Metab.* **2021**, *4*, e00291. [CrossRef]
34. Demeulemeester, F.; de Punder, K.; van Heijningen, M.; van Doesburg, F. Obesity as a Risk Factor for Severe COVID-19 and Complications: A Review. *Cells* **2021**, *10*, 933. [CrossRef]
35. Merad, M.; Blish, C.A.; Sallusto, F.; Iwasaki, A. The immunology and immunopathology of COVID-19. *Science* **2022**, *375*, 1122–1127. [CrossRef]
36. Akácsos-Szász, O.Z.; Pál, S.; Nyulas, K.I.; Nemes-Nagy, E.; Fárr, A.M.; Dénes, L.; Szilveszter, M.; Bán, E.G.; Tilinca, M.C.; Simon-Szabó, Z. Pathways of Coagulopathy and Inflammatory Response in SARS-CoV-2 Infection among Type2 Diabetic Patients. *Int. J. Mol. Sci.* **2023**, *24*, 4319. [CrossRef]
37. Docherty, A.B.; Harrison, E.M.; Green, C.A.; Hardwick, H.E.; Pius, R.; Norman, L.; Holden, K.A.; Read, J.M.; Dondelinger, F.; Carson, G.; et al. Featuresof 20133 UK patients in hospital with COVID-19 using the ISARICWHO Clinical Characterisation Protocol: Prospective observational cohort study. *BMJ* **2020**, *369*, m1985. [CrossRef]
38. Müller-Wieland, D.; Marx, N.; Dreher, M.; Fritzen, K.; Schnell, O. COVID-19 and Cardiovascular Comorbidities. *Exp. Clin. Endocrinol. Diabetes* **2022**, *130*, 178–189. [CrossRef] [PubMed]
39. Bader, F.; Manla, Y.; Atallah, B.; Starling, R.C. Heart failure and COVID-19. *Heart Fail. Rev.* **2021**, *26*, 1–10. [CrossRef] [PubMed]
40. Da Porto, A.; Tascini, C.; Colussi, G.; Peghin, M.; Graziano, E.; De Carlo, C.; Bulfone, L.; Antonello, M.; Sozio, E.; Fabris, M.; et al. Relationship between cytokine release and stress hyperglycemia in patients hospitalized with COVID-19infection. *Front. Med.* **2022**, *9*, 988686. [CrossRef]
41. Copaescu, A.; Smibert, O.; Gibson, A.; Phillips, E.J.; Trubiano, J.A. The role of IL-6 and other mediators in the cytokine storm associated with SARS-CoV-2 infection. *J. Allergy Clin. Immunol.* **2020**, *146*, 518–534.e1. [CrossRef] [PubMed]
42. Li, J.; Li, Y.; Wang, Z.; Liu, N.; He, L.; Zhang, H. Increased risk of new-onset diabetes in patients with COVID-19: A systematic review and meta-analysis. *Front. Public Health* **2023**, *11*, 1170156. [CrossRef] [PubMed]
43. Gerganova, A.; Assyov, Y.; Kamenov, Z. Stress Hyperglycemia, Diabetes Mellitus and COVID-19 Infection: RiskFactors, Clinical Outcomes and Post-Discharge Implications. *Front. Clin. Diabetes Healthc.* **2022**, *3*, 826006. [CrossRef]

biomedicines

MDPI

Review

The Role of Insulin Within the Socio-Psycho-Biological Framework in Type 2 Diabetes—A Perspective from Psychoneuroimmunology

Anne Wevers [1], Silvia San Roman-Mata [2], Santiago Navarro-Ledesma [3,4,*] and Leo Pruimboom [4]

1 Clinical Medicine and Public Health PhD Program, Faculty of Health Sciences, University of Granada, 18071 Granada, Spain; info@anne-wevers.com
2 Department of Nursing, Faculty of Health Sciences, Campus of Melilla, University of Granada, 52004 Melilla, Spain; silviasanroman@ugr.es
3 Department of Physical Therapy, Faculty of Health Sciences, Campus of Melilla, University of Granada, 52004 Melilla, Spain
4 University Chair in Clinical Psychoneuroimmunology, Campus of Melilla, University of Granada and PNI Europe, 52004 Melilla, Spain; leo@cpnieurope.com
* Correspondence: snl@ugr.es

Abstract: The interplay between socio-psychological factors and biological systems is pivotal in defining human health and disease, particularly in chronic non-communicable diseases. Recent advancements in psychoneuroimmunology and mitochondrial psychobiology have emphasized the significance of psychological factors as critical determinants of disease onset, progression, recurrence, and severity. These insights align with evolutionary biology, psychology, and psychiatry, highlighting the inherent social nature of humans. This study proposes a theory that expands insulin's role beyond traditional metabolic functions, incorporating it into the Mitochondrial Information Processing System (MIPS) and exploring it from an evolutionary medicine perspective to explore its function in processing psychological and social factors into biological responses. This narrative review comprises data from preclinical animal studies, longitudinal cohort studies, cross-sectional studies, machine learning analyses, and randomized controlled trials, and investigates the role of insulin in health and disease. The result is a proposal for a theoretical framework of insulin as a social substance within the socio-psycho-biological framework, emphasizing its extensive roles in health and disease. Type 2 Diabetes Mellitus (T2DM) with musculoskeletal disorders and neurodegeneration exemplifies this narrative. We suggest further research towards a comprehensive treatment protocol meeting evolutionary expectations, where incorporating psychosocial interventions plays an essential role. By supporting the concept of 'insulin resilience' and suggesting the use of heart rate variability to assess insulin resilience, we aim to provide an integrative approach to managing insulin levels and monitoring the effectiveness of interventions. This integrative strategy addresses broader socio-psychological factors, ultimately improving health outcomes for individuals with T2DM and musculoskeletal complications and neurodegeneration while providing new insights into the interplay between socio-psychological factors and biological systems in chronic diseases.

Keywords: psychoneuroimmunology; psychosocial factors; insulin; mitochondrial information processing system; type 2 diabetes mellitus with musculoskeletal disorders and neurodegeneration; insulin resistance; mitochondrial dynamics; insulin resilience; evolutionary medicine; integrative health interventions

1. Introduction

Insulin (INS), traditionally viewed merely as a metabolic regulator implicated in various diseases [1], might hold a more expansive role as a 'socio-psychological substance' within the body's biological systems. This narrative review explores incorporating INS into the Mitochondrial Information Processing System (MIPS), a model that redefines mitochondria not just as cellular powerhouses but as central processors of socio-psychological factors [2]. Such a conceptualization positions mitochondria as 'social organelles' essential in processing social and psychological factors through mechanisms of sensing, integration, and transduction—a cornerstone of mitochondrial psychobiology. We hypothesize that INS plays a pivotal role in this process—beyond its established metabolic actions—by cooperating with mitochondria in modulating biological responses to psychological and social factors. We adopt the MIPS [2] model as a theoretical framework for the exploration of INS's function as a socio-psycho-metabolic hormone with systemic influence.

To further support this hypothesis, we examine INS through an evolutionary lens, considering how its roles may have been shaped by ancient social, psychological and environmental stressors and survival mechanisms. This evolutionary perspective deepens our understanding of INS as a socio-psychological substance and informs the development of interventions that align with human biology's evolutionary adaptations.

This paradigm shift aims to contextualize INS within a broader socio-psycho-biological framework, enriching our understanding of its multifaceted functions. This narrative review, along with the presented theoretical framework and evolutionary perspective, aims to offer new directions for hypothesis building and establishes a foundation for more systematic experimental approaches. Ultimately, it seeks to contribute to the development of potential new strategies for managing health conditions where INS is a key factor, such as Type 2 Diabetes (T2DM) with associated musculoskeletal (MSK) and neurodegenerative complications.

2. Sensing, Integrating and Transducing—A Theoretical Role for Insulin

The MIPS model, as proposed by Picard and Shirihai [2], positions mitochondria as social organelles adept at a three-step process—sensing, integrating, and transducing psychological and social factors into cellular and molecular modifications, next to their classical role at the level of cell- and systemic metabolism. They highlight the dual role of mitochondria as both targets of stress and sources of signaling, essential for biologically embedding both stressful and other psycho-social experiences into our biology [3]. Accumulating evidence in both human and animal studies further underscores the pivotal role of mitochondria in the response to both acute and chronic stress and in the biological embedding of adversity [4]. Their functions are indicated as important mechanisms in understanding how stressful life events 'get under the skin' and impact health and physical well-being, recently also shown in studies examining human peripheral tissue [5].

Evolution generated multiple methods of communication between mitochondria and the rest of the cell [6]. The inherent plasticity and dynamic nature of mitochondria are important mitochondrial characteristics and facilitate their roles as processors and communication hubs, allowing them to adapt through functional and morphological changes such as alterations in size, shape, and distribution. These adaptations respond to both internal and external stimuli and are crucial for meeting various demands [7,8]. The adaptive capacity of mitochondria, known as mitochondrial dynamics, specifically involves processes such as fission, fusion, biogenesis, and mitophagy [9]. Mitochondria are pivotal in producing complex signals across biological domains, suggesting their importance as fundamental elements in both cellular and systemic communication networks [10].

Completing the understanding of the MIPS model seems to require the identification of key mediators within this system. Evolutionary pressure has led to the development of multiple communication pathways not only between mitochondria and other organelles [6] within the host cell but also across different cells [11]. Despite recent scientific advances, the construction of a coherent molecular map that fully integrates and delineates mitochondrial functions during psychological stress remains incomplete [12]. Specifically, the molecular mechanisms that control mitochondrial plasticity, dynamics, and their capacity to integrate and respond to a spectrum of cellular, environmental, and developmental stimuli are still to be fully understood [13]. Identifying the biological substrates and pathways that bridge psychological experiences with physiological processes seems important, as these links might be essential for elucidating the mechanisms behind observed biological changes [4]. Given these complexities, a detailed theoretical exploration of potential mediators like INS, and its relevant pathways, as well as elucidating its extensive roles within the MIPS model, seems valuable and relevant.

Insulin resistance (IR) is a central mechanism underlying most chronic diseases [14]. Mitochondrial dysfunction is frequently implicated as a precursor to IR; however, IR itself can also contribute to mitochondrial dysfunction [15]. When viewed through a psychosocial stress model, IR becomes a stronger predictor of the hypothalamus–pituitary–adrenal (HPA) axis response than obesity [16]. This suggests a complex interaction between psychosocial and physiological factors, with INS playing a critical role alongside mitochondria. The proposal to explore INS as a social-psychological substance within MIPS is further based on findings that psychosocial stress acts as an upstream event for IR, with mitochondria as downstream targets. This bidirectional relationship indicates that stress can influence INS sensitivity, which in turn impacts mitochondrial function [17].

The neurons in the arcuate nucleus of the hypothalamus (ARC) are activated by emotional stimuli and express INS receptors [18]. This might further illustrate INS's role in processing socio-psychological factors. The neurons in the ARC function as master regulators that integrate physiological signals with the energy state of the organism [19]. The melanocortin neurons within this nucleus receive peripheral metabolic information and mediate appropriate behavioral and metabolic responses to maintain energy homeostasis. By signaling energy availability, INS in the ARC coordinates metabolic functions and stress adaptation, reflecting its dual role in both biological and psychosocial processes. INS has also been used as a socio-psycho substance in a historical context, where INS shock therapy was used in psychiatric treatment, highlighting the hormone's significant impact on the central nervous system. While this practice is no longer in use, it underscores INS's profound effects on behavior and stress adaptation. This historical use of INS in psychiatric treatment, along with its role in the ARC regulating energy and stress responses, further encourages the exploration of INS as a socio-psychological substance within the MIPS model.

Integrating INS and IR into the MIPS model requires an in-depth understanding of the strong relationship between mitochondrial function and INS and INS receptor sensitivity, as well as an exploration of experimental findings [20]. In this review, we propose a theoretical framework and assess whether it aligns with existing empirical evidence by examining relevant experimental findings. While these findings may support, refine, or challenge the proposed mechanisms, it is important to note that our hypothesis remains speculative, and future research will be required to empirically validate the theory we are constructing.

A recent in vitro study on mouse and human-derived neurons [21], and another study conducting a series of ex vivo and in vivo experiments in obese IR human subjects either with or without T2DM, indicate that INS's actions directly impact mitochondrial health and efficiency [15,22]. INS plays a role in both the detection of cues and the subsequent adaptations within mitochondria [23]. Mitochondria possess their own genome, and the mitochondrial DNA copy number (mtDNA-CN) serves as a measure of the number of mitochondrial genomes per cell, thus providing possible insights into mitochondrial health [24]. A possible mechanism of INS influence is its ability to affect the regulation of mitochondrial DNA. A study in humans showed associations with INS sensitivity and mtDNA-CN [25]. Mutations and deletions in mtDNA or mitochondrion-related nuclear DNA genes have been indicated in mitochondrial dysfunction [26]. A recent study applying mitochondrial transplantation, in vitro and ex vivo, shows that DNA methyltransferase 1 (DNMT1) translocates to the mitochondrial D-loop region in vascular smooth muscle cells. This hypermethylation represses mitochondrial gene expression, leading to functional damage and reduced mitochondrial respiration [27]. Research in obese human subjects identifies a strong correlation between IR and alterations in methylation feedback loops, indicating that IR possibly leads to mitochondrial alterations through epigenetic mechanisms [28]. IR is strongly associated with a reduction in mtDNA numbers [28].

Often mentioned as a culprit in disease or merely positioned as a metabolic hormone, the above sets the stage to zoom out the microscope and theoretically examine INS's role as a psychosocial modulator.

Moving forward, the article will explore in greater detail the specific molecular pathways influenced by INS and how these pathways might impact mitochondrial dynamics, subsequently deepening our understanding of how INS might modulate mitochondrial sensing, integration, and transduction of psychosocial factors.

2.1. Sensing: The Role of Insulin

To strengthen our proposal of expanding INS's role beyond metabolism to a broader function as a socio-psycho-metabolic hormone, we will also apply the lens of evolutionary medicine. This approach highlights that, while INS is central to metabolic regulation, it may also play a role in managing stress and social behaviors—both evolutionary pressures that shaped human adaptation. Together, the MIPS model and evolutionary perspective provide a foundation for a theoretical proposal of interventions that consider our evolutionary origins and the psychosocial dimensions involved in conditions where INS is implicated.

The adage 'nothing in biology makes sense except in the light of evolution' aptly describes how human physiological responses still mirror those of our ancestors.

Ancient psychosocial stressors are defined as 'chronic demands that have persisted throughout human evolutionary history', while modern stressors are described as 'novel challenges that emerged with the advent of agriculture during the Neolithic period, approximately 10,000 to 12,000 years ago' [29]. The evolutionary mismatch hypothesis postulates that our behavioral and inflammatory responses, which evolved to help individuals manage ancient stressors (e.g., serious arguments within families or a child confronting frightening situations), are less suited to modern stressors (e.g., commuting to work, hospitalization, family members frequently away, or unemployment) [29].

Psychosocial stressors, whether novel or ancient (e.g., threats from lions), activate deeply ingrained, robust and well-coordinated stress, behavioral and immune responses shaped by natural selection, which likely provided early humans with an evolutionary advantage in dealing with pathogens, predators, and immediate survival threats [30–32].

This evolutionary legacy has resulted in an inflammatory bias, which is triggered not only by pathogens but also by psychosocial stressors [32]. These modern psychosocial stressors are recognized as 'danger signals', as they pose possible perturbations to homeostasis [18,33].

These non-specific biological responses of the robust IS are mediated by evolutionary conserved neuroendocrine networks of the hypothalamus–pituitary–adrenal (HPA) axis and the sympathetic nervous system (SAM) [34]. Without energy, stress adaptation is not possible [35], highlighting the critical role of these signals and stress axis in increasing the energy demand [30].

Activation of the HPA axis leads to glucocorticoid production such as cortisol (CORT), which in turn increases blood glucose levels through gluconeogenesis, enhancing the availability of energy needed to manage stressors [36]. As blood glucose levels rise, the pancreas detects this increase, and in physiological situations, it triggers the production and release of INS to help regulate and lower the blood glucose levels [37].

The sympathetic–adrenal–medullary (SAM) axis stimulates the release of catecholamines such as dopamine (DOP), norepinephrine (NE), and epinephrine (EPI) [38]. In vitro research has revealed that both human and mouse pancreatic β-cells contain the necessary machinery for catecholamine biosynthesis and signaling. These catecholamines, especially DOP, play a significant role in regulating pancreatic glucagon and INS secretion, showcasing a complex interplay between stress and metabolic regulation [39]. The β-cell stress hypothesis suggests that various factors such as psychological stress can indeed increase INS demand [40].

Physiologic INS secretion follows an oscillating pattern of secretion, marked by distinct periods of ligand and receptor activation [41]. Chronic exposure to INS, but also glucocorticoids (GC) [42], leptin and cytokines [43], triggers a negative feedback loop that over time down-regulates the receptor availability. This creates a state of, in the case of INS, relative hyperinsulinemia. This excess of INS leads to IR due to decreased receptor availability, with catecholamines also hypothesized to be involved in the induction of IR at the receptor level [40,41].

In light of INS's socio-psychological role, it is important to acknowledge the significant impact of psychological stress, inflammatory reactions and cytokines and chemokines on IR development as well.

In the same way that the stress response activates the cardiovascular, musculoskeletal, and neuroendocrine systems for fight-or-flight, it may also, under certain conditions, prime the immune system to face potential threats posed by the stressor [44].

This involves various mechanisms and mediators, such as the movement and function of dendritic cells, neutrophils, macrophages, and lymphocytes, along with significant local and systemic production of chemokines and cytokines [45].

Various stressors can trigger neuroinflammation responses. An example of immune activation in a psychosocial context is the activation of innate immune receptors known as pattern recognition receptors (PRRs), with the Toll-like receptor (TLR) family being a key example. TLRs are an evolutionary well-conserved family of innate sensors of danger.

These might have their origins as early as the dawn of animal evolution, more than 700 million years ago [33]. These receptors play a crucial role in the immune system by recognizing pathogenic molecules and initiating an immune response. However, research has indicated that TLRs can also be activated by non-infectious stimuli such as stress hormones and metabolic byproducts, which can be elevated in states of psychological stress. Indeed, in response to chronic stress paradigms in rodents, elevated levels of TLR expression in the hippocampus, prefrontal cortex, blood and serum are reported [46]. Exemplifying the latter and the influence of psychosocial factors, studies in macaques have shown low-status-associated polarization of the TLR4 pathway towards a pro-inflammatory response. The latter provides an indication of the (direct) biological effects of social inequity on immune function and the influence of social gradients in health [47]. Another mouse model studying the effects of 4 weeks of social isolation showed an elevated neuroinflammation response, medicated by TLR-4 [48].

The evolutionary theory of loneliness (ETL) posits that social isolation once posed life-threatening risks, leading to the development of robust biological responses [49]. Much like pain signals harm to the body, loneliness signals broken social bonds, triggering stress responses designed to restore connection [39,40]. The lack of social cohesion has also been mentioned in the literature as an evolutionary mismatch [38]. Indicating the contextual importance of the psychosocial environment—and the lack thereof—in health and disease management.

Subsequently, TLRs can stimulate pathways leading to the activation of NF-κB, a transcription factor that regulates the expression of inflammation-related genes, including cytokines. Chronic stress models in mice show a hyperactivation of the NF-κB pathway in brain regions involved in stress response and affect [46]. In rodent models, it has been shown that the TLR-NF-κB pathway is one of the main mechanisms contributing to inflammation in times of chronic stress [46]. The aforementioned mediators prompt both central and peripheral immune cells to release pro-inflammatory cytokines. Cytokines identified in chronic stress paradigms are IL-1β, IL-6, and TNF-α and, to a lesser extent, IL-10, interferon-gamma (IFN-γ), IL-17, IL-22, and IL-4 [46].

Whilst stress response mechanisms once enabled survival from environmental threats, modern-day stressors may fail to serve their original function. While adaptive in the short term, prolonged activation of stress mechanisms and cytokine and chemokine production can lead to a pro-inflammatory state, disrupting metabolic processes and inhibiting INS signal transduction processes (see Figure 1) [50].

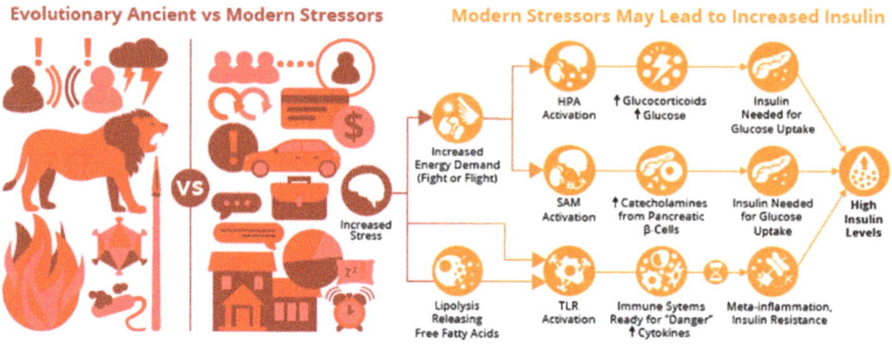

Figure 1. Evolutionary ancient vs. modern stressors and their impact on insulin (INS). Modern stressors activate the HPA and SAM axes, increasing glucocorticoids and catecholamines, leading to elevated glucose and INS demand. Chronic activation induces lipolysis, TLR activation, and meta-inflammation, contributing to hyperinsulinemia and INS resistance (IR).

So-called 'critical nodes' form an important part of the signalling network that functions downstream of the INS receptor (INSR) and the INS growth factor-1 receptor (IGF1R). Signaling pathways that are activated by cytokines through receptors such as the TNFR with affinity for tumour necrosis factor-α (TNFα), and the REC receptor, activated by cytokines such as interleukin-6 (IL-6) and leptin, interfere with INS signaling through crosstalk with the critical nodes [51]. Important examples in light of the communication between INS and mitochondria and in the context of this narrative review are the AKT and MAPK pathways discussed in the paragraphs hereafter.

Adipose tissue is part of the stress response as well. Stress, via multiple pathways, induces lipolysis, releasing free fatty acids (FFA) into the circulation. These can directly activate immune cells by TLR receptor activation, leading to further inflammation and cytokine release and influencing the above-described pathways. This is referred to as metainflammation, a portmanteau of metabolism and inflammation [43].

While stress, through the pathways discussed above, can induce IR, conversely, IR and the crosstalk between inflammatory pathways and neurocircuits in the brain can trigger behavioral responses, such as avoidance and heightened alarm [52]. Moreover, dopamine (DOP) and INS signaling systems have been shown to exhibit reciprocal regulatory relationships, emphasizing the interdependence of metabolic and neurochemical processes [53]. Additionally, INS and oxytocin (OXY) share a cross-talk mechanism in glucose homeostasis. OXY which plays a role in the stress response, has been demonstrated to stimulate INS secretion and improve pancreatic function through central regulation via vagal neurons that innervate β-cells [54].

The reciprocal regulation between INS, DOP, and OXY may demonstrate INS's broader function, beyond its metabolic role, in modulating psychosocial and behavioral processes. This PNI view highlights how INS operates at the intersection of metabolic, immune, neural, and endocrine pathways, emphasizing its relevance in the context of Type 2 Diabetes (T2DM).

Indeed, chronic stress impairs INS signaling (INSS) both in vitro and in vivo in laboratory animals [55], and stressful life events, traumatic experiences, general emotional stress, anger and hostility, distressed sleep, and workplace stress might induce IR [17]. In a longitudinal study with 12,844 Australian women initially free of DMT2, where IR is seen as a hallmark [56], those reporting moderate–high stress levels had a 2.3 times higher risk of developing later T2DM [57].

The psycho-physiological stress response remains one of nature's fundamental survival mechanisms [45]. While detrimental in the long term, the immune system is simply doing what it is designed to do: protect us [30]. Understanding the latter enables the proposal of theoretical interventions later in this review that support the original function and context of INS and mitochondria.

2.2. Sensing: The Role of INS Receptors

The physiological interactions between INS and INS-like growth factor (IGF-1) with cellular receptors such as INS receptors (INSRs), INS-like growth factor 1 receptors (IGF1Rs), and hybrid INS receptors/INS-like growth factor 1 receptors (INSR/IGF1Rs) initiate a cascade of responses that prepare mitochondria to sense and respond to environmental cues effectively, as shown in studies [58,59]. Recent research in mice highlights the significant role of the INS/IGF1 signaling pathways in regulating mitochondrial biogenesis, fusion, architecture, and functionality, underscoring the intricate link between INSS and mitochondrial dynamics [60]. This is setting the stage for an inclusion of INS in the theoretical MIPS model.

In vitro research in Human embryonic Stem Cells (HSCs) shows that when INS binds to its receptors, it triggers a series of signaling cascades, including the AKT-kinase (AKT) and Mitogen-Activated Protein Kinase (MAPK) pathways. Along with their downstream effectors, they facilitate a range of cellular and mitochondrial functions [61]. The AKT pathway predominantly mediates the metabolic effects of INS, whereas the MAPK pathway is crucial for regulating cell growth, proliferation, differentiation, mortality, and survival [62]. It interacts with the AKT pathway and others to modulate cell growth and differentiation [20].

The AKT and MAPK pathways operate in a sequence and context-dependent manner, demonstrating complex cooperation and interaction within cellular signaling networks [63]. Studies, including in rats, indicate that these pathways are not isolated; they work synergistically with each other but also other pathways. They can reciprocally influence each other, where the modification of one pathway can affect the other, either enhancing or inhibiting its functions [8,64,65]. This dynamic interaction is especially crucial in stressed conditions, where external stressors modulate INS levels and signaling, subsequently impacting mitochondrial dynamics [66]. An imbalance in mitochondrial dynamics and dysregulated opposing and counterbalancing processes can cause significant disruptions in mitochondrial function [9]. These disruptions are pivotal as they can precipitate abnormal cellular outcomes and contribute to the development of diseases such as Type 2 Diabetes Mellitus (T2DM), emphasizing the critical implications of INS Signaling (INSS) interplays in disease pathology [9,66]. Depending on their size and morphology, mitochondria exhibit distinct responses to incoming signals. For example, in vitro research shows that larger mitochondria, with a greater matrix volume and a lower surface-area-to-volume ratio, respond differently compared to smaller counterparts [67,68].

2.3. Sensing: INS, AKT-Pathway, and Mitochondrial Dynamics

INS and IGF-1 signaling, through their respective receptors, significantly enhance mitochondrial function in a PI3K/AKT-dependent manner, as shown in in vitro studies [69]. Under physiological conditions, INS promotes mitochondrial fusion, while IR triggers mitochondrial fission—the physiological interplay of both processes are crucial for mitochondrial quality control [70]. Furthermore, INS, via the AKT pathway, orchestrates a network of downstream effectors such as Glycogen synthase kinase 3 beta (GSK3β) [71], mammalian target of rapamycin 1 (mTORC1), Forkhead box protein O1 (FoxO1) [68,72], the mammalian target of rapamycin (mTOR), Peroxisome proliferator-activated receptor gamma coactivator 1-alpha (PGC-1α), Unc-51 Like Autophagy Activating Kinase (ULK1), and the pro-apoptotic proteins Bcl-2-associated X protein (BAX) and Bcl-2-associated death promoter (BAD) [72,73]. These effectors have been shown in mice studies [36,37] to collectively influence a range of mitochondrial functions, including biogenesis, mitophagy, fusion, fission, and apoptosis [20,62]. Through its impact on these effectors, INS might facilitate a complex interplay that maintains mitochondrial dynamics [20].

2.4. Sensing: INS, MAPK-Pathway and Mitochondrial Dynamics

INS modulates the MAPK pathway, which is pivotal for transmitting extracellular signals to cellular responses [20]. The key effectors of this pathway include extracellular signal-regulated kinases 1 and 2 (ERK1/2), which influence mitochondrial functions [74]; BCL2 proteins, involved in apoptosis regulation [74] and Rapidly Accelerated Fibrosarcoma kinase (RAF), as well as transcription factors such as cAMP response element-binding protein (CREB), Myelocytomatosis oncogene (MYC), and FBJ Murine osteosarcoma viral oncogene homolog (FOS), which contribute to mitochondrial biogenesis and mitophagy [20] (see Figure 2).

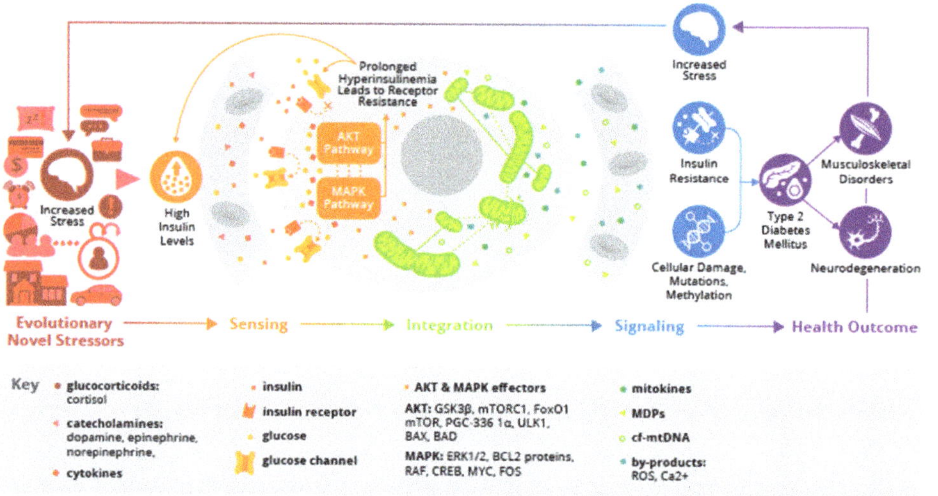

Figure 2. Incorporation of Insulin into the Mitochondrial Information Processing System (MIPS). This figure illustrates the potential role of insulin (INS) within the Mitochondrial Information Processing System (MIPS) in response to psychosocial and evolutionary novel stressors. Using the MIPS model and an evolutionary perspective, we propose that INS functions as a socio-psycho-metabolic hormone that cooperates with mitochondria to mediate the sensing, integration, and signaling of these stressors. This cooperation might affect mitochondrial dynamics through pathways such as AKT and MAPK. Prolonged hyperinsulinemia, driven by chronic stress, may lead to receptor resistance, impacting mitochondrial function. This figure highlights the hypothesized relationship between psychosocial stress, insulin resistance, and the development of complications associated with Type 2 Diabetes Mellitus (T2DM), such as neurodegeneration and musculoskeletal disorders (MSDs). By positioning insulin as a central modulator working in cooperation with mitochondria in the MIPS framework, we propose that it plays a key role in integrating psychosocial and metabolic signals, ultimately influencing health outcomes.

The above provides theoretical insights into how INS contributes to the sensing of psychosocial factors. However, further clinical studies are necessary to further explore this theory.

Insulin's Role in Sensing: Proof of Concept

In a series of studies involving rats subjected to four distinct models of stress-induced depression—chronic unpredictable mild stress, learned helplessness, chronic restraint, and social defeat—significant modifications were observed in the AKT and MAPK signaling pathways. Notably, phosphorylated AKT (p-AKT) levels were altered across all four depression models, demonstrating the extensive impact of stress on INSS mechanisms [65]. Another study in rats highlighted that social isolation could induce early-stage dysfunctions in the INSS pathways. This was evident through a reduction in AKT phosphorylation, potentially exacerbating an oxidative state and further complicating metabolic homeostasis [75]. The MAPK pathway, critical for cellular processes such as growth and response to stressors, showed significant changes in the context of social defeat stress in rats [76]. As this is a review, the discussed concepts remain theoretical. Further clinical research in humans is necessary to elucidate the role of INS in mitochondrial sensing of psychosocial factors.

2.5. Integrating—The Role of Insulin

As part of the sensing function, INS influences cellular dynamics through its receptors, affecting the strength and duration of AKT and MAPK pathway activities. Subsequently, mitochondria integrate these inputs together with information from interactions with other organelles facilitated by mitochondria-associated membranes (MAMs) [2,64]. These structural domains establish physical connections with the nucleus, lysosomes, endoplasmic reticulum (ER), and Golgi apparatus, enhancing cellular coordination and response to changes [77].

This integrative function strengthens our hypothesis that INS might be an important player in the MIPS framework; however, additional research is required.

Insulin's Role in Integration: Proof of Concept

Altered signaling through MAMs is a characteristic feature in various tissues exhibiting IR, such as muscles [78]. This alteration underscores the systemic impact of INS's regulatory role at the cellular level. A proteomic analysis in rats, which underwent chronic psychological stress, demonstrated significant changes in the MAM proteome [79]. Altogether, the above might serve as a proof of concept that psychological stress, through INSS, influences mitochondrial function. However, it remains theoretical, and further research is needed to confirm these findings.

2.6. Transduction—The Role of INS

Mitochondria systematically impact cellular and organismal behaviors through the release of signaling molecules [12]. Mitokines, for example, are released into the systemic circulation and mediate a non-autonomous stress response [24]. This process is suggested to be analogous to bacterial quorum sensing, where signaling molecules coordinate group behaviors in bacterial populations [80]. Similarly, mitokines facilitate intercellular communication, allowing mitochondria to influence distant cells and maintain homeostasis across the organism [81]. This process enhances inter-tissue communication of mitochondrial stress, playing a critical role in synchronizing and amplifying stress responses across the body, thereby maintaining more efficient organismal homeostasis [24]. The increase in mitokines might be an attempt at mitohormesis, enhancing stress resistance [82]. However, the outcomes of mitokine signaling can be both beneficial and detrimental, depending on the signal's magnitude and duration, indicating that mitokine production has dual aspects [83].

Additionally, the mitochondrial genome (mtDNA) is responsible for producing small mitochondrial DNA (mtDNA)-encoded peptides, such as the mitochondrial open reading frame of the twelve S-c (MOTS-c), and humanin and small HN-like peptides (SHLPs) are classified as mitochondrial-derived peptides (MDPs) [84]. An observational study indicates that INS signaling also influences mitochondrial integrity and immune responses by influencing the release of cell-free mitochondrial DNA (cf-mtDNA) [85]. A recent systematic review of human studies suggest that this cf-mtDNA, integral to mitochondrial damage-associated molecular patterns (mtDAMPs), acts as a potent immunological activator due to the bacterial origin of mitochondria. This activation marks cf-mtDNA as a significant indicator of inflammatory diseases and a predictor of mortality [86,87].

Dysfunctional mitochondria, and altered dynamics, can lead to increased production of reactive oxygen species (ROS) and other byproducts. A recent review from 2024 describes that mitochondrial ROS production can be both a normal function and a sign of dysfunction, depending on the context. In the case of dysfunction, excessive ROS can damage cellular structures, including nuclear DNA, potentially resulting in mutations [88].

Dysfunctional mitochondria also lead to the buildup of, for example, Calcium (Ca^{2+}), as per mitochondria's buffering function [64]. Ca^{2+} levels have quite narrow limits, and small changes can cause negative health outcomes, as will be shown later in the article.

Further to the above, mitochondria generate cellular and organismal behaviors through mitochondrial-nuclear crosstalk and interspecies epigenetic remodeling [12].

Mitochondrial metabolites serve as substrates for epigenetic marks in the nucleus, while others function as mediators that modulate nuclear gene expression. This dynamic interaction results in modifications to both the epigenome and gene expression, which, in turn, regulate mitochondrial function [89]. This systemic communication, possibly influenced by INS as elaborated on hereafter, is essential for regulating gene expression and happens via epigenetic mechanisms such as DNA methylation and histone modification [12,87]. In addition to nuclear DNA (nDNA) methylation, emerging evidence shows that mtDNA can undergo methylation [90]. Methylation of the D-loop region in mtDNA, which regulates both mtDNA replication and transcription, has been observed to increase in individuals with IR. Recent studies in IR obese humans have unveiled, for the first time, an INS signaling-epigenetic-genetic axis that may regulate mitochondria, suggesting that INS has the capability to directly modulate mitochondrial gene expression and mitochondrial function [28]. This may suggest that INS signaling could modulate both nuclear and mitochondrial gene expression, potentially through epigenetic regulation of genes encoded by both mtDNA and nDNA. Data demonstrate impaired mitochondrial structure and function in IR muscle, which may be caused by epigenetic regulation of genes encoded by mtDNA and nuclear DNA [90].

Research on C. elegans has shown perturbations in INSS to possibly lead to changes in mitochondrial function, resulting in significant alterations in gene expression at both transcriptional and translational levels [91]. It is hypothesized that mitochondrial abnormalities may arise from the epigenetic regulation of both mitochondrial and nuclear-encoded genes responsible for mitochondrial structure and function, with INS potentially playing a critical role in modulating these epigenetic changes, particularly through its influence on mitochondrial DNA (mtDNA) methylation and gene expression pathways [92].

Epigenetic modifications are suggested to be key intermediaries in the interactions between environmental stimuli, such as stress, and the genome. These modifications can trigger inflammatory responses that promote metabolic disorders [62].

Ultimately, it might come down to communication. Based on the information above, we hypothesize that INS might act as a socio-psychological communication substance, possibly supporting mitochondria to sense, integrate, and transduce psychosocial signals. This dynamic dialogue between the environment, INS, mitochondria, and the rest of the organism enables maintaining homeostasis, though it might lead to adverse health outcomes if dysregulated. To further validate these findings and hypotheses, additional research involving human subjects is necessary.

INS's Role in Integration: Proof of Concept

Summarizing the above, recent evidence underscores INS's role in the integration and transduction of psychosocial signals through mitochondrial pathways. Acute mental stress has been shown to elevate levels of circulating mitochondrial DNA (mtDNA), with psychological factors amplifying these effects, suggesting potential mediation by INS. A systematic review of human studies mentions higher cf-mtDNA levels in suicide attempters to correlate with increased CORT response during the dexamethasone suppression test (DST), indicating a possible link between HPA hyperactivity and cf-mtDNA levels [87]. While this suggests an interaction between stress and mitochondrial dynamics, the role of INS remains speculative. Other factors may also contribute to cf-mtDNA release, and further studies are required to explore these potential mechanisms.

Machine learning analyses on human serum suggests that psychological factors, rather than inherent personal traits, predict stress-induced changes in circulating cell-free mtDNA (ccf-mtDNA). Major depression and other conditions linked to psychological stress have been shown to lead to a rise in serum ccf-mtDNA levels [60]. In a study involving 46 healthy middle-aged adults exposed to a brief psychological stressor—a public speaking simulation—a significant surge in serum circulating cell-free mtDNA was documented shortly afterward [93], with potential mediation by INS.

The mechanisms of cf-mtDNA release extend beyond cell death and can also be triggered by psychological stress [94]. A study in 20 healthy young men indeed shows cf-mtDNA release in response to psychosocial stress, suggesting an active release mechanism resulting from psychosocial challenges [95], possibly mediated by INS. Nuancing and further research are important, as variations in cf-mtDNA responses to stressors indicate that not all forms of cf-mtDNA are pro-inflammatory, adding complexity to INS's role as a social substance affecting physiological responses [56,96].

In lower levels of MOTS-c, a mitochondrial-derived peptide, in T2D patients, INS was found to regulate and attenuate the MOTS-c response in a study in humans [54,64,97]. Moreover, conditions like major depression are known to alter mitokine production and cf-mtDNA, as shown in human studies [98].

A recent study performed among older adults indicates that early life stress impacts mitochondrial functionality by altering mtDNA content, affecting cellular respiration and bioenergetics. Adults who suffered childhood maltreatment or experienced parental loss before age 18 typically exhibit reduced mtDNA-CN compared to those without adverse childhood events (ACE) [5].

While the above advances the understanding of INS as a socio-psychological substance and its potential place in the MIPS model, it remains theoretical. Further research is needed to confirm these findings and explore their practical applications.

2.7. Type 2 Diabetes Mellitus with Musculoskeletal Problems and Neurodegeneration

Further to the above, we hypothesize that INS acts as a potential key modulator within the MIPS model, orchestrating the interplay between psychosocial risk factors, INS, mitochondrial dynamics, and various health outcomes. Two significant examples that reinforce the role of INS as a social substance and the need for integrative interventions, including those in the psychosocial realm, are Type 2 Diabetes Mellitus (T2DM) with musculoskeletal disorders (MSDs) and T2DM with neurodegeneration.

In the sections that follow, we will explore how the models discussed earlier could theoretically contribute to the knowledge about the development of T2DM with MSDs and neurodegeneration. We will highlight the role of psychosocial factors in shaping health and disease, consider INS's role as a 'social substance' within the MIPS model, and illustrate how the function of the MS system might extend beyond mere movement, potentially acting—under the influence of INS and mitochondria—as a component in the psychosocial-biological axis or as a psychobiological interface. To better understand this interplay, we look at recent research and studies that demonstrate the effects of psychosocial stressors, INS and mitochondrial function in T2DM and subsequent musculoskeletal- and neurological health and complications.

2.7.1. Type 2 Diabetes Mellitus with Musculoskeletal Disorders

Studies in rodent models have demonstrated that adverse childhood experiences (ACE) lead to altered mitochondrial structure and bioenergetics in peripheral muscle. Duchowny's research revealed compromised maximal ATP production in skeletal muscle (SM) mitochondria among individuals who experienced ACEs, with each additional adverse event associated with modestly lower ATPmax, a measure of maximal capacity for ATP production [5]. A systematic review and meta-analysis from 2024 on human cohort studies indicates that Musculoskeletal Disorders (MSDs) are prevalent in individuals with T2DM [99]. There seems to exist a vicious cycle where T2DM and MSDs mutually exacerbate each other. This interconnection is largely driven by skeletal muscle (SM) IR and mitochondrial dysfunction, which are identified as the key pathophysiological links between T2DM and MSDs [100]. A significant reduction in mtDNA-CN has been documented in critical tissues such as skeletal muscle (SM), adipose tissue, and peripheral blood in individuals with obesity and T2DM. A population-based follow-up study suggests that this decrease in mtDNA-CN often precedes the clinical onset of T2DM, which might show its potential as an early biomarker for disease prediction and a target for therapeutic intervention [28,101].

IR can lead to mitochondrial dysfunction, which in turn results in hyperglycemia and its metabolic consequences [102]. This hyperglycemia contributes to the glycosylation of collagen structures, reducing bone flexibility. Advanced glycation end-products (AGEs) accumulate in musculoskeletal (MSK) tissues, adversely affecting biomechanical properties by altering charges and forming collagen cross-linkages. Such mechanisms are linked to various T2DM-related MSD, including osteoporosis, osteoarthritis, sarcopenia, tendinopathy, neuropathy, and joint stiffness [103]. Additionally, AGEs induce structural changes in myofibrillar proteins of muscles, further impacting the MS system [100]. Integrating psychosocial factors into this narrative, recent studies in adult mice exposed to social isolation for four weeks showed significant reductions in bone quality, including reduced bone mineral density [104]. This indicates an impact of psychosocial stressors on MS health, further highlighting the intricate interplay between INS, psychosocial factors, and the musculoskeletal system.

Under conditions of glucose overload, mitochondria experience an increase in ROS production and oxidative stress (OS), which can significantly reduce ATP production [100]. In the context of hyperglycemia, mitochondrial fragmentation precedes ROS production induced by high glucose levels. Hyperglycemia increases ROS production within approximately 30 min, and fragmented mitochondria produce about 50% more ROS compared to their filamentous counterparts in the same cell [2]. This might suggest an important role of mitochondrial dynamics in ROS production and suggests the potential effects of psychosocial factors and INS on mitochondrial function and subsequent MSD.

ROS can both activate and repress the nuclear factor kappa-light-chain-enhancer of activated B cells (NF-κB), signaling in a phase- and context-dependent manner [105]. This factor plays a pivotal role in driving the increased expression of inflammatory cytokines and chemokines, exacerbating inflammation [106]. This inflammatory response further contributes to the cycle earlier described and MS deterioration seen in T2DM. Muscle cells, with their relatively high-energy demands, possess a notably high concentration of mitochondria to meet these demands [107]. As such, IR and impaired glucose uptake, but also more chances of high ROS levels in SM, contribute to a spectrum of adverse conditions, including mitochondrial dysfunction [100]. Indeed, in the SM of individuals with IR or T2DM, mitochondria tend to be smaller and fewer [20,108]. This mitochondrial insufficiency in SM correlates with decreased muscle performance, reduced mobility, and increased susceptibility to frailty and muscle atrophy [5].

Additionally, a recent review from 2024 reports elevated production of lipid intermediates such as diacylglycerol (DAG) and ceramides, as well as pro-inflammatory cytokines resulting from intramyocellular lipid deposition. Moreover, the myomitokine GDF15 is extensively studied as a biomarker for various diseases, including those affecting the MSS, further emphasizing the wide-ranging impacts of IR, mitochondrial dysfunction and its subsequent transduction substances such as mitokines [83].

Following the cascade of IR and mitochondrial dysfunction, mitochondrial abnormalities significantly influence muscle and multisystem diseases through various interconnected mechanisms. Mitochondrial defects can lead to muscle diseases due to a loss of oxidative phosphorylation (OXPHOS), abnormalities in mitochondrial dynamics, atypical mitochondrial structures, and morphologies, disrupted energy metabolism, mitophagy, and apoptosis [109]. Specifically, certain mitochondrial mutations or dysfunctions have been identified and as triggers for muscular dystrophy [106]. The literature describes that in SM fibers, mitochondria are strategically positioned between myofibrils, encircle the nucleus, and are densely packed within the sarcolemma [110]. Dysfunction often originates from the loss of structural integrity during Mitochondrial Outer Membrane Permeabilization (MOMP) and Mitochondrial Inner Membrane Permeabilization (MIMP), which are typically triggered by the activation of BAX and BAK proteins [111]—earlier elucidated as effectors of INS pathways. Such events lead to the release of mitochondrial byproducts such as cytochrome c (CYTC), apoptosis-inducing factor (AIF), caspase-9, and Ca^{2+} into the cytosol, thereby initiating programmed cell death pathways [106]. Mitochondrial defects or abnormalities can precipitate muscle and multisystem diseases through various mechanisms, notably including dysregulated Ca^{2+} signaling [106]. SM mitochondria play a crucial role in the storage and regulation of Ca^{2+}, essential for maintaining cellular functions [107]. Marchioretti and colleagues show in their study on skeletal muscle of mice and patients that dysfunctions such as excitation–contraction coupling (ECC) deregulation and impaired mitochondrial respiration often precede shifts in muscle force, Ca^{2+} imbalances, and the breakdown of triad structures. Ca^{2+} overload, resulting from leakage from the sarcoplasmic reticulum (SR), impaired Ca^{2+} reuptake into the SR, or increased Ca^{2+} influx through the cell membrane, can activate Ca^{2+}-dependent proteins such as calpains, which then degrade intracellular proteins, cellular membranes, and nuclear DNA [112]. A study in mice demonstrated that intramuscular injections of allogenic mitochondria from healthy animals into the hind limbs of mdx mice alleviated SM damage and reduced Ca^{2+} deposits [113]. Additionally, high glucocorticoid doses, often associated with stress and subsequent IR, are known to influence mitochondria in a biphasic manner with high glucocorticoid doses reducing Ca^{2+} buffering capacity, increase ROS production, and heighten susceptibility to cell death [35], which is confirmed as well in an in vitro study [114]. Research further shows that IR and T2DM are associated with dysregulated Ca^{2+} homeostasis, with higher serum Ca^{2+} levels correlating positively with fasting blood glucose and the IR index in humans [115]. The regulation of mitochondrial Ca^{2+} is particularly significant in excitable cells such as skeletal and smooth muscle, where insufficient mitochondrial Ca^{2+} uptake can impair cell function, while Ca^{2+} overload may lead to cellular injury and apoptosis [116]. Notably, an in vitro study showed that, compared to smaller fragmented mitochondria, larger tubular mitochondria in the same cell exhibit similar Ca^{2+} uptake rates but recover more quickly, highlighting how mitochondrial dynamics influence their capacity to modulate Ca^{2+} levels and buffering [117].

Furthermore, macrophages within SM exhibit significant phenotypic diversity, adapting their behavior by switching between M1 and M2 phenotypes in response to environmental changes [118]. A recent review explains that macrophages are not only crucial for tissue homeostasis and the response to injury but are also linked to IR in SM. The concentration of macrophages in SM is intricately linked to INS sensitivity; a negative correlation exists, where higher macrophage presence often signifies lower INS sensitivity [119]. Mitochondrial metabolic alterations significantly influence gene expression, leading to varied responses in immune cells. Specifically, M1 macrophages, which are compromised in their ability to complete the tricarboxylic acid (TCA) cycle, tend to adopt a pro-inflammatory state. In contrast, M2 macrophages engage in β-oxidation, exhibiting anti-inflammatory responses, highlighting their role in maintaining homeostasis and promoting healing [120,121]. During the healing of tendon injuries in mice, tendons of T2DM mice exhibit an increased expression of markers associated with pro-inflammatory M1 macrophages, alongside a prolonged and elevated expression of markers for anti-inflammatory M2 macrophages, which are involved in the decomposition of the extracellular matrix (ECM) [122]. The dysfunction of mitochondria can lead to an accumulation of metabolites, which in turn promotes a shift toward pro-inflammatory M1 phenotypes. This shift is pivotal in the context of SM IR, where macrophages play a significant role [118].

Additionally, recent studies in humans have identified a link between mitochondrial dysfunction and INS sensitivity in conditions like fibromyalgia (FM), indicating that similar INS and mitochondrial impairments could be underlying factors in various MS and metabolic disorders [123]. A review summarizing studies in animals as well as a few in humans describes that hyperglycemia-induced aberrant levels of INS or INS growth factors (IGF) may lead to neuropathic complications, intensifying pain through mechanisms such as central sensitization. Commonly, neuropathic joints manifest in the foot and ankle of patients, and conditions like diabetic polyneuropathy and rheumatoid arthritis (RA)-associated pain are complications [124]. Oxidative stress, driven by elevated ROS and prolonged hyperglycemia in T2DM, is known to contribute to nerve damage, which plays a role in the development of diabetic neuropathy. The latter might manifest as pain [125]. Alternatively, these effects can be mediated indirectly through mitochondrial damage and heightened inflammation [126]. This dynamic might ultimately illustrate how psychosocial 'pain', via INS and mitochondria, can exacerbate physical pain and possibly lead to additional complications at the physiological level.

2.7.2. Type 2 Diabetes Mellitus with Neurodegeneration

People suffering from Type 2 Diabetes Mellitus (T2DM) often experience a cluster of symptoms, including pain, chronic fatigue, depression, and circadian disruptions [127]. Besides the role of the musculoskeletal (MSK) system, these health issues likely share another common factor: hippocampal atrophy [128]. The hippocampus is particularly vulnerable to uncontrollable stress [129]. Research in rats has shown for the first time that social defeat exposure, psychosocial threat of attack, and severe psychological stress are combined with divergent structural remodeling of dendrites in hippocampal neurons [130]. Furthermore, another study in rats indicated that the rhythmic expression of the hippocampal transcriptome, as well as the circadian regulation of synaptic plasticity, was misaligned with natural light/dark circadian-entraining [131].

A human study showed changes in the structure, perfusion, and function of the hippocampus in T2DM [132]. Moreover, IR-induced abnormalities in the hippocampus of obese/T2DM patients include inflammatory stress, oxidative stress, mitochondrial stress, and increased generation of advanced glycated end products [133]. Meanwhile, the hippocampus is particularly vulnerable to uncontrollable stress [129], such as emotional, cognitive, social, and metabolic stress, showing another example of how T2DM and its diverse set of complications could be seen in light of the socio-psycho-biological framework.

Altogether, SM exhibits remarkable adaptability to changing metabolic demands, a characteristic that extends to its response to psychological stressors [134]. Indeed, emerging research in human peripheral tissue supports a hypothesis that mitochondria within SM might be integrators of these adverse experiences, effectively linking metabolic responses with broader social and environmental factors [5]. This adaptability can be explained by looking at muscles, the brain, INS and psychosocial factors, from an evolutionary point of view, as we will attempt hereafter.

Under normal physiological conditions, SM is responsible for approximately 80% of postprandial glucose uptake [135]. However, in the presence of IR, this process is inhibited as the IS prioritizes its own energy needs, described as acting 'selfishly' [136]. This shift in glucose allocation might be a strategic response by the IS to harness more resources during periods of stress, reflecting an evolutionary mechanism designed to enhance survival. Consequently, IR might redirect glucose away from SMs towards immune functions, supporting the body's immediate defense mechanisms but leading to reduced glucose availability for muscle activity. For this reason, muscle has been referred to as the 'forgotten' organ of the IS [137]. This adaptation, while beneficial in short-term immune responses, might lead to chronic MSDs and chronic pain if the IS remains continuously activated without actual threats, as is often the case with modern psychological stressors [138]. The same goes for the brain. While the brain and immune system might be the only two systems that can dominate all others by extracting resources, including glucose, the selfish immune system has been hypothesized to have the capacity to override the selfish brain. The adagio 'prima vivere e dopo filosofare' (first live and then philosophize) summarizes this situation well [30]. In times of stress, inhibiting the hippocampus's function of regulating the hypothalamus–pituitary–adrenal (HPA) axis might be beneficial. This inhibition facilitates the release of energy-demanding substances necessary for an immediate stress response. However, when the stressor becomes chronic, as is often the case with modern life stressors, prolonged activation of the HPA axis can have detrimental effects. One significant consequence is hippocampal atrophy, which might impair cognitive functions and overall brain health [139].

Although clinical studies are necessary and the jury remains out, the above emphasizes the importance of further investigating the psychosocial factors in the treatment of type 2 diabetes mellitus (T2DM) and the relevance of taking its interrelated evolutionary biology into account while designing prevention as well as treatment protocols for T2DM and other INS implicated conditions. It underscores the need for further research towards an integrative treatment approach in T2DM and highlights the importance of future research to deepen our understanding of the evolutionary-determined socio-psycho-biological cascade. This includes examining the interconnected mechanisms of psychological factors, insulin resistance, mitochondrial dysfunction, and T2DM with musculoskeletal- and/or neurological complications, as well as the role of evolutionary expectations. The latter will be further elaborated on in the following section.

3. Discussion: Zooming Out the Microscope on INS-Implicated Diseases and Treatments

This article has explored the socio-psycho-biological framework and INS's potential place herein. Hereafter, we will theoretically explore interventions and possible parameters that might have an impact at different layers in the proposed socio-psycho-biological framework, and specifically INS, considering its evolutionary origins, enabling the exploration of an integrative approach towards mechanisms involved in T2DM with MSD and neurodegeneration. It needs to be highlighted that it remains a theoretical exploration; further studies are needed to validate the theoretical framework proposed throughout this article and the following paragraphs.

3.1. Expectations of Evolution

Evolutionary medicine suggests that many chronic diseases might stem from a mismatch between our evolved bodies and modern human-induced environments [140]. This theoretical framework, combined with the previously proposed model of insulin (INS) as a social substance within the MIPS, is used to explore interventions at multiple levels of this model, as well as methods for measuring their effectiveness, altogether providing a theoretical yet comprehensive overview to guide future research.

Within the evolutionary framework, we assume the existence of 'expectations of evolution', which we define as the set of conditions, behaviors, and environmental factors that human bodies have evolved to thrive under, based on the selective pressures experienced by our ancestors. By aligning interventions with these 'evolutionary expectations', we might potentially enhance health outcomes by addressing the root causes of these mismatches.

Within the definition 'expectations of evolution' we distinguish between evolutionary stressors and evolutionary buffers. Interventions based on stressors are challenges that required adaptation for survival and often had beneficial effects on health through hormesis. Evolutionary buffers, on the other hand, are natural factors that were consistently present in the environment and are essential for optimal functioning and health.

It is important to note that the applications of the theory of evolutionary mismatch might have limitations and should be used with caution, considering that ancestral conditions should not be oversimplified [141]. Careful monitoring and scientific research are necessary to address these concerns and prove the use of this theoretical framework.

3.2. Evolutionary Stressors

We propose resilience to embody a system's capacity to adjust to alterations, encompassing both tolerance and adaptability to a spectrum of stresses—spanning physical, chemical, biological, and psychological domains. Mitochondria, pivotal entities in both health and disease paradigms, emerge as principal focal points in hormetic methodologies, commonly referred to as mitohormesis [142]. These strategies aim to fortify mitochondrial resilience, fostering what has been termed mitoresilience [143]. Hormesis is characterized by a biphasic dose-response to specific mild stressors, such as fasting, intake of polyphenols, exercising, physical and chemical stress, and mental engagement [143]. These stimuli elicit beneficial cellular metabolic pathways influenced by INS signaling (INS), such as the down-regulation of mTOR and IGF-1 [143].

Coping with 'ancient mild stress factors'—including intermittent fasting, exposure to diverse environmental stresses like cold, heat, hypoxia, and hypercapnia, alongside strategies such as calorie restriction and time-based food intake—has shown significant impacts on various mitochondrial parameters and INS levels [64,144]. This has been demonstrated in a study on human subjects who followed a 10-day protocol including a combination of 'ancient stress factors' and hermetic interventions. This study showed an improvement in anthropometrics and metabolic indices, including INS [145].

In the context of T2DM with metabolic syndrome (MS) and hippocampal atrophy, aerobic training has been shown in a clinical trial of 100 patients with T2DM to increase total and right hippocampal volume and protect cognitive function [146]. Exercise also induces adaptations in the MSS, which is beneficial in the prevention and treatment of T2DM [147]. Implementing a 'ketogenic status', intermittently steering the system in and out of ketosis, has also demonstrated benefits. Recent studies have shown a ketogenic diet to improve muscle mass and function in mice [148] and influence brain gene expression involved in neurodegenerative disease in T2DM mice [149]. An intervention study in nine patients with T2DM showed that cold acclimatization improves skeletal muscle insulin sensitivity by 43%, comparable to the effects of exercise training [150]. In a recent study in mice, cold exposure was shown to affect the brain peptidome and gut microbiome [151]. A study involving 14 patients with T2DM showed that therapeutic intermittent hypoxia influences multiple mechanisms in T2DM, including blood glucose regulation [152]. Although nutritional interventions have been extensively studied, breath work and temperature interventions, with their diverse forms and mechanisms, remain less systematically explored. Their specific effects on T2DM with MSD and neurodegeneration warrant further research.

It is important to mention there are critics of hormesis and subsequent interventions as well. There seems to be controversy on the interpretation and a lack of standardization, such as the definition and application of hormesis, leading to inconsistent use across different studies and contexts. There seems to be individual variability of the responses to doses, the biological mechanisms are not yet fully understood, and there is a dependence on the context, making it difficult to generalize findings [153]. To rectify the uncertainties, further research is needed in both healthy and specific populations such as T2DM patients, and careful monitoring with tools (such as HRV), which are discussed later, could improve these uncertainties.

3.3. Evolutionary Buffers

In addition to stressors, there is another category we propose to introduce as 'evolutionary buffers'—factors that have been consistently present during evolution. An example is varied food intake, which has been shown to improve INS sensitivity and mitochondrial health.

The plant diversity of homo sapiens' early diet was composed of over 3000 species [144]. Low nutrient variety is apparent in modern life where people eat an average of twenty ingredients or fewer, which is associated with several chronic diseases, including T2DM. Perhaps the most intruding factor of food variety is provided when the food is fermented [144]. Indeed, a study including in vitro and in vivo experiments in a variety of human cell types shows the activation of Nrf2 cell defense pathways by ancient foods, including fermented vegetables [154], as well as fermented vegetables and spices as NRF2-induced enzyme agonists [64] influencing mitochondria. Another literature study summarizes in vitro and in vivo and clinical studies about the antidiabetic properties of fermented foods [155]. Another case-control study has shown that a higher dietary diversity score might diminish the odds of complications in T2DM [156].

Another evolutionary support might be the maintenance of a healthy circadian rhythm. The circadian timing system includes a central clock in the suprachiasmatic nucleus (SCN) and tissue-specific clocks in peripheral tissues [157]. Desynchronization between the central and peripheral clocks is linked to a higher incidence of insulin resistance (IR) and related diseases [158]. A cross-sectional study in patients indicated that disruptions in the circadian clock may be linked to the disruption of several mechanisms and conditions mentioned earlier, including desynchronization of the SNS and the HPA-axis, IR but also mitochondrial dysfunction and chronic musculoskeletal pain and hippocampal atrophy [159]. Evidence from experimental animal studies as well as controlled human subjects has shown that sleep deprivation and circadian misalignment can both directly drive metabolic dysfunction, possibly causing diabetes [160]. A recent review summarizes that sleep interventions such as sleep education and cognitive therapy have been shown to improve glucose homeostasis [161]. Also, stimulus control, sleep restriction, relaxation and sleep hygiene, as well as bright light therapy and timed melatonin administration are currently being studied with a focus on their effects on glucose metabolism [162]. While there are studies showing the benefits of sleep interventions in T2DM, research is still in its infancy and more research is necessary [163]. A newly proposed circadian rhythm-based intervention might be photobiomodulation (PBM). A recent randomized controlled trial has shown the impact of photobiomodulation of circadian variation in blood pressure, pain pressure threshold and elasticity of tissue as well as improvement in musculoskeletal and neuropathic pain in fibromyalgia (FM) patients [159], a condition in which IR is thought to play a role, with FM being a common comorbidity in individuals with T2DM [164].

A recent systematic review describes that the hippocampus has a unique metabolism requiring high energy for optimal function, especially in humans. PBM is proposed to upregulate mitochondrial activity. It also reports the improvement of self-efficacy and pain catastrophizing, as well as psychological factors [165]. Thereby, PBM, including transcranial PBM, has been suggested to enhance neuronal bioenergetics, cerebral blood flow, oxidative stress, neuroinflammation, neural cell survival, neurotrophic factors, neurogenesis, and brain circuit functions [166]. A study in sleep-deprived mice shows improvement of hippocampal function by the use of PBM [167]. This, in turn, regulates the central nervous system and, subsequently, the peripheral nervous system, which via the earlier discussed cascade could improve central and peripheral sensitization symptoms in individuals with DMT2 with MSD and chronic pain [168]. An RCT, in 34 patients with major depressive disorder, showed that using hyperthermia (WBH) in individuals with depression might be effective [169]. WBH improves IR as well [170]. Similarly, whole-body PBM has recently shown promising results in an RCT, reducing pain and improving quality of life, as well as psychological factors like kinesiophobia, pain catastrophizing, and self-efficacy in patients with fibromyalgia [171]. The proposed underlying mechanisms in T2DM might be similar, ultimately promoting hippocampal neurogenesis; however, further research is necessary to confirm this hypothesis. PBM, thus, could be a valuable treatment modality, emerging as a promising multifactorial intervention [171] spanning a major part of the extended MIPS model and fitting into the evolutionary framework as per the evolutionary mechanisms of photon–biological tissue interactions. As it is improving psychological factors, as well as multiple mechanisms in the previously proposed model, it is therefore a valuable option in the treatment of T2DM with MSD. It also shows the potential of modern technology being able to fulfill evolutionary expectations.

As discussed earlier, human physiological responses still mirror those of our ancestors, even though modern 'threats' like academic exams do not require physical action.

Indeed, a meta-analysis shows that these threats can lead to physical consequences as if the stressor should be solved by movement [172]. This might suggest that movement could serve as a buffer, aligning with the system's evolutionary design to release built-up energy after a threat or as a signal to move away to avoid becoming prey [173]. Although humans evolved for regular physical activity, they were also selected to avoid unnecessary exertion due to energy limitations in early environments. This creates a paradox: despite the known health benefits of exercise, people tend to avoid it unless it is either necessary or enjoyable. To overcome this inertia, but also to facilitate movement as an intervention in conditions where INS is implicated, nudging and altering environments might be of importance, making it more integrated into daily life as it was for our ancestors [173].

Given the integrative nature of the socio-psycho-biological framework, the focus of this study and discussing evolutionary expectations, the recognition of the role of psychosocial factors and subsequent interventions in shaping glycemic control and overall health may be the most important.

A systematic review, as well as a systematic review and meta-analysis, demonstrated the effectiveness of mindfulness-based interventions (MBI) in enhancing glycemic control for individuals with T2DM [174,175]. These interventions, which include mindfulness-based stress reduction (MBSR) and mindfulness-based cognitive therapy (MBCT), not only improve glycemic control but also enhance psychological well-being, illustrating the profound interaction between psychological health and metabolic regulation mediated by INS as a social substance [175]. As the included studies sometimes lack methodological quality, further research is necessary to elucidate the effects of MBI.

Similarly, yoga might support autonomic balance, vagal modulation, hormonal regulation, and glycemic control through mechanisms that involve neurophysiological, neuroendocrinological, and psychophysiological systems [176]. These systems are intricately connected with INS's role in cellular signaling and energy metabolism, further emphasizing the substance's broad impact on health beyond its traditional metabolic functions [176].

Additionally, an RCT on Baduanjin, a form of Qigong, shows promising results in preventing and improving hyperlipidemia, primarily by promoting glucose decomposition and consumption. This practice might not only improve the psychological state but also relieve anxiety and depression, spread knowledge of health maintenance, and change dietary customs, demonstrating the possible wide-reaching effects of lifestyle interventions on INS-related pathways [177].

Mindful exercise programs such as Tai Chi, Qigong, and yoga might provide long-term benefits for chronic pain management, particularly in conditions like fibromyalgia [177,178]. They offer pain relief while improving glycemic control.

A randomized controlled pilot study suggests that Qigong may serve as a possible complementary therapy for individuals with T2DM, providing a holistic approach to managing this condition through INS modulation and psychosocial improvements [179].

A prospective study in 100 patients with T2DM shows that diaphragmatic breathing and systematic relaxation techniques, when practiced consistently, can amplify the effectiveness of conventional medication and enhance glycemic control and mental health in T2DM patients [180]. By influencing the autonomic nervous system, these practices optimize heart rate variability (HRV) and reduce diabetes distress.

A prospective mediation study in 440 diabetes patients (both type 1 and type 2) showed that meta-cognitive beliefs (such as 'worrying about the future keeps me prepared' or 'worry is uncontrollable') are associated with anxiety as well as depression and T2DM. Metacognitive beliefs predict rumination and psychological distress independently of illness representations in adults with T2DM [181]. This suggests that metacognitive therapy might be an effective complementary intervention.

The literature describes that faith-based interventions (FBIs) involve leveraging personal resources like knowledge, self-efficacy, spiritual beliefs, and symptom management skills to promote self-management attitudes (dieting, exercising, emotion regulation) and integrate health with spirituality. FBIs might provide an important framework for enhancing T2DM management through increased social support, strengthened spiritual beliefs and cognition, and improved emotion regulation [182].

Furthermore, psychoeducation about emotions and their evolutionary significance might be an interesting avenue to explore, addressing the psycho-socio-biological framework for conditions where INS is implicated. Emotions like fear, stress and loneliness trigger physiological and behavioral responses designed to protect and guide the organism [183]. By understanding emotions from an evolutionary standpoint, interventions can be aligned with our biological and psychological needs—an example being loneliness.

Early in human history, survival and prosperity depended on banding together—in couples, families, or tribes—for mutual protection and assistance. The pain of loneliness served as a prompt to renew social connections necessary for survival, fostering social trust, cohesiveness, and collective action. Although loneliness can feel like a negative emotion without value, it may have evolved as an aversive state, similar to hunger or pain, to drive behavior change [184]. This understanding of emotional drivers—of which loneliness is one of multiple examples—can offer actionable insights for individuals managing INS-implicated diseases, as psychoeducation empowers people to recognize emotional states and make informed decisions. This, in turn, might support immune function and overall health [184]. This can inform as well on the need of mindfulness interventions or support networks and social interventions, which will be discussed hereafter.

Lastly, it has been suggested for decades that social networks are causally related to disease and mortality risk, and tribe/clan interventions have been recognized as important in the improvement of mitochondrial health [64]. Social interactions are fundamental human needs, and the literature suggests that humans have evolved the need for social connection [185]. Ignoring these evolutionary expectations might impair the IS and diminish INS's efficacy. However, this field of research and its potential for implementation into T2DM care is still in its infancy. Research indicates that social networks play a crucial role in the prevention of T2DM. Social ties significantly influence individuals' perceptions, behaviors, and norms related to health behaviors, highlighting the importance of incorporating social networks into lifestyle interventions and T2DM management [186]. While this field is emerging, there is a notable need for more detailed studies that assess the specific benefits of integrating social networks into health interventions. However, as discussed earlier, there is strong longitudinal evidence that social isolation, particularly in men, and a general lack of social support in both genders are associated with an increased risk of developing T2DM [187]. The literature suggests that insufficient social support is linked to a heightened risk of severe T2D complications and that social support can significantly enhance T2DM self-management efforts [186].

Social support might serve as a crucial buffer in T2DM, promoting glycemic control. Social network intervention showed improved integration of patients within their existing networks, leading to a greater reduction in HbA1c and blood glucose, as well as improved behavior-mediating outcomes, as described in a prospective observational study [188].

We propose that in an environment with evolutionary expectations, such as acute stressors and evolutionary buffers proposed in this study, even individuals carrying genes that contribute to diabetes when food is plentiful and sedentary lifestyles are common, are less likely to develop DMT2. However, further studies need to be carried out to prove this hypothesis.

As an outcome measure, building upon the concept of mitoresilience previously discussed [143], we propose introducing 'insulin resilience' as an additional dimension within the psycho-social-biological framework aimed at addressing insulin-related conditions. This concept shifts the perception of INS from being merely a culprit in disease to a beneficial player in health management. By focusing on INS resilience, we could improve health communication with health-enhancing messages that align with the theory of regulatory focus [189].

The term 'INS resilience' aligns well with proposed interventions designed to be health-promoting rather than merely treating disease or IR. However, it is important to note the limitations of regulatory focus theory, particularly its complexity in real clinical settings and its relevance in the specific context of patients with T2DM [190]. Therefore, the use of the term 'INS resilience' requires further research to fully understand its applicability and impact in managing T2DM.

3.4. Complementary Tools to Measure the Impact of Interventions for Insulin Resilience

Furthermore, we advocate for the incorporation of Heart Rate Variability (HRV), previously proposed as a parameter for mitoresilience and individual resilience, into this comprehensive approach [143]. IR might be a hallmark of T2DM [56]. The literature states IR is closely linked to the performance of the autonomic nervous system (ANS) [191]. A systematic review and meta-analysis mentioned that IR is closely associated with a heightened sympathetic tone or vagal imbalance and reduced HRV values [192]. This autonomic impairment might be due to hyperinsulinemia alone or with hyperglycemia, potentially damaging peripheral nerves [193]. An observational study on overweight individuals with IR exhibited increased central activation of the HPA during hypoglycemia and showed that IR is a stronger predictor of the HPA response than obesity [16]. This suggests that factors beyond the classical nutritional risk factors might play a role in IR, which could support the hypothesis proposed in this article of INS functioning as—amongst others—a social substance. HRV has shown a correlation with HbA1c levels, suggesting its potential as a possible metric for monitoring glycemic control [194].

A meta-analysis and review of HRV suggests that the current neurobiological evidence informs HRV to be impacted by stress and supports its use for the objective assessment of psychological health and stress [195]. A recent observational study on 197 participants indicated that RSI—an HRV-based stress index—reacts to physiological changes related to psychosocial stress and recovery [16,196]. HRV has emerged as an important tool to measure the physiological response to stress, both in adults and children, as well as in research fields of psychiatric conditions and biological psychology [197].

Lastly, there might be a connection between HRV and mitochondria, as explained in a recent review from 2024. A bidirectional relationship seems to exist between the ANS and mitochondria where autonomic activity is thought to directly impact mitochondrial function, while mitochondria participate in and modulate ANS function and signaling [198]. Examples given are co-enzyme Q—a mitochondrial enzyme—enhancing ANS function in healthy humans [199], while mitochondria-derived ROS might mediate sympathetic activity [200]. Thereby, one of the first studies of a potential autonomic mechanism directly linking stress to mitochondrial dysfunction, which was a study in rats, showed that chronic stress results in persistent sympathetically mediated effects that subsequently alter mitochondrial function [201].

There are limitations on the use of HRV, and to the best of our knowledge, there is currently no consensus on normal ranges for these parameters, neither for healthy individuals nor for T2DM patients [197]. Furthermore, HRV is influenced by factors beyond stress and autonomic function, making it challenging to isolate the impact of single factors. For these reasons, the use of HRV in the specific context of this article requires further research.

Given the heterogeneity in the etiology of T2DM [56] and the subsequent need for personalized interventions and measurement tools, HRV emerges as a promising, affordable, and non-invasive tool. HRV shows sensitivity to psychosocial factors as well as T2DM hallmarks and parameters related to mitochondrial health, making it a valuable and complementary addition to existing clinical practices. Unlike parameters such as HbA1c and the Homeostatic Model Assessment (HOMA) index, which require professional evaluation and may limit patients' self-management capabilities, HRV allows for regular self-monitoring. This enables patients to actively participate in their health management, facilitating more frequent measurements and tracking the impact of various interventions on their condition.

It might also allow validation of the theoretical framework and subsequent interventions proposed in this article, given its sensitivity to IR, hyperglycemia, mitochondrial health, and psychological stress factors. This comprehensive sensitivity supports measuring the effects of personalized treatment methods, helping to detect trends and assess the effectiveness of specific interventions for individual patients. This approach is especially beneficial for patients seeking to actively engage in their self-care and therapeutic processes and with their supporting healthcare professionals.

The proposed theoretical framework, as well as the interventions and measurement tools proposed, needs further validation, and we, therefore, recommend quality research to confirm the above. A full overview of our theoretical framework and subsequent interventions can be found in Figure 3.

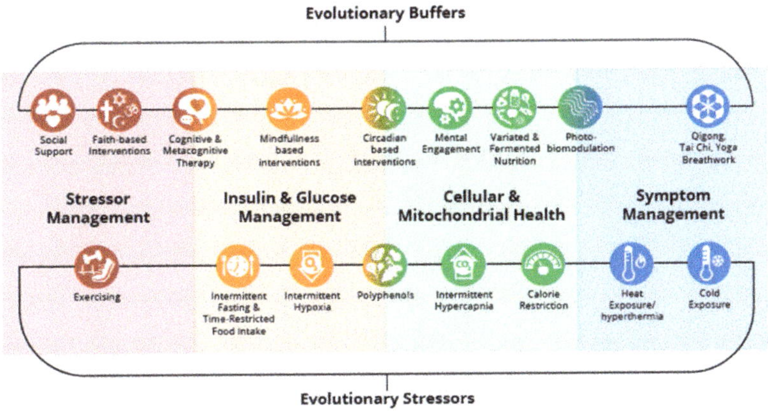

Figure 3. Evidence-based interventions within the mitochondrial information processing (MIPS) framework can enhance insulin resilience, a newly proposed health outcome resulting from the improvement of psychosocial factors and the implementation of evolutionary interventions. This ultimately contributes to positive health outcomes in conditions such as Type 2 Diabetes Mellitus (T2DM) with musculoskeletal (MS) problems and subsequent Chronic Non-Communicable Diseases (CNCDs), where the occurrence of one chronic condition increases the likelihood of developing additional diseases over time. Heart Rate Variability (HRV) is proposed as an additional parameter in the diagnostic toolbox, alongside existing parameters.

4. Conclusions

This article proposed an expanded view of INS as a metabolic-socio-psychological substance within the MIPS framework, suggesting its roles beyond metabolism, particularly in cooperating with mitochondria in processing psychosocial factors into the biological fabric. By exploring INS's potential involvement in mitochondrial sensing, integration, and transduction of psychosocial factors, we explored a theoretical framework that might link INS to a broader socio-psycho-biological approach to health.

Additionally, we adopted an evolutionary perspective, considering how modern psychosocial stressors may misalign with human evolutionary expectations. Mismatches between ancient evolutionary stressors (such as acute physical threats) and modern chronic stressors (such as social isolation or workplace pressures) might lead to chronic diseases, including T2DM with musculoskeletal and neurological complications.

Conversely, we proposed that integrative interventions aligned with evolutionary expectations—such as hormesis, intermittent fasting, physical exercise, breath work, and environmental stress exposure—might improve insulin resilience. Evolutionary buffers like diverse plant-based diets, fermentation, and maintaining circadian rhythms could also support metabolic and mitochondrial health.

Modern therapies, including photobiomodulation (PBM), but above all, psychosocial interventions such as mindfulness-based interventions, social network support and psychoeducation, meta-cognitive therapy and faith-based interventions, might offer integrative approaches to managing INS-implicated conditions. To evaluate these interventions, Heart Rate Variability (HRV) was proposed as a potential complementary diagnostic tool, alongside traditional clinical markers like HbA1c and insulin sensitivity indices. HRV's sensitivity to psychosocial stress and metabolic changes suggests that it might be a useful, non-invasive method for tracking intervention outcomes, especially in patients with T2DM and related complications.

Ultimately, viewing INS as a social substance within the MIPS framework suggests that addressing psychosocial factors and evolutionary expectations might be essential in managing INS-related diseases. This comprehensive perspective could enhance our understanding of INS beyond its metabolic functions and promote a more integrative, evidence-based approach to chronic disease management. However, this theoretical framework and the proposed interventions need further empirical validation through clinical studies to assess their effectiveness and practical application.

By incorporating psychosocial, biological, and evolutionary components, future research might focus on testing the proposed interventions and frameworks, with the goal of creating more holistic approaches to managing T2DM and other INS-implicated conditions. Addressing upstream psychosocial needs, alongside downstream metabolic processes, might improve patient outcomes and treatment efficacy.

Author Contributions: Study conception: A.W. and S.N.-L.; design: A.W. and S.N.-L.; acquisition of data: A.W. and S.N.-L.; analysis and interpretation of data: A.W., S.S.R.-M., L.P. and S.N.-L.; drafting of manuscript: A.W. and S.N.-L.; critical revision: S.N.-L., S.S.R.-M. and L.P. All authors have read and agreed to the published version of the manuscript.

Funding: This research received no external funding.

Conflicts of Interest: The authors declare no conflicts of interest.

Abbreviations

ACE	Adverse childhood events
AGEs	Advanced glycation end-products
AIF	Apoptosis-inducing factor
AKT	AKT-kinase (Protein Kinase B)
BAD	Bcl-2-associated death promoter
BAX	Bcl-2-associated X protein
BCL2	B-cell lymphoma 2
Ca^{2+}	Calcium ions
CAMP	Cyclic adenosine monophosphate
CNCDs	Chronic non-communicable diseases
CORT	Cortisol
cf-mtDNA	Cell-free mitochondrial DNA
CREB	cAMP response element-binding protein
CYTC	Cytochrome c
DAG	Diacylglycerol
Drp1	Dynamin-related protein 1
DST	Dexamethasone suppression test
ECC	Excitation-contraction coupling
ECM	Extracellular matrix
ER	Endoplasmic reticulum
ERK1/2	Extracellular signal-regulated kinases 1 and 2
FBIs	Faith-based interventions
FM	Fibromyalgia
FoxO1	Forkhead box protein O1
FOS	FBJ murine osteosarcoma viral oncogene homolog
GDF15	Growth differentiation factor 15
GSK-3β	Glycogen synthase kinase 3 beta

HPA	Hypothalamus-pituitary-adrenal axis
HRV	Heart rate variability
IGF-1	Insulin-like growth factor 1
IGF1Rs	Insulin-like growth factor 1 receptors
INS	Insulin
INR	Insulin receptor
INSR/IGF1Rs	Hybrid insulin receptors/insulin-like growth factor 1 receptors
INSRs	Insulin receptors
INSS	Insulin signaling
IR	Insulin resistance
MAPK	Mitogen-Activated Protein Kinase
MAMs	Mitochondria-associated membranes
MIPS	Mitochondrial Information Processing System
MDPs	Mitochondrial-derived peptides
MIPs	Mitochondrial Information Processors
mTOR	Mechanistic target of rapamycin
mtDNA	Mitochondrial DNA
MOTS-c	Mitochondrial Open Reading Frame of the 12S rRNA-c
MOMP	Mitochondrial outer membrane permeabilization
MIMP	Mitochondrial inner membrane permeabilization
MSD	Musculoskeletal disorders
MSDs	Musculoskeletal disorders
MSK	Musculoskeletal
MSS	Musculoskeletal system
mTORC1	Mechanistic target of rapamycin complex 1
MYC	Myelocytomatosis oncogene
NAD(+)/NADH	Nicotinamide adenine dinucleotide (oxidized form)/ Nicotinamide adenine dinucleotide (reduced form)
NF-kB	Nuclear factor kappa-light-chain-enhancer of activated B cells
OXPHOS	Oxidative phosphorylation
PI3K	Phosphoinositide 3-kinase
PGC-1α	Peroxisome proliferator-activated receptor gamma coactivator 1-alpha
PNI	Psychoneuroimmunology
RAS	Rat sarcoma
RAF	Rapidly Accelerated Fibrosarcoma kinase
RCT	Randomized Controlled Trial
ROS	Reactive oxygen species
SAM	Sympathetic-adrenomedullary axis
SHLPs	Small HN-like peptides
SM	Skeletal muscle
SR	Sarcoplasmic reticulum
T2DM	Type 2 Diabetes Mellitus
TCA	Tricarboxylic acid cycle
ULK1	Unc-51 like autophagy activating kinase 1

References

1. Norton, L.; Shannon, C.; Gastaldelli, A.; DeFronzo, R.A. Insulin: The master regulator of glucose metabolism. *Metabolism* **2022**, *129*, 155142. [CrossRef] [PubMed]
2. Picard, M.; Shirihai, O.S. Mitochondrial signal transduction. *Cell Metab.* **2022**, *34*, 1620–1653. [CrossRef] [PubMed]
3. Picard, M.; Sandi, C. The social nature of mitochondria: Implications for human health. *Neurosci. Biobehav. Rev.* **2021**, *120*, 595–610. [CrossRef] [PubMed]
4. Daniels, T.E.; Olsen, E.M.; Tyrka, A.R. Stress and Psychiatric Disorders: The Role of Mitochondria. *Annu. Rev. Clin. Psychol.* **2020**, *16*, 165–186. [CrossRef]
5. Duchowny, K.A.; Marcinek, D.J.; Mau, T.; Diaz-Ramierz, L.G.; Lui, L.Y.; Toledo, F.G.S.; Cawthon, P.M.; Hepple, R.T.; Kramer, P.A.; Newman, A.B.; et al. Childhood adverse life events and skeletal muscle mitochondrial function. *Sci. Adv.* **2024**, *10*, eadj6411. [CrossRef]
6. Stoolman, J.S.; Porcelli, A.M.; Martínez-Reyes, I. Editorial: Mitochondria as a hub in cellular signaling. *Front. Cell Dev. Biol.* **2022**, *10*, 981464. [CrossRef]

7. Bahat, A.; Gross, A. Mitochondrial plasticity in cell fate regulation. *J. Biol. Chem.* **2019**, *294*, 13852–13863. [CrossRef]
8. Tilokani, L.; Nagashima, S.; Paupe, V.; Prudent, J. Mitochondrial dynamics: Overview of molecular mechanisms. *Essays Biochem.* **2018**, *62*, 341–360.
9. Chen, W.; Zhao, H.; Li, Y. Mitochondrial dynamics in health and disease: Mechanisms and potential targets. *Signal Transduct. Target. Ther.* **2023**, *8*, 333. [CrossRef]
10. Aguilar-López, B.A.; Moreno-Altamirano, M.M.B.; Dockrell, H.M.; Duchen, M.R.; Sánchez-García, F.J. Mitochondria: An Integrative Hub Coordinating Circadian Rhythms, Metabolism, the Microbiome, and Immunity. *Front. Cell Dev. Biol.* **2020**, *8*, 51. [CrossRef]
11. Shen, K.; Pender, C.L.; Bar-Ziv, R.; Zhang, H.; Wickham, K.; Willey, E.; Durieux, J.; Ahmad, Q.; Dillin, A. Mitochondria as Cellular and Organismal Signaling Hubs. *Annu. Rev. Cell Dev. Biol.* **2022**, *38*, 179–218. [CrossRef] [PubMed]
12. Liu, X.; Zhang, X.; Zhao, L.; Long, J.; Feng, Z.; Su, J.; Gao, F.; Liu, J. Mitochondria as a sensor, a central hub and a biological clock in psychological stress-accelerated aging. *Ageing Res. Rev.* **2024**, *93*, 102145. [CrossRef] [PubMed]
13. Barabino, S.; Lombardi, S.; Zilocchi, M. Keep in touch: A perspective on the mitochondrial social network and its implication in health and disease. *Cell Death Discov.* **2023**, *9*, 417. [CrossRef] [PubMed]
14. Ruiz-Núñez, B.; Pruimboom, L.; Dijck-Brouwer, D.A.J.; Muskiet, F.A.J. Lifestyle and nutritional imbalances associated with Western diseases: Causes and consequences of chronic systemic low-grade inflammation in an evolutionary context. *J. Nutr. Biochem.* **2013**, *24*, 1183–1201. [CrossRef]
15. Sadeghi, A.; Niknam, M.; Momeni-Moghaddam, M.A.; Shabani, M.; Aria, H.; Bastin, A.; Teimouri, m.; Meshkani, R.; Akbar, H. Crosstalk between autophagy and insulin resistance: Evidence from different tissues. *Eur. J. Med. Res.* **2023**, *28*, 456. [CrossRef]
16. Lundqvist, M.H.; Almby, K.; Wiklund, U.; Abrahamsson, N.; Kamble, P.G.; Pereira, M.J.; Eriksson, J.W. Altered hormonal and autonomic nerve responses to hypo- and hyperglycaemia are found in overweight and insulin-resistant individuals and may contribute to the development of type 2 diabetes. *Diabetologia* **2021**, *64*, 641–655. [CrossRef]
17. Yaribeygi, H.; Maleki, M.; Butler, A.E.; Jamialahmadi, T.; Sahebkar, A. Molecular mechanisms linking stress and insulin resistance. *EXCLI J.* **2022**, *21*, 317–334.
18. Fang, X.; Jiang, S.; Wang, J.; Bai, Y.; Kim, C.S.; Blake, D.; Weintraub, N.L.; Lei, Y.; Lu, X. Chronic unpredictable stress induces depression-related behaviors by suppressing AgRP neuron activity. *Mol. Psychiatry* **2021**, *26*, 2299–2315. [CrossRef]
19. Jais, A.; Brüning, J.C. Arcuate Nucleus-Dependent Regulation of Metabolism—Pathways to Obesity and Diabetes Mellitus. *Endocr. Rev.* **2022**, *43*, 314–328. [CrossRef]
20. Galizzi, G.; Di Carlo, M. Insulin and Its Key Role for Mitochondrial Function/Dysfunction and Quality Control: A Shared Link between Dysmetabolism and Neurodegeneration. *Biology* **2022**, *11*, 943. [CrossRef]
21. Hees, J.T.; Wanderoy, S.; Lindner, J.; Helms, M.; Murali Mahadevan, H.; Harbauer, A.B. Insulin signalling regulates Pink1 mRNA localization via modulation of AMPK activity to support PINK1 function in neurons. *Nat. Metab.* **2024**, *6*, 514–530. [CrossRef] [PubMed]
22. Goodpaster, B.H.; Coen, P.M. Improved Mitochondrial Function Is Linked with Improved Insulin Sensitivity Through Reductions in FFA. *Diabetes* **2014**, *63*, 2611–2612. [CrossRef] [PubMed]
23. Cheng, Z.; Tseng, Y.; White, M.F. Insulin signaling meets mitochondria in metabolism. *Trends Endocrinol. Metab.* **2010**, *21*, 589–598. [CrossRef] [PubMed]
24. Zhang, H.; Li, X.; Fan, W.; Pandovski, S.; Tian, Y.; Dillin, A. Inter-tissue communication of mitochondrial stress and metabolic health. *Life Metab.* **2023**, *2*, load001. [CrossRef]
25. Constantin-Teodosiu, D.; Constantin, D.; Pelsers, M.M.; Verdijk, L.B.; van Loon, L.; Greenhaff, P.L. Mitochondrial DNA copy number associates with insulin sensitivity and aerobic capacity, and differs between sedentary, overweight middle-aged males with and without type 2 diabetes. *Int. J. Obes.* **2020**, *44*, 929–936. [CrossRef] [PubMed]
26. Schaefer, A.M.; Taylor, R.W.; Turnbull, D.M.; Chinnery, P.F. The epidemiology of mitochondrial disorders—Past, present and future. *Biochim. Et Biophys. Acta (BBA)—Bioenerg.* **2004**, *1659*, 115–120. [CrossRef] [PubMed]
27. Liu, Y.F.; Zhu, J.J.; Yu Tian, X.; Liu, H.; Zhang, T.; Zhang, Y.P.; Xie, S.A.; Zhen, M.; Kong, W.; Yao, W.J.; et al. Hypermethylation of mitochondrial DNA in vascular smooth muscle cells impairs cell contractility. *Cell Death Dis.* **2020**, *11*, 35. [CrossRef] [PubMed]
28. Zheng, L.D.; Linarelli, L.E.; Liu, L.; Wall, S.S.; Greenawald, M.H.; Seidel, R.W.; Estabrooks, P.; Almeida, F.A.; Cheng, Z. Insulin resistance is associated with epigenetic and genetic regulation of mitochondrial DNA in obese humans. *Clin. Epigenet.* **2015**, *7*, 60. [CrossRef]
29. Katsampouris, E.; Turner-Cobb, J.M.; Barnett, J.C.; Arnold, R.S. Can ancient and modern stressors be distinguished? A mixed-methods exploration of psychosocial characteristics and health symptoms in young and older adults. *J. Health Psychol.* **2022**, *27*, 624–636. [CrossRef]
30. Pruimboom, L. The Selfish Immune System when the Immune System Overrides the 'Selfish' Brain. *J. Immunol. Clin. Microbiol.* **2020**, *5*, 1–34.
31. Raison, C.L.; Miller, A.H. The evolutionary significance of depression in Pathogen Host Defense (PATHOS-D). *Mol. Psychiatry* **2013**, *18*, 15–37. [CrossRef] [PubMed]
32. Raison, C.L.; Miller, A.H. Malaise, melancholia and madness: The evolutionary legacy of an inflammatory bias. *Brain Behav. Immun.* **2013**, *31*, 1–8. [CrossRef]

33. Leulier, F.; Lemaitre, B. Toll-like receptors—Taking an evolutionary approach. *Nat. Rev. Genet.* **2008**, *9*, 165–178. [CrossRef] [PubMed]
34. Ortega, V.A.; Mercer, E.M.; Giesbrecht, G.F.; Arrieta, M.C. Evolutionary Significance of the Neuroendocrine Stress Axis on Vertebrate Immunity and the Influence of the Microbiome on Early-Life Stress Regulation and Health Outcomes. *Front. Microbiol.* **2021**, *12*, 634539. [CrossRef] [PubMed]
35. Picard, M.; McEwen, B.S. Psychological Stress and Mitochondria: A Conceptual Framework. *Psychosom. Med.* **2018**, *80*, 126–140. [CrossRef] [PubMed]
36. Navarro-Ledesma, S.; Gijon-Nogueron, G.; Reina-Martín, I.; Ortega-Avila, A.B.; Pruimboom, L. Patellar and Achilles Tendon Thickness Differences among Athletes with Different Numbers of Meals per Day: A Cross-Sectional Study. *Int. J. Environ. Res. Public Health* **2022**, *19*, 2468. [CrossRef]
37. Rorsman, P.; Ashcroft, F.M. Pancreatic β-Cell Electrical Activity and Insulin Secretion: Of Mice and Men. *Physiol. Rev.* **2018**, *98*, 117–214. [CrossRef]
38. Godoy, L.D.; Rossignoli, M.T.; Delfino-Pereira, P.; Garcia-Cairasco, N.; de Lima Umeoka, E.H. A Comprehensive Overview on Stress Neurobiology: Basic Concepts and Clinical Implications. *Front. Behav. Neurosci.* **2018**, *12*, 127. [CrossRef]
39. Aslanoglou, D.; Bertera, S.; Sánchez-Soto, M.; Benjamin Free, R.; Lee, J.; Zong, W.; Xue, X.; Shrestha, S.; Brissova, M.; Logan, R.W.; et al. Dopamine regulates pancreatic glucagon and insulin secretion via adrenergic and dopaminergic receptors. *Transl. Psychiatry* **2021**, *11*, 59. [CrossRef]
40. Afrisham, R.; Paknejad, M.; Soliemanifar, O.; Sadegh-Nejadi, S.; Meshkani, R.; Ashtary-Larky, D. The Influence of Psychological Stress on the Initiation and Progression of Diabetes and Cancer. *Int. J. Endocrinol. Metab.* **2019**, *in press*. [CrossRef]
41. Lewis, S.T.; Greenway, F.; Tucker, T.R.; Alexander, M.; Jackson, L.K.; Hepford, S.A.; Loveridge, B.; Lakey, J.R.R. A Receptor Story: Insulin Resistance Pathophysiology and Physiologic Insulin Resensitization's Role as a Treatment Modality. *Int. J. Mol. Sci.* **2023**, *24*, 10927. [CrossRef] [PubMed]
42. Zefferino, R.; Di Gioia, S.; Conese, M. Molecular links between endocrine, nervous and immune system during chronic stress. *Brain Behav.* **2021**, *11*, e01960. [CrossRef] [PubMed]
43. Muskiet, F.; Carrera-Bastos, P.; Pruimboom, L.; Lucia, A.; Furman, D. Obesity and Leptin Resistance in the Regulation of the Type I Interferon Early Response and the Increased Risk for Severe COVID-19. *Nutrients* **2022**, *14*, 1388. [CrossRef] [PubMed]
44. Dhabhar, F.S. Effects of stress on immune function: The good, the bad, and the beautiful. *Immunol. Res.* **2014**, *58*, 193–210. [CrossRef] [PubMed]
45. Dhabhar, F.S. The short-term stress response—Mother nature's mechanism for enhancing protection and performance under conditions of threat, challenge, and opportunity. *Front. Neuroendocrinol.* **2018**, *49*, 175–192. [CrossRef]
46. White, A.G.; Elias, E.; Orozco, A.; Robinson, S.A.; Manners, M.T. Chronic Stress-Induced Neuroinflammation: Relevance of Rodent Models to Human Disease. *Int. J. Mol. Sci.* **2024**, *25*, 5085. [CrossRef]
47. Snyder-Mackler, N.; Sanz, J.; Kohn, J.N.; Brinkworth, J.F.; Morrow, S.; Shaver, A.O.; Grenier, J.C.; Pique-Regi, R.; Johnson, Z.P.; Wilson, M.E.; et al. Social status alters immune regulation and response to infection in macaques. *Science* **2016**, *354*, 1041–1045. [CrossRef]
48. Matrisciano, F.; Pinna, G. PPAR-α Hypermethylation in the Hippocampus of Mice Exposed to Social Isolation Stress Is Associated with Enhanced Neuroinflammation and Aggressive Behavior. *Int. J. Mol. Sci.* **2021**, *22*, 10678. [CrossRef]
49. Cacioppo, J.T.; Cacioppo, S. Loneliness in the modern age: An evolutionary theory of loneliness (ETL). In *Advances in Experimental Social Psychology*; Elsevier Academic Press: Cambridge, MA, USA, 2018; Volume 58, pp. 127–197.
50. de Luca, C.; Olefsky, J.M. Inflammation and insulin resistance. *FEBS Lett.* **2008**, *582*, 97–105. [CrossRef]
51. Taniguchi, C.M.; Emanuelli, B.; Kahn, C.R. Critical nodes in signalling pathways: Insights into insulin action. *Nat. Rev. Mol. Cell Biol.* **2006**, *7*, 85–96. [CrossRef]
52. Miller, A.H.; Raison, C.L. The role of inflammation in depression: From evolutionary imperative to modern treatment target. *Nat. Rev. Immunol.* **2016**, *16*, 22–34. [CrossRef] [PubMed]
53. Nash, A.I. Crosstalk between insulin and dopamine signaling: A basis for the metabolic effects of antipsychotic drugs. *J. Chem. Neuroanat.* **2017**, *83–84*, 59–68. [CrossRef] [PubMed]
54. Bhatt, N. Oxytocin as a Metabolic Modulator. In *Oxytocin and Health*; IntechOpen: London, UK, 2021.
55. Woo, H.; Hong, C.J.; Jung, S.; Choe, S.; Yu, S.W. Chronic restraint stress induces hippocampal memory deficits by impairing insulin signaling. *Mol. Brain* **2018**, *11*, 37. [CrossRef] [PubMed]
56. Larsen, J.; Stocks, B.; Henderson, J.; Andersson, D.; Backdahl, J.; Eriksson-Hogling, D.; Stidsen, J.; Sakamoto, K.; Hojlund, K.; Ryden, M.; et al. Personalized Molecular Signatures of Insulin Resistance and Type 2 Diabetes. *bioRxiv* **2024**. [CrossRef]
57. Harris, M.L.; Oldmeadow, C.; Hure, A.; Luu, J.; Loxton, D.; Attia, J. Stress increases the risk of type 2 diabetes onset in women: A 12-year longitudinal study using causal modelling. *PLoS ONE* **2017**, *12*, e0172126. [CrossRef] [PubMed]
58. Navarro-Ledesma, S.; Hamed-Hamed, D.; González-Muñoz, A.; Pruimboom, L. Physical Activity, Insulin Resistance and Cancer: A Systematic Review. *Cancers* **2024**, *16*, 656. [CrossRef]
59. Guan, X.; Yan, Q.; Wang, D.; Du, G.; Zhou, J. IGF-1 Signaling Regulates Mitochondrial Remodeling during Myogenic Differentiation. *Nutrients* **2022**, *14*, 1249. [CrossRef]

60. Radovic, S.M.; Starovlah, I.M.; Capo, I.; Miljkovic, D.; Nef, S.; Kostic, T.S.; Andric, S.A. Insulin/IGF1 signaling regulates the mitochondrial biogenesis markers in steroidogenic cells of prepubertal testis, but not ovary. *Biol. Reprod.* **2019**, *100*, 253–267. [CrossRef]
61. Ren, Z.; Zhong, H.; Song, C.; Deng, C.; Hsieh, H.T.; Liu, W.; Chen, G. Insulin Promotes Mitochondrial Respiration and Survival through PI3K/AKT/GSK3 Pathway in Human Embryonic Stem Cells. *Stem Cell Rep.* **2020**, *15*, 1362–1376. [CrossRef]
62. Klimczak, S.; Śliwińska, A. Epigenetic regulation of inflammation in insulin resistance. *Semin. Cell Dev. Biol.* **2024**, *154*, 185–192. [CrossRef]
63. Manning, B.D.; Toker, A. AKT/PKB Signaling: Navigating the Network. *Cell* **2017**, *169*, 381–405. [CrossRef] [PubMed]
64. Casanova, A.; Wevers, A.; Navarro-Ledesma, S.; Pruimboom, L. Mitochondria: It is all about energy. *Front. Physiol.* **2023**, *14*, 1114231. [CrossRef] [PubMed]
65. Li, X.; Teng, T.; Yan, W.; Fan, L.; Liu, X.; Clarke, G.; Zhu, D.; Jiang, Y.; Xiang, Y.; Yu, Y.; et al. AKT and MAPK signaling pathways in hippocampus reveals the pathogenesis of depression in four stress-induced models. *Transl. Psychiatry* **2023**, *13*, 200. [CrossRef] [PubMed]
66. Liu, Y.J.; McIntyre, R.L.; Janssens, G.E.; Houtkooper, R.H. Mitochondrial fission and fusion: A dynamic role in aging and potential target for age-related disease. *Mech. Ageing Dev.* **2020**, *186*, 111212. [CrossRef]
67. Leonard, A.P.; Cameron, R.B.; Speiser, J.L.; Wolf, B.J.; Peterson, Y.K.; Schnellmann, R.G.; Beeson, C.C.; Rohrer, B. Quantitative analysis of mitochondrial morphology and membrane potential in living cells using high-content imaging, machine learning, and morphological binning. *Biochim. Et Biophys. Acta (BBA)—Mol. Cell Res.* **2015**, *1853*, 348–360. [CrossRef]
68. Xie, K.; Tan, K.; Naylor, M.J. Transcription Factors as Novel Therapeutic Targets and Drivers of Prostate Cancer Progression. *Front. Oncol.* **2022**, *12*, 854151. [CrossRef]
69. Ribeiro, M.; Rosenstock, T.R.; Oliveira, A.M.; Oliveira, C.R.; Rego, A.C. Insulin and IGF-1 improve mitochondrial function in a PI-3K/Akt-dependent manner and reduce mitochondrial generation of reactive oxygen species in Huntington's disease knock-in striatal cells. *Free Radic. Biol. Med.* **2014**, *74*, 129–144. [CrossRef]
70. Andres, A.M.; Stotland, A.; Queliconi, B.B.; Gottlieb, R.A. A time to reap, a time to sow: Mitophagy and biogenesis in cardiac pathophysiology. *J. Mol. Cell Cardiol.* **2015**, *78*, 62–72. [CrossRef]
71. Yang, K.; Chen, Z.; Gao, J.; Shi, W.; Li, L.; Jiang, S.; Hu, H.; Liu, Z.; Xu, D.; Wu, L. The Key Roles of GSK-3β in Regulating Mitochondrial Activity. *Cell. Physiol. Biochem.* **2017**, *44*, 1445–1459. [CrossRef]
72. Cheng, Z. FoxO transcription factors in mitochondrial homeostasis. *Biochem. J.* **2022**, *479*, 525–536. [CrossRef]
73. Xie, X.; Shu, R.; Yu, C.; Fu, Z.; Li, Z. Mammalian AKT, the Emerging Roles on Mitochondrial Function in Diseases. *Aging Dis.* **2022**, *13*, 157. [CrossRef] [PubMed]
74. Cook, S.J.; Stuart, K.; Gilley, R.; Sale, M.J. Control of cell death and mitochondrial fission by ERK1/2 MAP kinase signalling. *FEBS J.* **2017**, *284*, 4177–4195. [CrossRef] [PubMed]
75. Bove, M.; Lama, A.; Schiavone, S.; Pirozzi, C.; Tucci, P.; Sikora, V.; Trinchese, G.; Corso, G.; Morgese, M.G.; Trabace, L. Social isolation triggers oxidative status and impairs systemic and hepatic insulin sensitivity in normoglycemic rats. *Biomed. Pharmacother.* **2022**, *149*, 112820. [CrossRef] [PubMed]
76. Iio, W.; Matsukawa, N.; Tsukahara, T.; Kohari, D.; Toyoda, A. Effects of chronic social defeat stress on MAP kinase cascade. *Neurosci. Lett.* **2011**, *504*, 281–284. [CrossRef] [PubMed]
77. Lv, Y.; Cheng, L.; Peng, F. Compositions and Functions of Mitochondria-Associated Endoplasmic Reticulum Membranes and Their Contribution to Cardioprotection by Exercise Preconditioning. *Front. Physiol.* **2022**, *13*, 910452. [CrossRef]
78. Cheng, H.; Gang, X.; He, G.; Liu, Y.; Wang, Y.; Zhao, X.; Wang, G. The Molecular Mechanisms Underlying Mitochondria-Associated Endoplasmic Reticulum Membrane-Induced Insulin Resistance. *Front. Endocrinol.* **2020**, *11*, 592129. [CrossRef]
79. Xu, H.; Zhou, W.; Zhan, L.; Bi, T.; Lu, X. Liver mitochondria-associated endoplasmic reticulum membrane proteomics for studying the effects of ZiBuPiYin recipe on Zucker diabetic fatty rats after chronic psychological stress. *Front. Cell Dev. Biol.* **2022**, *10*, 995732. [CrossRef]
80. Williams, C.F.; George, C.H. Connect and Conquer: Collectivized Behavior of Mitochondria and Bacteria. *Front. Physiol.* **2019**, *10*, 340. [CrossRef]
81. Burtscher, J.; Soltany, A.; Visavadiya, N.P.; Burtscher, M.; Millet, G.P.; Khoramipour, K.; Khamoui, A.V. Mitochondrial stress and mitokines in aging. *Aging Cell* **2023**, *22*, e13770. [CrossRef]
82. Klaus, S.; Ost, M. Mitochondrial uncoupling and longevity—A role for mitokines? *Exp. Gerontol.* **2020**, *130*, 110796. [CrossRef]
83. Johann, K.; Kleinert, M.; Klaus, S. The Role of GDF15 as a Myomitokine. *Cells* **2021**, *10*, 2990. [CrossRef] [PubMed]
84. Mohtashami, Z.; Singh, M.K.; Salimiaghdam, N.; Ozgul, M.; Kenney, M.C. MOTS-c, the Most Recent Mitochondrial Derived Peptide in Human Aging and Age-Related Diseases. *Int. J. Mol. Sci.* **2022**, *23*, 11991. [CrossRef] [PubMed]
85. Yuzefovych, L.V.; Pastukh, V.M.; Ruchko, M.V.; Simmons, J.D.; Richards, W.O.; Rachek, L.I. Plasma mitochondrial DNA is elevated in obese type 2 diabetes mellitus patients and correlates positively with insulin resistance. *PLoS ONE* **2019**, *14*, e0222278. [CrossRef] [PubMed]
86. Thurairajah, K.; Briggs, G.D.; Balogh, Z.J. The source of cell-free mitochondrial DNA in trauma and potential therapeutic strategies. *Eur. J. Trauma. Emerg. Surg.* **2018**, *44*, 325–334. [CrossRef] [PubMed]

87. Trumpff, C.; Michelson, J.; Lagranha, C.J.; Taleon, V.; Karan, K.R.; Sturm, G.; Lindqvist, D.; Fernström, J.; Moser, D.; Kaufman, B.A.; et al. Stress and circulating cell-free mitochondrial DNA: A systematic review of human studies, physiological considerations, and technical recommendations. *Mitochondrion* **2021**, *59*, 225–245. [CrossRef]
88. Palma, F.R.; Gantner, B.N.; Sakiyama, M.J.; Kayzuka, C.; Shukla, S.; Lacchini, R.; Cunniff, B.; Boini, M.G. ROS production by mitochondria: Function or dysfunction? *Oncogene* **2024**, *43*, 295–303. [CrossRef]
89. Zhang, C.; Meng, Y.; Han, J. Emerging roles of mitochondrial functions and epigenetic changes in the modulation of stem cell fate. *Cell. Mol. Life Sci.* **2024**, *81*, 26. [CrossRef]
90. Low, H.C.; Chilian, W.M.; Ratnam, W.; Karupaiah, T.; Md Noh, M.F.; Mansor, F.; Xiang, Z.; Pung, Y.F. Changes in Mitochondrial Epigenome in Type 2 Diabetes Mellitus. *Br. J. Biomed. Sci.* **2023**, *80*, 10884. [CrossRef]
91. Lan, J.; Rollins, J.A.; Zang, X.; Wu, D.; Zou, L.; Wang, Z.; Ye, C.; Wu, Z.; Kapahi, P.; Rogers, A.N.; et al. Translational Regulation of Non-autonomous Mitochondrial Stress Response Promotes Longevity. *Cell Rep.* **2019**, *28*, 1050–1062.e6. [CrossRef]
92. Rautenberg, E.K.; Hamzaoui, Y.; Coletta, D.K. Mini-review: Mitochondrial DNA methylation in type 2 diabetes and obesity. *Front. Endocrinol.* **2022**, *13*, 968268. [CrossRef]
93. Trumpff, C.; Marsland, A.L.; Sloan, R.P.; Kaufman, B.A.; Picard, M. Predictors of ccf-mtDNA reactivity to acute psychological stress identified using machine learning classifiers: A proof-of-concept. *Psychoneuroendocrinology* **2019**, *107*, 82–92. [CrossRef] [PubMed]
94. Picard, M.; Trumpff, C.; Burelle, Y. Mitochondrial psychobiology: Foundations and applications. *Curr. Opin. Behav. Sci.* **2019**, *28*, 142–151. [CrossRef] [PubMed]
95. Hummel, E.M.; Hessas, E.; Müller, S.; Beiter, T.; Fisch, M.; Eibl, A.; Wolf, O.T.; Giebel, B.; Platen, P.; Kumsta, R.; et al. Cell-free DNA release under psychosocial and physical stress conditions. *Transl. Psychiatry* **2018**, *8*, 236. [CrossRef] [PubMed]
96. Lima, T.; Li, T.Y.; Mottis, A.; Auwerx, J. Pleiotropic effects of mitochondria in aging. *Nat. Aging* **2022**, *2*, 199–213. [CrossRef] [PubMed]
97. Ramanjaneya, M.; Jerobin, J.; Bettahi, I.; Bensila, M.; Aye, M.; Siveen, K.S.; Satyapalan, T.; Skarulis, M.; Abou-Samra, A.B.; Atkin, S.L. Lipids and insulin regulate mitochondrial-derived peptide (MOTS-c) in PCOS and healthy subjects. *Clin. Endocrinol.* **2019**, *91*, 278–287. [CrossRef]
98. Lindqvist, D.; Wolkowitz, O.M.; Picard, M.; Ohlsson, L.; Bersani, F.S.; Fernström, J.; Westrin, A.; Hough, C.M.; Lin, J.; Reus, V.I.; et al. Circulating cell-free mitochondrial DNA, but not leukocyte mitochondrial DNA copy number, is elevated in major depressive disorder. *Neuropsychopharmacology* **2018**, *43*, 1557–1564. [CrossRef]
99. Azami, M.; Moradkhani, A.; Afraie, M.; Saed, L.; Tapak, M.A.; Khoramipoor, K.; Khateri, S.; Moradi, Y. The association between diabetes mellitus and musculoskeletal disorders: A systematic review and meta-analysis. *Front. Endocrinol.* **2024**, *15*, 1320468. [CrossRef]
100. Lopez-Pedrosa, J.M.; Camprubi-Robles, M.; Guzman-Rolo, G.; Lopez-Gonzalez, A.; Garcia-Almeida, J.M.; Sanz-Paris, A.; Rueda, R. The Vicious Cycle of Type 2 Diabetes Mellitus and Skeletal Muscle Atrophy: Clinical, Biochemical, and Nutritional Bases. *Nutrients* **2024**, *16*, 172. [CrossRef]
101. Memon, A.A.; Sundquist, J.; Hedelius, A.; Palmér, K.; Wang, X.; Sundquist, K. Association of mitochondrial DNA copy number with prevalent and incident type 2 diabetes in women: A population-based follow-up study. *Sci. Rep.* **2021**, *11*, 4608. [CrossRef]
102. Freeman, A.M.; Acevedo, L.A.; Pennings, N. Insulin Resistance. In *StatPearls [Internet]*; StatPearls Publishing: Treasure Island, FL, USA, 2024.
103. Csonka, V.; Varjú, C.; Lendvay, M. Diabetes mellitus-related musculoskeletal disorders: Unveiling the cluster of diseases. *Prim. Care Diabetes* **2023**, *17*, 548–553. [CrossRef]
104. Mountain, R.V.; Langlais, A.L.; Hu, D.; Baron, R.; Lary, C.W.; Motyl, K.J. Social Isolation Causes Cortical and Trabecular Bone Loss in Adult Male, but not Female, C57BL/6J Mice. *bioRxiv* **2023**. [CrossRef]
105. Lingappan, K. NF-κB in oxidative stress. *Curr. Opin. Toxicol.* **2018**, *7*, 81–86. [CrossRef] [PubMed]
106. Chen, T.H.; Koh, K.Y.; Lin, K.M.C.; Chou, C.K. Mitochondrial Dysfunction as an Underlying Cause of Skeletal Muscle Disorders. *Int. J. Mol. Sci.* **2022**, *23*, 12926. [CrossRef] [PubMed]
107. Dong, H.; Tsai, S.Y. Mitochondrial Properties in Skeletal Muscle Fiber. *Cells* **2023**, *12*, 2183. [CrossRef]
108. Genders, A.J.; Holloway, G.P.; Bishop, D.J. Are Alterations in Skeletal Muscle Mitochondria a Cause or Consequence of Insulin Resistance? *Int. J. Mol. Sci.* **2020**, *21*, 6948. [CrossRef]
109. Di Leo, V.; Bernardino Gomes, T.M.; Vincent, A.E. Interactions of mitochondrial and skeletal muscle biology in mitochondrial myopathy. *Biochem. J.* **2023**, *480*, 1767–1789. [CrossRef]
110. Willingham, T.B.; Ajayi, P.T.; Glancy, B. Subcellular Specialization of Mitochondrial Form and Function in Skeletal Muscle Cells. *Front. Cell Dev. Biol.* **2021**, *9*, 757305. [CrossRef]
111. Riley, J.S.; Quarato, G.; Cloix, C.; Lopez, J.; O'Prey, J.; Pearson, M.; Chapman, J.; Sesaki, H.; Carlin, L.M.; Passos, J.F.; et al. Mitochondrial inner membrane permeabilisation enables mtDNA release during apoptosis. *EMBO J.* **2018**, *37*, e99238. [CrossRef]
112. Marchioretti, C.; Zanetti, G.; Pirazzini, M.; Gherardi, G.; Nogara, L.; Andreotti, R.; Martini, P.; Marcucci, L.; Canato, M.; Nath, S.R.; et al. Defective excitation-contraction coupling and mitochondrial respiration precede mitochondrial Ca^{2+} accumulation in spinobulbar muscular atrophy skeletal muscle. *Nat. Commun.* **2023**, *14*, 602. [CrossRef]

113. Dubinin, M.V.; Mikheeva, I.B.; Stepanova, A.E.; Igoshkina, A.D.; Cherepanova, A.A.; Semenova, A.A.; Sharapov, V.A.; Kireev, I.I.; Belosludtsev, K.N. Mitochondrial Transplantation Therapy Ameliorates Muscular Dystrophy in mdx Mouse Model. *Biomolecules* **2024**, *14*, 316. [CrossRef]
114. Du, J.; Wang, Y.; Hunter, R.; Wei, Y.; Blumenthal, R.; Falke, C.; Khairova, R.; Zhou, R.; Yuan, P.; Machado-Vieira, R.; et al. Dynamic regulation of mitochondrial function by glucocorticoids. *Proc. Natl. Acad. Sci. USA* **2009**, *106*, 3543–3548. [CrossRef] [PubMed]
115. Wang, C.H.; Wei, Y.H. Role of mitochondrial dysfunction and dysregulation of Ca^{2+} homeostasis in the pathophysiology of insulin resistance and type 2 diabetes. *J. Biomed. Sci.* **2017**, *24*, 70. [CrossRef] [PubMed]
116. Yuan, Q.; Zeng, Z.L.; Yang, S.; Li, A.; Zu, X.; Liu, J. Mitochondrial Stress in Metabolic Inflammation: Modest Benefits and Full Losses. *Oxid. Med. Cell Longev.* **2022**, *2022*, 8803404. [CrossRef] [PubMed]
117. Kowaltowski, A.J.; Menezes-Filho, S.L.; Assali, E.A.; Gonçalves, I.G.; Cabral-Costa, J.V.; Abreu, P.; Miller, N.; Nolasco, P.; Laurindo, F.R.M.; Bruni-Cardoso, A.; et al. Mitochondrial morphology regulates organellar Ca^{2+} uptake and changes cellular Ca^{2+} homeostasis. *FASEB J.* **2019**, *33*, 13176–13188. [CrossRef] [PubMed]
118. Walton, R.G.; Kosmac, K.; Mula, J.; Fry, C.S.; Peck, B.D.; Groshong, J.S.; Finlin, B.S.; Zhu, B.; Kern, P.A.; Peterson, C.A. Human skeletal muscle macrophages increase following cycle training and are associated with adaptations that may facilitate growth. *Sci. Rep.* **2019**, *9*, 969. [CrossRef]
119. Lee, M.K.; Ryu, H.; Van, J.Y.; Kim, M.J.; Jeong, H.H.; Jung, W.K.; Jun, J.Y.; Lee, B. The Role of Macrophage Populations in Skeletal Muscle Insulin Sensitivity: Current Understanding and Implications. *Int. J. Mol. Sci.* **2023**, *24*, 11467. [CrossRef]
120. Wang, Y.; Li, N.; Zhang, X.; Horng, T. Mitochondrial metabolism regulates macrophage biology. *J. Biol. Chem.* **2021**, *297*, 100904. [CrossRef]
121. Di Benedetto, G.; Lefkimmiatis, K.; Pozzan, T. The basics of mitochondrial cAMP signalling: Where, when, why. *Cell Calcium.* **2021**, *93*, 102320. [CrossRef]
122. Ackerman, J.E.; Geary, M.B.; Orner, C.A.; Bawany, F.; Loiselle, A.E. Obesity/Type II diabetes alters macrophage polarization resulting in a fibrotic tendon healing response. *PLoS ONE* **2017**, *12*, e0181127. [CrossRef]
123. Gerdle, B.; Ghafouri, B.; Lund, E.; Bengtsson, A.; Lundberg, P.; van Ettinger-Veenstra, H.; Leinhard, O.D.; Forsgren, M.F. Evidence of Mitochondrial Dysfunction in Fibromyalgia: Deviating Muscle Energy Metabolism Detected Using Microdialysis and Magnetic Resonance. *J. Clin. Med.* **2020**, *9*, 3527. [CrossRef]
124. Gupta, V.; Ezhilarasan Santhi, S.S.; Ravi, S.; Ramanan, E.A. Rheumatological and Musculoskeletal Complications in Diabetes Patients. *J. Endocrinol. Metab.* **2022**, *12*, 117–124. [CrossRef]
125. Caturano, A.; D'Angelo, M.; Mormone, A.; Russo, V.; Mollica, M.P.; Salvatore, T.; Galiero, F.; Rinaldi, L.; Betrani, E.; Marfella, R.; et al. Oxidative Stress in Type 2 Diabetes: Impacts from Pathogenesis to Lifestyle Modifications. *Curr. Issues Mol. Biol.* **2023**, *45*, 6651–6666. [CrossRef] [PubMed]
126. Ye, D.; Fairchild, T.J.; Vo, L.; Drummond, P.D. Painful diabetic peripheral neuropathy: Role of oxidative stress and central sensitisation. *Diabet. Med.* **2022**, *39*, e14729. [CrossRef] [PubMed]
127. Peng, X.; Fan, R.; Xie, L.; Shi, X.; Dong, K.; Zhang, S.; Tao, J.; Xu, W.; Ma, D.; Chen, J.; et al. A Growing Link between Circadian Rhythms, Type 2 Diabetes Mellitus and Alzheimer's Disease. *Int. J. Mol. Sci.* **2022**, *23*, 504. [CrossRef] [PubMed]
128. Navarro-Ledesma, S.; Hamed-Hamed, D.; Pruimboom, L. A new perspective of frozen shoulder pathology; the interplay between the brain and the immune system. *Front. Physiol.* **2024**, *15*, 1248612. [CrossRef]
129. Kim, E.J.; Pellman, B.; Kim, J.J. Stress effects on the hippocampus: A critical review. *Learn. Mem.* **2015**, *22*, 411–416. [CrossRef]
130. Patel, D.; Anilkumar, S.; Chattarji, S.; Buwalda, B. Repeated social stress leads to contrasting patterns of structural plasticity in the amygdala and hippocampus. *Behav. Brain Res.* **2018**, *347*, 314–324. [CrossRef]
131. Birnie, M.T.; Claydon, M.D.B.; Troy, O.; Flynn, B.P.; Yoshimura, M.; Kershaw, Y.M.; Zhao, Z.; Demski-Allen, R.C.R.; Barker, G.R.R.; Warburton, E.C.; et al. Circadian regulation of hippocampal function is disrupted with corticosteroid treatment. *Proc. Natl. Acad. Sci. USA* **2023**, *120*, e2211996120. [CrossRef]
132. Li, M.; Li, Y.; Zhao, K.; Tan, X.; Chen, Y.; Qin, C.; Qiu, S.; Liang, Y. Changes in the structure, perfusion, and function of the hippocampus in type 2 diabetes mellitus. *Front. Neurosci.* **2023**, *16*, 1070911. [CrossRef]
133. Yonamine, C.Y.; Michalani, M.L.E.; Moreira, R.J.; Machado, U.F. Glucose Transport and Utilization in the Hippocampus: From Neurophysiology to Diabetes-Related Development of Dementia. *Int. J. Mol. Sci.* **2023**, *24*, 16480. [CrossRef]
134. Zhang, W.; Liu, H.T. MAPK signal pathways in the regulation of cell proliferation in mammalian cells. *Cell Res.* **2002**, *12*, 9–18. [CrossRef] [PubMed]
135. Merz, K.E.; Thurmond, D.C. Role of Skeletal Muscle in Insulin Resistance and Glucose Uptake. In *Comprehensive Physiology*; Wiley: Hoboken, NJ, USA, 2020; pp. 785–809.
136. Pruimboom, L. The Multiple Faces of the Human Immune System: Modern Life Causes Low-Grade Inflammation and Thereby Provokes Conflict Between the Selfish Immune System and the Selfish Brain. Ph.D. Thesis, Rijksuniversiteit Groningen, Groningen, The Netherlands, 2017.
137. Pruimboom, L.; Raison, C.L.; Muskiet, F.A.J. Physical Activity Protects the Human Brain against Metabolic Stress Induced by a Postprandial and Chronic Inflammation. *Behav. Neurol.* **2015**, *2015*, 569869. [CrossRef] [PubMed]
138. Zhou, W.B.S.; Meng, J.; Zhang, J. Does Low Grade Systemic Inflammation Have a Role in Chronic Pain? *Front. Mol. Neurosci.* **2021**, *14*, 785214. [CrossRef] [PubMed]

139. Levone, B.R.; Cryan, J.F.; O'Leary, O.F. Role of adult hippocampal neurogenesis in stress resilience. *Neurobiol. Stress.* **2015**, *1*, 147–155. [CrossRef] [PubMed]
140. Nesse, R.M.; Williams, G.C. *Why We Get Sick*; Vintage: New York, NY, USA, 1996.
141. Gurven, M.D.; Lieberman, D.E. WEIRD bodies: Mismatch, medicine and missing diversity. *Evol. Human. Behav.* **2020**, *41*, 330–340. [CrossRef]
142. Bordon, Y. Protect the species with mitohormesis? *Nat. Rev. Immunol.* **2021**, *21*, 407. [CrossRef]
143. Cavezzi, A.; Colucci, R.; d'Errico, G. Mitoresilience: Hormesis, Psycho-physical Resilience, Mitochondria and Heart Rate Variability as Relevant Interplaying Elements in Longevity Medicine. *Curr. Aging Sci.* **2023**, *16*, 25–32. [CrossRef]
144. Pruimboom, L.; Muskiet, F.A.J. Intermittent living; the use of ancient challenges as a vaccine against the deleterious effects of modern life—A hypothesis. *Med. Hypotheses* **2018**, *120*, 28–42. [CrossRef]
145. Pruimboom, L.; Ruiz-Núñez, B.; Raison, C.L.; Muskiet, F.A.J. Influence of a 10-Day Mimic of Our Ancient Lifestyle on Anthropometrics and Parameters of Metabolism and Inflammation: The "Study of Origin". *Biomed. Res. Int.* **2016**, *2016*, 6935123. [CrossRef]
146. Wang, Y.; Wang, L.; Yan, J.; Yuan, X.; Lou, Q.Q. Aerobic Training Increases Hippocampal Volume and Protects Cognitive Function for Type 2 Diabetes Patients with Normal Cognition. *Exp. Clin. Endocrinol. Diabetes* **2023**, *131*, 605–614. [CrossRef]
147. Stanford, K.I.; Goodyear, L.J. Exercise and type 2 diabetes: Molecular mechanisms regulating glucose uptake in skeletal muscle. *Adv. Physiol. Educ.* **2014**, *38*, 308–314. [CrossRef] [PubMed]
148. Park, S.B.; Yang, S.J. Ketogenic diet preserves muscle mass and strength in a mouse model of type 2 diabetes. *PLoS ONE* **2024**, *19*, e0296651. [CrossRef] [PubMed]
149. Ren, Q.; Fu, J.; Duan, X.; Sun, L.; Mu, Z.; Liang, W.; Li, Y.; Wang, Z.; Xiu, S. The Effects of Ketogenic Diet on Brain Gene Expressions in Type 2 Diabetes Background. *Neuroscience* **2024**, *549*, 101–109. [CrossRef] [PubMed]
150. Remie, C.M.E.; Moonen, M.P.B.; Roumans, K.H.M.; Nascimento, E.B.M.; Gemmink, A.; Havekes, B.; Schaart, B.; Kornips, E.; Joris, P.J.; Schrauwen-Hinderlnig, V.B.; et al. Metabolic responses to mild cold acclimation in type 2 diabetes patients. *Nat. Commun.* **2021**, *12*, 1516. [CrossRef]
151. Wang, X.; Wang, Q.; Zhao, M.; Xu, Y.; Fu, B.; Zhang, L.; Wu, S.; Yang, D.; Jia, C. Cold Exposure–induced Alterations in the Brain Peptidome and Gut Microbiome Are Linked to Energy Homeostasis in Mice. *Mol. Cell. Proteom.* **2023**, *22*, 100525. [CrossRef]
152. Duennwald, T.; Gatterer, H.; Groop, P.H.; Burtscher, M.; Bernardi, L. Effects of a single bout of interval hypoxia on cardiorespiratory control and blood glucose in patients with type 2 diabetes. *Diabetes Care* **2013**, *36*, 2183–2189. [CrossRef]
153. Bondy, S.C. The Hormesis Concept: Strengths and Shortcomings. *Biomolecules* **2023**, *13*, 1512. [CrossRef]
154. Senger, D.R.; Li, D.; Jaminet, S.C.; Cao, S. Activation of the Nrf2 Cell Defense Pathway by Ancient Foods: Disease Prevention by Important Molecules and Microbes Lost from the Modern Western Diet. *PLoS ONE* **2016**, *11*, e0148042. [CrossRef]
155. Sivamaruthi, B.; Kesika, P.; Prasanth, M.; Chaiyasut, C. A Mini Review on Antidiabetic Properties of Fermented Foods. *Nutrients* **2018**, *10*, 1973. [CrossRef]
156. Rezazadegan, M.; Mirjalili, F.; Jalilpiran, Y.; Aziz, M.; Jayedi, A.; Setayesh, L.; Yekaninejad, M.S.; Casazza, K.; Mirzaei, K. The Association Between Dietary Diversity Score and Odds of Diabetic Nephropathy: A Case-Control Study. *Front. Nutr.* **2022**, *9*, 767415. [CrossRef]
157. Mieda, M. The central circadian clock of the suprachiasmatic nucleus as an ensemble of multiple oscillatory neurons. *Neurosci. Res.* **2020**, *156*, 24–31. [CrossRef]
158. Catalano, F.; De Vito, F.; Cassano, V.; Fiorentino, T.V.; Sciacqua, A.; Hribal, M.L. Circadian Clock Desynchronization and Insulin Resistance. *Int. J. Environ. Res. Public Health* **2022**, *20*, 29. [CrossRef]
159. Navarro-Ledesma, S.; Carroll, J.; González-Muñoz, A.; Pruimboom, L.; Burton, P. Changes in Circadian Variations in Blood Pressure, Pain Pressure Threshold and the Elasticity of Tissue after a Whole-Body Photobiomodulation Treatment in Patients with Fibromyalgia: A Tripled-Blinded Randomized Clinical Trial. *Biomedicines* **2022**, *10*, 2678. [CrossRef]
160. Parameswaran, G.; Ray, D.W. Sleep, circadian rhythms, and type 2 diabetes mellitus. *Clin. Endocrinol.* **2022**, *96*, 12–20. [CrossRef]
161. Henson, J.; Covenant, A.; Hall, A.P.; Herring, L.; Rowlands, A.V.; Yates, T.; Davies, M.J. Waking Up to the Importance of Sleep in Type 2 Diabetes Management: A Narrative Review. *Diabetes Care* **2024**, *47*, 331–343. [CrossRef]
162. Rutters, F.; Nefs, G. Sleep and Circadian Rhythm Disturbances in Diabetes: A Narrative Review. *Diabetes Metab. Syndr. Obes.* **2022**, *15*, 3627–3637. [CrossRef]
163. Kothari, V.; Cardona, Z.; Chirakalwasan, N.; Anothaisintawee, T.; Reutrakul, S. Sleep interventions and glucose metabolism: Systematic review and meta-analysis. *Sleep. Med.* **2021**, *78*, 24–35. [CrossRef]
164. Salman, S.; Abdali, H. P094 Prevalence of fibromyalgia syndrome among patients with type 2 diabetes mellitus. *Rheumatology* **2023**, *62* (Suppl. S2), kead104.135. [CrossRef]
165. Navarro-Ledesma, S.; Hamed-Hamed, D.; Gonzalez-Muñoz, A.; Pruimboom, L. Impact of physical therapy techniques and common interventions on sleep quality in patients with chronic pain: A systematic review. *Sleep. Med. Rev.* **2024**, *76*, 101937. [CrossRef]
166. Shen, Q.; Guo, H.; Yan, Y. Photobiomodulation for Neurodegenerative Diseases: A Scoping Review. *Int. J. Mol. Sci.* **2024**, *25*, 1625. [CrossRef]

167. Salehpour, F.; Farajdokht, F.; Erfani, M.; Sadigh-Eteghad, S.; Shotorbani, S.S.; Hamblin, M.R.; Karimi, P.; Rasta, S.H.; Mahmoudi, J. Transcranial near-infrared photobiomodulation attenuates memory impairment and hippocampal oxidative stress in sleep-deprived mice. *Brain Res.* **2018**, *1682*, 36–43. [CrossRef]
168. González-Muñoz, A.; Cuevas-Cervera, M.; Pérez-Montilla, J.J.; Aguilar-Núñez, D.; Hamed-Hamed, D.; Aguilar-García, M.; Pruimboom, L.; Navarro-Ledesma, S. Efficacy of Photobiomodulation Therapy in the Treatment of Pain and Inflammation: A Literature Review. *Healthcare* **2023**, *11*, 938. [CrossRef]
169. Janssen, C.W.; Lowry, C.A.; Mehl, M.R.; Allen, J.J.B.; Kelly, K.L.; Gartner, D.E.; Medrano, A.; Begay, T.K.; Rentscher, K.; White, J.J.; et al. Whole-Body Hyperthermia for the Treatment of Major Depressive Disorder. *JAMA Psychiatry* **2016**, *73*, 789. [CrossRef]
170. Kokura, S.; Adachi, S.; Manabe, E.; Mizushima, K.; Hattori, T.; Okuda, T.; Nakabe, N.; Handa, O.; Takagi, T.; Naito, Y.; et al. Whole body hyperthermia improves obesity-induced insulin resistance in diabetic mice. *Int. J. Hyperth.* **2007**, *23*, 259–265. [CrossRef]
171. Navarro-Ledesma, S.; Carroll, J.D.; González-Muñoz, A.; Burton, P. Outcomes of whole-body photobiomodulation on pain, quality of life, leisure physical activity, pain catastrophizing, kinesiophobia, and self-efficacy: A prospective randomized triple-blinded clinical trial with 6 months of follow-up. *Front. Neurosci.* **2024**, *18*, 1264821. [CrossRef]
172. Segerstrom, S.C.; Miller, G.E. Psychological Stress and the Human Immune System: A Meta-Analytic Study of 30 Years of Inquiry. *Psychol. Bull.* **2004**, *130*, 601–630. [CrossRef]
173. Lieberman, D.E. Is Exercise Really Medicine? An Evolutionary Perspective. *Curr. Sports Med. Rep.* **2015**, *14*, 313–319. [CrossRef]
174. Noordali, F.; Cumming, J.; Thompson, J.L. Effectiveness of Mindfulness-based interventions on physiological and psychological complications in adults with diabetes: A systematic review. *J. Health Psychol.* **2017**, *22*, 965–983. [CrossRef]
175. Hamasaki, H. The Effects of Mindfulness on Glycemic Control in People with Diabetes: An Overview of Systematic Reviews and Meta-Analyses. *Medicines* **2023**, *10*, 53. [CrossRef]
176. Kurian, J.; Mohanthy, S.; Nanjumdaiah, R.M. Mechanism of action of yoga on prevention and management of type 2 diabetes mellitus: Narrative review. *J. Bodyw. Mov. Ther.* **2022**, *29*, 134–139. [CrossRef]
177. Ma, Q.; Li, H.; Gao, Y.; Zou, Y. Effects of Baduanjin on glucose and lipid metabolism in diabetic patients A protocol for systematic review and meta-analysis. *Medicine* **2021**, *100*, e23532. [CrossRef]
178. Cardle, P.; Kumar, S.; Leach, M.; McEvoy, M.; Veziari, Y. Mindfulness and Chronic Musculoskeletal Pain: An Umbrella Review. *J. Multidiscip. Healthc.* **2023**, *16*, 515–533. [CrossRef]
179. Sun, G.C.; Lovejoy, J.C.; Gillham, S.; Putiri, A.; Sasagawa, M.; Bradley, R. Effects of Qigong on Glucose Control in Type 2 Diabetes. *Diabetes Care* **2010**, *33*, e8. [CrossRef]
180. Yadav, A.; Kaushik, R.M.; Kaushik, R. Effects of Diaphragmatic Breathing and Systematic Relaxation on Depression, Anxiety, Stress, and Glycemic Control in Type 2 Diabetes Mellitus. *Int. J. Yoga Ther.* **2021**, *31*, 13. [CrossRef]
181. Cherry, M.G.; Brown, S.L.; Purewal, R.; Fisher, P.L. Do metacognitive beliefs predict rumination and psychological distress independently of illness representations in adults with diabetes mellitus? A prospective mediation study. *Br. J. Health Psychol.* **2023**, *28*, 814–828. [CrossRef]
182. Onyishi, C.N.; Ilechukwu, L.C.; Victor-Aigbodion, V.; Eseadi, C. Impact of spiritual beliefs and faith-based interventions on diabetes management. *World J. Diabetes* **2021**, *12*, 630–641. [CrossRef]
183. Al-Shawaf, L.; Conroy-Beam, D.; Asao, K.; Buss, D.M. Human Emotions: An Evolutionary Psychological Perspective. *Emot. Rev.* **2016**, *8*, 173–186. [CrossRef]
184. Cacioppo, J.T.; Cacioppo, S.; Boomsma, D.I. Evolutionary mechanisms for loneliness. *Cogn. Emot.* **2014**, *28*, 3–21. [CrossRef]
185. Matthew, D.L. *Social*; Crown: New York, NY, USA, 2013.
186. Schram, M.T.; Assendelft, W.J.J.; van Tilburg, T.G.; Dukers-Muijrers, N.H.T.M. Social networks and type 2 diabetes: A narrative review. *Diabetologia* **2021**, *64*, 1905–1916. [CrossRef]
187. Rosenkilde, S.; Hoffmann, S.H.; Thorsted, A.B.; Horsbøl, T.A.; Madsen, K.R.; Lehn, S.F.; Kafoed-Enevoldsen, A.; Iversen, P.B.; Grønkjær, M.S.; Thygesen, L.C. Loneliness and the risk of type 2 diabetes. *BMJ Open Diabetes Res. Care* **2024**, *12*, e003934. [CrossRef]
188. Baek, R.N.; Tanenbaum, M.L.; Gonzalez, J.S. Diabetes Burden and Diabetes Distress: The Buffering Effect of Social Support. *Ann. Behav. Med.* **2014**, *48*, 145–155. [CrossRef]
189. Fridman, I.; Higgins, E.T. Regulatory Focus and Regulatory Fit in Health Messaging. In *Oxford Research Encyclopedia of Communication*; Oxford University Press: Oxford, UK, 2017.
190. Watling, C.; Driessen, E.; van der Vleuten, C.P.M.; Vanstone, M.; Lingard, L. Understanding responses to feedback: The potential and limitations of regulatory focus theory. *Med. Educ.* **2012**, *46*, 593–603. [CrossRef]
191. Fan, Y.; Yan, Z.; Li, T.; Li, A.; Fan, X.; Qi, Z.; Zhang, J. Primordial Drivers of Diabetes Heart Disease: Comprehensive Insights into Insulin Resistance. *Diabetes Metab. J.* **2024**, *48*, 19–36. [CrossRef]
192. Mirzohreh, S.T.; Panahi, P.; Heidari, F. Exploring heart rate variability in polycystic ovary syndrome: Implications for cardiovascular health: A systematic review and meta-analysis. *Syst. Rev.* **2024**, *13*, 194. [CrossRef]
193. Carnethon, M.R.; Jacobs, D.R.; Sidney, S.; Liu, K. Influence of Autonomic Nervous System Dysfunction on the Development of Type 2 Diabetes. *Diabetes Care* **2003**, *26*, 3035–3041. [CrossRef]
194. Huang, Y.; Chen, H.; Hu, D.; Wan, R. Blood hemoglobin A1c might predict adverse differences in heart rate variability in a diabetic population: Evidence from the Midlife in the United States (MIDUS) study. *Front. Endocrinol.* **2022**, *13*, 921287. [CrossRef]

195. Kim, H.G.; Cheon, E.J.; Bai, D.S.; Lee, Y.H.; Koo, B.H. Stress and Heart Rate Variability: A Meta-Analysis and Review of the Literature. *Psychiatry Investig.* **2018**, *15*, 235–245. [CrossRef]
196. Seipäjärvi, S.M.; Tuomola, A.; Juurakko, J.; Rottensteiner, M.; Rissanen, A.P.E.; Kurkela, J.L.O.; Kujala, U.M.; Laukkanen, J.A.; Wikgren, J. Measuring psychosocial stress with heart rate variability-based methods in different health and age groups. *Physiol. Meas.* **2022**, *43*, 055002. [CrossRef]
197. Kristiansen, E.; Wanby, P.; Åkesson, K.; Blomstrand, P.; Brudin, L.; Thegerström, J. Assessing heart rate variability in type 1 diabetes mellitus—Psychosocial stress a possible confounder. *Ann. Noninvasive Electrocardiol.* **2020**, *25*, e12760. [CrossRef]
198. Ciubuc-Batcu, M.T.; Stapelberg, N.J.C.; Headrick, J.P.; Renshaw, G.M.C. A mitochondrial nexus in major depressive disorder: Integration with the psycho-immune-neuroendocrine network. *Biochim. Et Biophys. Acta (BBA)—Mol. Basis Dis.* **2024**, *1870*, 166920. [CrossRef]
199. Zheng, A.; Moritani, T. Influence of CoQ10 on Autonomic Nervous Activity and Energy Metabolism during Exercise in Healthy Subjects. *J. Nutr. Sci. Vitaminol.* **2008**, *54*, 286–290. [CrossRef]
200. Nozoe, M.; Hirooka, Y.; Koga, Y.; Araki, S.; Konno, S.; Kishi, T.; Ide, T.; Sunagawa, K. Mitochondria-derived reactive oxygen species mediate sympathoexcitation induced by angiotensin II in the rostral ventrolateral medulla. *J. Hypertens.* **2008**, *26*, 2176–2184. [CrossRef]
201. Kullmann, F.A.; McDonnell, B.M.; Wolf-Johnston, A.S.; Kanai, A.J.; Shiva, S.; Chelimsky, T.; Rodriguez, L.; Birder, L.A. Stress-induced autonomic dysregulation of mitochondrial function in the rat urothelium. *Neurourol. Urodyn.* **2019**, *38*, 572–581. [CrossRef]

biomedicines

MDPI

Review

Diabetes and Osteoarthritis: Exploring the Interactions and Therapeutic Implications of Insulin, Metformin, and GLP-1-Based Interventions

Iryna Halabitska [1,*], Liliia Babinets [1], Valentyn Oksenych [2,*] and Oleksandr Kamyshnyi [3]

[1] Department of Therapy and Family Medicine, I. Horbachevsky Ternopil National Medical University, Voli Square, 1, 46001 Ternopil, Ukraine

[2] Broegelmann Research Laboratory, Department of Clinical Science, University of Bergen, 5020 Bergen, Norway

[3] Department of Microbiology, Virology, and Immunology, I. Horbachevsky Ternopil National Medical University, 46001 Ternopil, Ukraine; alexkamyshnyi@gmail.com

* Correspondence: halabitska@tdmu.edu.ua (I.H.); valentyn.oksenych@uib.no (V.O.)

Abstract: Diabetes mellitus (DM) and osteoarthritis (OA) are prevalent chronic conditions with shared pathophysiological links, including inflammation and metabolic dysregulation. This study investigates the potential impact of insulin, metformin, and GLP-1-based therapies on OA progression. Methods involved a literature review of clinical trials and mechanistic studies exploring the effects of these medications on OA outcomes. Results indicate that insulin, beyond its role in glycemic control, may modulate inflammatory pathways relevant to OA, potentially influencing joint health. Metformin, recognized for its anti-inflammatory properties via AMPK activation, shows promise in mitigating OA progression by preserving cartilage integrity and reducing inflammatory markers. GLP-1-based therapies, known for enhancing insulin secretion and improving metabolic profiles in DM, also exhibit anti-inflammatory effects that may benefit OA by suppressing cytokine-mediated joint inflammation and supporting cartilage repair mechanisms. Conclusions suggest that these medications, while primarily indicated for diabetes management, hold therapeutic potential in OA by targeting common underlying mechanisms. Further clinical trials are warranted to validate these findings and explore optimal therapeutic strategies for managing both DM and OA comorbidities effectively.

Keywords: cartilage; insulin resistance; obesity; inflammation

1. Introduction

Diabetes mellitus (DM) encompasses a variety of disorders that all involve elevated blood glucose levels. The current classification of DM is outlined, with a comparison of the key characteristics of type 1 and type 2 diabetes. Additionally, the criteria for accurate biochemical diagnosis during fasting and oral glucose tolerance tests, as well as the use of hemoglobin A1c (HbA1c), are summarized. The rising prevalence of DM necessitates targeted screening to identify diabetes and prediabetes in at-risk groups. This screening is essential for the early implementation of measures to prevent the onset of diabetes and to slow its progression in these groups [1]. The incidence of DM is rising quickly, often leading to severe metabolic disorders and complications [2]. In recent decades, the prevalence of DM has increased significantly in almost every country, and it can be regarded as a growing epidemic. Urbanization and income status are key factors affecting current prevalence rates, revealing notable differences among various population groups [3].

Type 1 diabetes mellitus (T1DM) is a significant subtype of diabetes, typically diagnosed in youth and characterized by insulin deficiency. The life expectancy of individuals with T1DM has markedly improved over the past three decades due to the availability of exogenous insulin; however, it remains lower than that of the general healthy population [4].

Type 2 diabetes mellitus (T2DM), a prevalent metabolic disorder, arises from two primary factors: impaired insulin secretion by pancreatic β-cells and the reduced responsiveness of insulin-sensitive tissues to insulin [5].

The prevalence of obesity and DM has been steadily increasing worldwide. Both conditions share significant genetic and environmental factors in their development. Obesity enhances the impact of genetic predisposition and environmental influences on DM. The abnormal growth of adipose tissue and the excessive accumulation of certain nutrients and metabolites disrupt metabolic balance through insulin resistance, impaired autophagy, and disturbances in the microbiome–gut–brain axis. This disruption leads to low-grade systemic inflammation, which further destabilizes immunometabolism, accelerates the loss of functional β-cells, and gradually increases blood glucose levels. Due to these complex connections, most treatments for obesity and DM affect both conditions [6].

Osteoarthritis (OA) is recognized as a degenerative joint disease marked by inflammation, chronic pain, and functional impairment [7]. OA is a progressive disease characterized by cartilage degradation, subchondral bone remodeling, and synovial inflammation. The disease is linked to factors such as obesity, mechanical load, and aging. Additionally, various pro-inflammatory immune mediators influence the expression of metalloproteinases, which play a role in cartilage breakdown. Genetic factors also contribute to the susceptibility to OA [8]. The prevailing understanding of osteoarthritis depicts it as a "comprehensive joint ailment", emphasizing the engagement of not just the articular cartilage but also the synovium, subchondral bone, ligaments, and muscles. Obesity and metabolic syndrome are linked to elevated levels of pro-inflammatory cytokines, heightened secretion of adipokines possessing both protective and detrimental impacts on articular cartilage, an increase in proteolytic enzymes like matrix metalloproteinases and aggrecanases, and a rise in free fatty acids and reactive oxygen species prompted by dyslipidemia [9].

DM and OA are prevalent conditions expected to become even more common [10]. The coexistence of OA and DM is often coincidental, attributed to their high prevalence and shared risk factors [11]. For instance, there is a well-established link between OA and obesity, and most individuals with type 2 diabetes mellitus (T2DM) are also affected by obesity [11,12].

However, there is a lack of information regarding the influence of various forms of diabetes, along with the medications utilized for diabetes treatment, on the progression of osteoarthritis. This review aims to address this gap to offer potential new treatment options and a more comprehensive understanding of the underlying mechanisms. By exploring these connections, this review could both clarify why these diseases often coexist, and also aid in developing future treatments for patients.

2. Understanding the Coexistence of Diabetes Mellitus and Osteoarthritis: Pathogenic Links and Therapeutic Consideration

Hyperglycemia is regarded as the primary instigator of joint deterioration by enhancing the production of advanced glycation end products (AGEs), which stimulate chondrocytes and synoviocytes to generate pro-degradative and pro-inflammatory agents, inciting a mild systemic inflammation that triggers local joint inflammation, exacerbating OA progression in different joint components, and leading to neuromuscular impairments that destabilize the joint and exacerbate OA symptoms [13].

In conditions of elevated extracellular glucose levels, the capacity to regulate glucose uptake through the downregulation of glucose transporters is compromised in chondrocytes affected by OA. This leads to the buildup of glucose and increased production of reactive oxygen species (ROS), fostering degenerative alterations and advancing the development of OA [13–15].

2.1. Intersection of Type 1 Diabetes Mellitus and Osteoarthritis: Shared Mechanisms and Therapeutic Challenges

Type 1 diabetes mellitus (T1DM) impacts 9.5% of the population and is marked by a severe insulin deficiency, resulting in hyperglycemia and various systemic effects. T1DM is considered a potential risk factor for damage and loss of articular cartilage, which could accelerate the onset of OA. The relationship between T1DM and OA remains largely unexplored [16,17].

Furthermore, recent research investigating the relationship between T1DM and OA has yielded conflicting findings, with some studies indicating a positive correlation while others did not. One study conducted histological assessments of joints in T1DM and control subjects, revealing that T1DM mice exhibited measurements of cartilage degeneration consistent with mild OA characteristics. RNA sequencing analyses identified a notable upregulation of genes associated with matrix-degrading enzymes in T1DM, which are known to contribute to cartilage matrix degradation, suggesting their involvement in OA development. Subsequently, the study examined whether preexisting T1DM affects the development of post-traumatic OA following injury. Results at the 6-week mark post-injury revealed that T1DM-injured joints exhibited considerably less cartilage damage and joint degeneration compared to injured non-diabetic joints, indicating a significant delay in the progression of post-traumatic OA. At a cellular level, an increased number of cells expressing chondrocyte markers Col2a1, Acan, and Cytl1 were identified in the T1DM-injured group [17,18].

The significance of glucose metabolism and its derivatives, such as AGEs, sorbitol, and diacylglycerol (DAG), in the pathogenesis of OA and DM is emphasized, as these derivatives activate inflammatory pathways. The potential link between DM and OA is indicated by the inflammatory response due to increased pro-inflammatory cytokine expression [19]. Recent research has illuminated immune cell populations' temporal dynamics and activation statuses, including macrophages, localized within joints or originating systemically, contributing to inflammatory responses in osteoarthritis. Their complex interactions may explain varying pain and symptom manifestations observed during osteoarthritis exacerbations. Additionally, investigations into biological and environmental factors such as exercise, age, and diet have explored their potential roles in mitigating or exacerbating osteoarthritis-related inflammation. However, despite these advancements, effective disease-modifying treatments targeting inflammation in osteoarthritis have yet to be developed [20]. Mitochondrial dysfunction, characterized by impaired mitophagy resulting in the release of mitochondrial reactive oxygen species (mtROS) and mitochondrial DNA (mtDNA), plays a critical role in initiating inflammation in T1DM. This process involves upregulating pro-inflammatory cytokines and engaging receptors akin to those involved in pathogen-associated responses. Furthermore, mtROS and mtDNA activate pathways that contribute to the progression of chronic inflammation, which is closely linked to autoimmunity in T1DM [21]. Therapeutic agents capable of influencing inflammation show promise for both T1DM and OA.

2.2. Insulin Resistance, Obesity, and Osteoarthritis: Intersecting Pathways and Clinical Implications

Obesity is linked to various diseases, particularly insulin resistance and T2DM. Evidence-based studies indicate that adipose tissue (AT) is highly adaptable in its metabolic functions, responding to the body's energy needs and managing the balance between fasting and feeding throughout the day. It also adjusts to long-term changes in energy balance through tissue expansion and reduction [22–24]. This adaptability, especially the ability to expand and contract, is crucial for AT health and overall metabolic balance, and changes in these responses may contribute to the varying metabolic health seen in people with obesity [25–27]. A significant discovery in mice revealed that AT produces pro-inflammatory cytokines, which lead to insulin resistance, and that AT macrophages accumulate in obese individuals, supporting the hypothesis that adipose inflammation is a key driver of insulin resistance in obesity [28–30]. Although there is a marked increase in inflammatory macrophages and pro-inflammatory protein gene expression in the subcutaneous abdominal AT of individuals with metabolically unhealthy obesity compared to those with metabolically healthy obesity, it remains challenging to determine if this inflammation is a cause or effect of insulin resistance [31–33]. Metabolically healthy obesity denotes a state in which individuals possess excessive body fat without manifesting the usual metabolic dysfunctions linked to obesity, such as insulin resistance, dyslipidemia, or hypertension [34]. Metabolically unhealthy obesity is characterized by the presence of metabolic dysfunctions such as insulin resistance, dyslipidemia, or hypertension in individuals with excess body fat, indicating heightened health risks associated with obesity [35].

The concentration of free fatty acids associated with obesity and T2DM can negatively impact pancreatic beta cells. Basal levels of plasma free fatty acids contributed to hyperinsulinemia in normoglycemic obese patients [36–38]. There is a strong link between obesity and increased rates of free fatty acids in the bloodstream, which are then delivered to body tissues [39–41]. Although numerous studies show that elevated plasma free fatty acid levels are a significant cause of liver and muscle insulin resistance, conflicting data from real-world scenarios challenge these findings. Several studies indicate that the breakdown of AT triglycerides is highly sensitive to insulin [42,43]. Postprandial suppression of lipolysis and plasma free fatty acid concentrations is generally similar in both lean and obese individuals, as the greater postprandial increase in plasma insulin in obese individuals may compensate for their increased fat mass [44–46]. The relationship between insulin resistance and obesity remains complex and requires a clear understanding of the pathways linking T2DM to the increase in inflammatory macrophages in subcutaneous adipose tissue.

Obesity is the most significant risk factor for the onset and progression of osteoarthritis, with recent research highlighting additional contributing factors such as adipose tissue accumulation, insulin resistance, and the misalignment of innate and adaptive immune responses, wherein various inflammatory cells, particularly polarized macrophages and their mediators, play a crucial role in the pathological changes of the synovial joint [37]. Obesity, a major and modifiable risk factor for osteoarthritis, not only increases mechanical stress on tibiofemoral cartilage but also correlates with higher OA prevalence in non-weight-bearing areas due to its role in systemic inflammation, driven by adipose tissue-derived cytokines and adipokines like adiponectin and leptin, which regulate inflammatory immune responses and contribute to elevated levels of pro-inflammatory cytokines such as TNF-α, IL-1β, and IL-6, produced by adipose tissue macrophages [47]. In individuals suffering from knee osteoarthritis and exhibiting overweight or obesity, dietary adjustments and exercise, when compared to an attention control group, resulted in a statistically significant albeit modest reduction in knee pain over an 18-month period [48]. Nutritional interventions can potentially impact adipose tissue mass and the secretion of inflammatory mediators, which may, in turn, exert effects on other tissues in the body, including bone and articular cartilage [49]. Emphasizing BMI in osteoarthritis research could potentially perpetuate weight bias in clinical settings and exacerbate disparities in accessing effective treatments for osteoarthritis [50].

2.3. *Type 2 Diabetes Mellitus and Osteoarthritis: Synergistic Impact on Musculoskeletal Health and Treatment Strategies*

Numerous studies have documented the increased occurrence of OA in patients with diabetes. Meta-analyses have confirmed an epidemiological link between T2DM and OA, indicating that individuals with diabetes have a higher risk of developing OA [51–53]. However, the strength of this association can differ based on factors such as age, ethnicity, duration of T2DM, body weight, and the specific joints affected by OA [54].

Various studies have shown a link between long-term T2DM and faster progression of OA, with increased rates of synovial inflammation and joint pain [55,56]. This connection is even stronger in younger diabetic individuals with hand OA, who are more likely to develop the erosive form of the disease [57,58]. Interestingly, the relationship between T2DM and OA appears to be bidirectional. A cohort study found that joint pain and reduced mobility in the knee and hip, leading to a sedentary lifestyle, significantly increased the risk of developing T2DM in individuals over 55 years of age [59,60].

Traditionally, age-related joint degeneration and biomechanical stress from being overweight were seen as the primary risk factors for OA in diabetic individuals. However, recent advancements in understanding OA and T2DM have highlighted the influence of systemic factors such as dyslipidemia, hyperglycemia, and inflammation—collectively known as metabolic syndrome—that may directly contribute to OA. This has led to the recognition of a new clinical phenotype called metabolic OA [61–63]. This form of OA affects both load-bearing joints (like the hip and knee) and non-load-bearing joints (such as the hand), indicating that factors beyond just biomechanical stress are at play [64,65]. T2DM and OA are interconnected through the chronic systemic inflammation associated with metabolic syndrome. Under hyperglycemic conditions, OA patients' chondrocytes fail to downregulate glucose transport [66–68]. High glucose levels trigger the production of ROS in OA cartilage [69]. The catabolic activity of ROS generates inflammatory mediators like IL-1β and NF-κB, which lead to chondrocyte degradation and apoptosis, thus damaging the chondrocytes [70,71]. Additionally, OA chondrocytes in a hyperglycemic environment express higher levels of matrix metalloproteinases than normal chondrocytes [72–74]. An in vivo cohort study found that elevated fasting serum glucose levels are linked to increased cartilage damage, indicated by bone marrow lesions and loss of tibial cartilage volume, particularly in post-menopausal women compared to men [75]. This gender disparity may stem from estrogen levels, which are known to have a protective effect on cartilage. These findings highlight the detrimental effects of hyperglycemia on articular cartilage and suggest that disrupted glucose metabolism may directly link OA and T2DM [76]. Another harmful effect of hyperglycemia is the induction of AGEs [77,78]. The age-related accumulation of AGEs in articular cartilage creates a pathogenic environment, leading to symptoms of OA, such as stiffness and cartilage degradation. High glucose levels in diabetics result in increased AGEs formation. AGEs and their receptor initiate the inflammatory cascade, primarily through the production of pro-inflammatory TNF-α and the activation of the transcription factor NF-κB [79,80].

Human chondrocytes have functional insulin receptors that respond to physiological insulin levels, but the expression and activity of these receptors are lower in OA chondrocytes compared to normal chondrocytes [81–83]. Insulin treatment increases the expression of metalloproteinases-13 and IL-1β, and reduces autophagy, a crucial homeostatic process, in chondrocytes by decreasing LC3 II expression and increasing phosphorylation of Akt and rpS6. This suggests that the excess insulin seen in T2DM patients may harm cartilage and contribute to OA [11]. Insulin is an essential negative regulator of synovial inflammation and catabolism, so the development of insulin resistance in obese individuals would impair insulin's ability to suppress the production of inflammatory and catabolic mediators that promote OA [84,85].

3. The Potential Impact of Diabetes Therapies on Osteoarthritis

The management of diabetes mellitus, particularly T2DM, often necessitates a multifaceted pharmacological approach to achieve optimal glycemic control and mitigate complications. Insulin therapy, fundamental for both T1DM and advanced T2DM, compensates for insufficient endogenous insulin production, helping to regulate blood glucose levels with various formulations tailored to address basal and prandial needs. Metformin, a first-line oral anti-hyperglycemic agent, enhances peripheral glucose uptake, decreases hepatic glucose production through AMPK activation, and improves insulin sensitivity while also reducing cardiovascular events and mortality. GLP-1 agonists mimic the incretin hormone GLP-1 to enhance glucose-dependent insulin secretion, suppress glucagon release, slow gastric emptying, and promote satiety, contributing to both glycemic control and weight loss [86].

The primary objectives in managing OA include mitigating pain, improving joint mobility, and maintaining overall joint function. Recent strides in comprehending OA's underlying pathophysiology have spurred investigations into a wide array of therapeutic strategies, including advancements in tissue engineering, manipulation of the immune system, refinement of surgical techniques, and the development of pharmacological and non-pharmacological treatments. However, despite these advancements, a definitive cure for OA remains elusive, underscoring the need for personalized treatment approaches tailored to the specific stage and manifestations of the disease [87]. Focusing on BMI in osteoarthritis research has the potential to perpetuate weight bias within clinical practice settings, influencing treatment decisions and patient outcomes based on weight alone. This approach may exacerbate disparities in accessing effective treatments for osteoarthritis, particularly for individuals with higher BMIs who may face barriers to receiving optimal care. Addressing these biases is crucial to ensure equitable healthcare delivery and improved outcomes for all patients with osteoarthritis [50].

3.1. Insulin Use and Osteoarthritis: Evaluating Effects and Therapeutic Implications

It has been observed that insulin, either independently or in conjunction with inflammatory factors, can promote synovial inflammation during the advancement of osteoarthritis. Insulin demonstrates significant capability in enhancing the inflammatory characteristics of fibroblast-like synoviocytes (FLSs), increasing cell viability, and boosting the production of inflammatory cytokines. Additionally, insulin fosters chemokine production and augments macrophage chemotaxis. Moreover, insulin activates the PI3K/mTOR/Akt/NF-κB signaling pathway while concurrently inhibiting autophagy in FLSs. Data suggest that preblocking three specific signaling pathways with pathway inhibitors in FLSs significantly diminishes insulin-induced inflammatory responses. Furthermore, insulin is shown to elevate levels of inflammatory cytokine receptors in FLSs, with PI3K/mTOR/Akt/NF-κB signaling inhibitors capable of reversing this effect. Notably, insulin sensitizes synovial inflammation mediated by inflammatory factors (including metalloproteinases production and activation of intracellular signaling pathways). Collectively, these findings suggest that insulin may exacerbate synovial inflammatory conditions, thereby contributing to the progression of OA [88,89]. Insulin might stimulate the generation of several pro-inflammatory substances (such as interleukins, tumor necrosis factor-alpha, and metalloproteinase-13) linked with OA [11]. In vitro studies have shown that insulin has the potential to hinder chondrocyte maturation and enhance cartilage degradation, thereby exacerbating the pathological progression of OA [90]. It was indicated that the PI3K/AKT and mTOR signaling pathways play a role in the pathophysiological impacts of insulin in OA [81,90]. NF-κB is responsible for regulating the expression of inflammatory factors and metalloproteinases within the joints, and it is widely recognized to have a crucial involvement in the development of OA (Figure 1) [88,91,92].

The research has demonstrated that insulin can induce the loss of proteoglycan components, and elevate levels of inflammatory cytokines and metalloproteinases in chondrocytes, and these effects may be attributed to the inhibition of chondrocyte autophagy. Furthermore, clinical observations from this study revealed decreased autophagy in the knee cartilage of diabetic patients compared to non-diabetic counterparts, evidenced by a significant reduction in the expression of the autophagy-related protein LC3II. Notably, the study unveiled that rapamycin, acting as an autophagy activator and an inhibitor of the mTOR signaling pathway, can mitigate insulin-induced suppression of autophagy and subsequent cartilage degradation [90]. The research has indicated that the biological effects of insulin vary depending on the dose and the specific type of cell involved [93]. In addition to the effects on FLSs observed in this study, insulin was also found to impact chondrocytes [90,93]. However, insulin's role in chondrocyte differentiation has been reported to be either promotive or inhibitory [93,94], thereby either improving or worsening cartilage degeneration depending on its concentration [90]. Moreover, at the molecular level, insulin's influence varies significantly when its concentration is extremely high or low [95–97]. It was discovered that low and supraphysiological insulin levels have varying impacts on aggrecan and proteoglycan synthesis in chondrocytes, likely due to different insulin receptors. Additionally, it was found that high insulin levels (1 μM) decreased FoxO transcriptional activity, while low insulin levels (0.1 μM) also reduced FoxO transcriptional activity in

SZ95 sebocytes in vitro [97]. It was demonstrated that insulin selectively influences specific downstream responses of the Akt pathway in a dose-dependent manner. Therefore, it was concluded that varying insulin concentrations are linked to different mechanisms of insulin action, which can modulate cellular responses [95,98]. Previous studies have indicated that specific cellular responses can be triggered only by high concentrations of insulin [99–101]. Collectively, these studies highlight that different effector cells involved in the complex pathophysiological processes of various diseases exhibit distinct sensitivities to insulin [99–101].

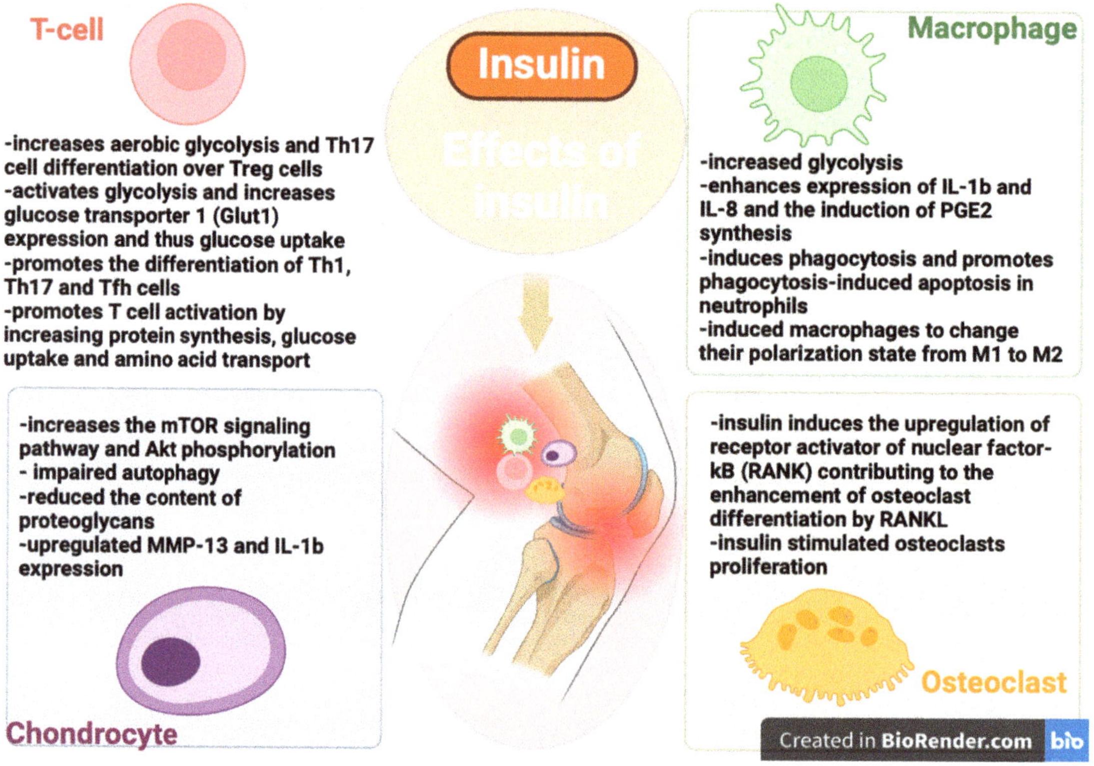

Figure 1. Illustration depicting the multifaceted effects of insulin on immune cells (T cells and macrophages), chondrocytes, and osteoclasts, emphasizing its regulatory role in immune response modulation, cartilage maintenance, and bone metabolism. Th17—T helper 17 cells, Glut1—Glucose transporter 1, mTOR—mammalian target of rapamycin, MMP-13—Matrix metalloproteinase-13, IL-1β—Interleukin-1 beta, IL-8—Interleukin-8, PGE2—Prostaglandin E2, M1—M1 macrophages (classically activated macrophages), M2—M2 macrophages (alternatively activated macrophages), RANK—Receptor activator of nuclear factor kappa-B, RANKL—RANK ligand. Figure 1 has been created in BioRender.com (accessed on 2 July 2024).

Immune cells require glucose for energy production [102]. Like adipose, muscle, and liver cells, they have insulin receptors (IRs) on their surfaces [103,104]. Insulin, functioning as a glucose-regulating hormone through IRs, also acts as a growth factor and cytokine regulator, thereby influencing immune modulation [105–107]. Insulin influences the immune response both indirectly by lowering glucose levels and directly by affecting immune cells, impacting their proliferation and signal transduction [108,109]. High blood sugar negatively impacts the immune system by causing cell stress and producing AGEs and ROS, which trigger the release of pro-inflammatory mediators. Thus, insulin's role in lowering glucose can reduce "glucose toxicity" and cell stress, providing an anti-inflammatory effect [110,111].

Insulin, beyond its metabolic role, exerts anti-inflammatory effects via PI3K/Akt pathway activation, suppressing TLR4 signaling and NF-κB activity in leukocytes, thus modulating immune responses and inflammation [112–114].

The precise regulation of insulin secretion by pancreatic β-cells is crucial for maintaining metabolic balance. β-cell mass must dynamically adjust to metabolic demands and can undergo significant changes in response to various conditions. The mTOR complexes, specifically mTORC1 and mTORC2, play pivotal roles in modulating β-cell mass. In states of systemic insulin resistance, mTORC1/mTORC2 signaling in β-cells is essential for increasing β-cell mass and enhancing insulin secretion. However, the failure of these compensatory mechanisms contributes to the development of type 2 diabetes, highlighting the complex and still incompletely understood role of mTOR complexes in β-cell dysfunction [115,116].

Some studies indicate insulin's potential pro-inflammatory role, affecting PMN leukocyte functions without increasing ROS production [117,118]. Insulin reduces ROS production in monocytes and dose-dependently inhibits tissue factor procoagulant activity via regulatory mechanisms [119,120].

While IRs are found on the surface of B cells, monocytes, and resting neutrophils, they are not present on resting T cells [121,122]. However, IR expression is significantly increased on activated T cells [123,124], which is crucial for meeting the high glucose demand necessary for T cells to achieve full effector functions. Insulin signaling in T cells enhances their activation by promoting protein synthesis, glucose uptake, and amino acid transport [123]. It was demonstrated in vitro that insulin shifts the response toward Th2, reducing the Th1 to Th2 ratio. This shift results in a change in cytokine secretion, with a decreased interferon-gamma to IL-4 ratio and increased phosphorylation of extracellular signal-regulated kinase (ERK), one of the four MAPK signaling pathways [125,126]. Experiments on mice lacking IRs demonstrated impaired polyclonal activation of CD4+ T cells, as well as deficiencies in cytokine production, migration, and proliferation [127]. Similar impairments were observed in CD8+ T cells, which showed reduced cytotoxicity in response to alloantigens. Studies on obese patients have shown that insulin resistance and related disorders are characterized by a cytokine imbalance, with elevated levels of TNF-α, IL-6, IL-1β, CRP, and NF-κB [128]. Th17 and Treg cells are two subsets of CD4+ T cells that share some developmental pathways but have different phenotypes and opposite functions. Th17 cells are pro-inflammatory, while Treg cells are anti-inflammatory [129]. An altered balance between Treg and Th17 cells is implicated in arthritis and other immune-mediated conditions [130]. Activation of quiescent T cells occurs through the stimulation of the T cell receptor (TCR) complex and the binding of the co-receptor CD28 to co-stimulatory molecules (Acuto). TCR engagement triggers intracellular signaling via the ERK/MAPK pathways, while CD28 signaling activates the PI3K-Akt-mTOR pathway [131,132].

PI3K-Akt signaling promotes glycolysis and increases the expression of glucose transporter 1 (Glut1), thereby enhancing glucose uptake. Overexpression of Glut1 facilitates the differentiation of T follicular helper (Tfh) cells, a T cell subset involved in B cell regulation, which may contribute to autoimmunity in both type 1 diabetes and arthritis [133,134]. Additionally, PI3K-Akt activation leads to mTOR activation, which supports the differentiation of Th1, Th17, and Tfh cells [135]. Moreover, mTOR can inhibit the formation of long-lived Tregs while favoring effector Tregs [136]. Tregs lacking mTOR exhibit reduced frequency, resulting in spontaneous activation of effector T cells and inflammation [137]. AMPK can inhibit cellular growth by suppressing the mTORC1 pathway [138]. Activation of AMPK and disruption of mTOR signaling have been shown to reduce inflammation in experimental arthritis. AMPK's control over fatty acid metabolism can also influence cell fate decisions in CD4+ T cells, particularly affecting the balance between Th17 and Treg lineages [139,140]. Additionally, growth factors like insulin, IGF-1, and IL-2 can stimulate PI3K-Akt-mTOR signaling. Insulin and insulin-like growth factors (IGFs) utilize common PI3K-AKT-mTOR and

RAS-RAF-MEK-ERK pathways. Activation of IGF-1 receptor (IGF1R) promotes Akt-mTOR signaling, enhances glycolysis, and favors Th17 differentiation, impacting inflammatory processes such as arthritis through IL-6 modulation [141].

In insulin resistance, Akt signaling becomes impaired, leading to the hyperactivation of mTORC1 and increased glycolysis. This heightened glycolysis in macrophages impacts their responses to pathogens and danger signals [142]. Insulin significantly boosts the LPS-dependent expression of IL-1β and IL-8, as well as the induction of enzymes involved in prostaglandin E2 (PGE2) synthesis by macrophages [143]. Both in vivo and in vitro studies suggest that insulin restores phagocytosis and promotes phagocytosis-induced apoptosis in neutrophils. Additionally, insulin treatment prompts macrophages to transition from an M1 to an M2 polarization state [142].

Previous research has highlighted the significance of insulin signaling in the biology and pathology of the joint, particularly in its ability to regulate bone architecture by affecting osteoblasts and osteoclasts [144–146]. In vitro experiments have shown that insulin increases IR expression and stimulates cell proliferation and differentiation in MG-63 cells through the MAPK and PI3K pathways, leading to enhanced alkaline phosphatase activity, secretion of type I collagen, and expression of osteocalcin [147,148]. Activation of mTORC1 by insulin-like growth factor 1 (IGF-1), released during bone resorption, promotes osteoblast differentiation of mouse bone marrow stromal cells (BMSCs), playing a critical role in the transition from pre-osteoblasts to mature osteoblasts [149,150].

However, insulin also affects osteoclasts. Through the ERK1/2 pathway, insulin upregulates receptor activator of nuclear factor-kB (RANK), contributing to enhanced osteoclast differentiation by RANK ligand (RANKL) [151]. The precise effects of mTORC1 on osteoclasts are not fully understood. Deletion of raptor, leading to mTORC1 inactivation in osteoclast precursors, or activation of mTORC1 by deletion of tuberous sclerosis complex 1 (Tsc1), can, respectively, increase or decrease osteoclastogenesis. Mechanistically, this is attributed to mTORC1's inhibition of NF-kB and nuclear factor of activated T cells 1 (NFATc1), both critical transcription factors for osteoclastogenesis [152]. Furthermore, RANKL-dependent osteoclastogenesis is impaired in Tsc1-deficient bone marrow macrophages, where TSC1 negatively regulates mTORC1 [153]. It was suggested that mTORC1 inhibition by rapamycin treatment or genetic deletion suppressed in vitro osteoclast differentiation, which was rescued by upregulation of the mTOR downstream target S6K1 [154].

Insulin resistance and hyperinsulinemia have been implicated in the development of OA and metabolic syndrome [155,156]. In human chondrocytes, insulin dose-dependently activates the mTOR signaling pathway and phosphorylates Akt, resulting in impaired cellular autophagy, a crucial mechanism for removing and degrading damaged intracellular components [90]. Additionally, insulin decreased the content of proteoglycans and increased the expression of metalloproteinase-13 and IL-1β, both of which play significant roles in chondrocytes and in the degradation of cartilage [90,91].

3.2. *Metformin's Influence on Osteoarthritis: Mechanisms and Therapeutic Implications*

Since diabetic patients face a higher risk of bone degradation, anti-diabetic medications may offer protective effects against bone disorders [157,158]. Metformin, an oral anti-hyperglycemic drug and the first-line treatment for T2DM, primarily works by inhibiting hepatic gluconeogenesis. Metformin, through the activation of AMPK, inhibits mTOR, which plays a crucial role in regulating lymphocyte immunometabolism and the balance of pro-inflammatory and anti-inflammatory cell populations within joints. When mTOR is inhibited, the production of pro-inflammatory Th1, Th17 cells, and M1 macrophages decreases, leading to a predominance of anti-inflammatory Treg cells and M2 macrophages (Figure 2). Therefore, the inhibition of mTOR via AMPK activation by metformin may have potential therapeutic effects in the treatment of inflammatory diseases, reducing the activity of pro-inflammatory cells while promoting the predominance of anti-inflammatory cell populations [159].

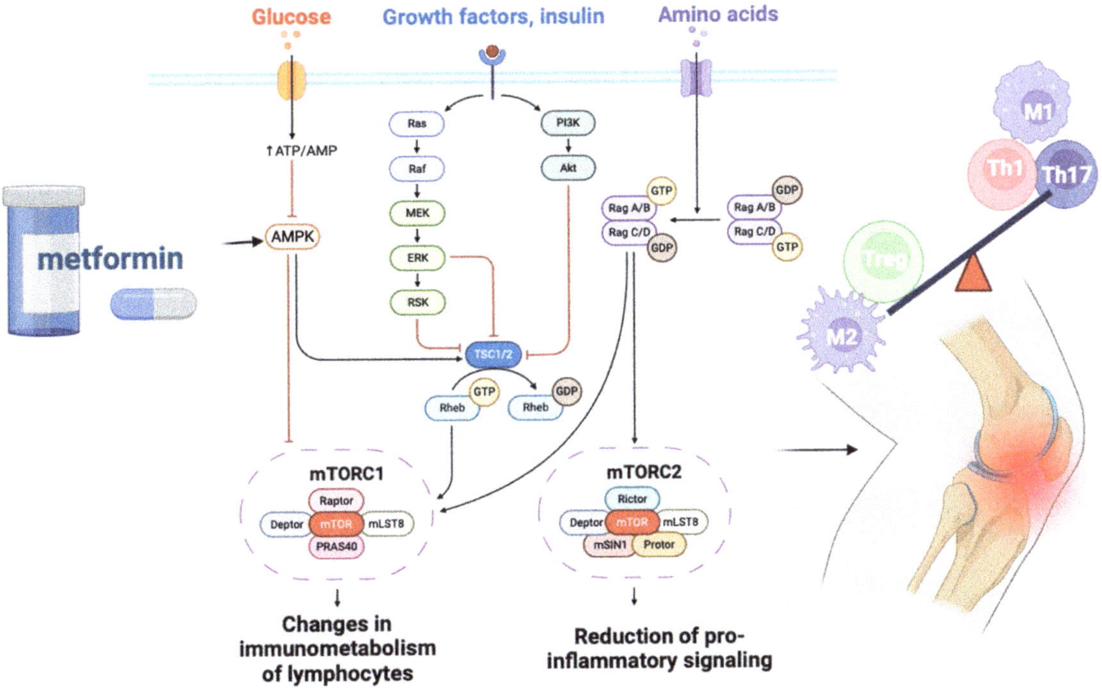

Figure 2. Metformin's activation of AMP-activated protein kinase (AMPK) leads to the inhibition of mTOR (mammalian target of rapamycin), a pivotal regulator of lymphocyte immunometabolism and the equilibrium between pro-inflammatory and anti-inflammatory cell populations within joint tissues. This inhibition results in decreased production of pro-inflammatory Th1 and Th17 cells, along with M1 macrophages, thereby promoting a predominance of anti-inflammatory Treg cells and M2 macrophages. ATP—Adenosine triphosphate, AMP—Adenosine monophosphate, AMPK—AMP-activated protein kinase, mTORC1—Mechanistic target of rapamycin complex 1, mTORC2—Mechanistic target of rapamycin complex 2, MLST8 (MLST8 protein)—mammalian lethal with SEC13 protein 8, PRAS40—Proline-rich AKT substrate 40 kDa, Ras—Rat sarcoma protein, Raf—Rapidly accelerated fibrosarcoma protein, MEK—mitogen-activated protein kinase kinase, ERK—extracellular signal-regulated kinase, RSK—Ribosomal S6 kinase, PI3K—phosphoinositide 3-kinase, Akt—protein kinase B (Akt), TSC1/2—tuberous sclerosis complex 1/2, Rheb—Ras homolog enriched in brain, GDP—Guanosine diphosphate, MSIN1—MAPK (mitogen-activated protein kinase)-interacting protein 1, MLSTS (MLSTS protein)—mammalian lethal with SEC13 protein, Reg A/B (regulatory proteins A/B), GTP—Guanosine triphosphate, Reg C/D (regulatory proteins C/D), Treg—regulatory T cells, M1—M1 macrophages (classically activated macrophages), M2—M2 macrophages (alternatively activated macrophages), Th1—T helper 1 cells, Th17—T helper 17 cells. Figure 2 has been created in BioRender.com (accessed on 2 July 2024).

The ability of metformin to regulate immune responses and improve gut microbiota diversity presents an encouraging opportunity for therapeutic interventions in individuals with type 2 diabetes who are at a higher risk of experiencing severe outcomes from COVID-19 [160,161]. The influence of type 2 diabetes, metformin, and insulin on COVID-19 was individually assessed. Among patients who received metformin, the CRP level was notably reduced compared to those who did not receive metformin [162–164]. Metformin's ability to influence immune responses and improve gut microbiota diversity indicates a promising path for therapeutic strategies in individuals with type 2 diabetes [163,165]. The administration of the type 2 diabetes medication metformin holds promise for treating this comorbidity, as it not only lowers blood sugar levels but also boosts the population of gut bacteria that stimulate regulatory T cell responses [166,167].

Metformin targets mitochondria, which produce ATP through oxidative phosphorylation [168]. This process generates ROS, which can cause oxidative stress and mitochondrial dysfunction, both associated with insulin resistance in skeletal muscle, liver, fat, and pancreas [158,169].

Metformin's metabolic effects are mainly due to its inhibition of the mitochondrial respiratory chain (complex 1), leading to ATP depletion and increased cytosolic AMP production [170]. This indirectly activates AMPK by phosphorylating Thr-172 in its alpha subunit, reducing gluconeogenesis in the liver. Elevated AMP levels also inhibit adenylate cyclase, decreasing cAMP production. Consequently, protein kinase A activity and its target, cyclic AMP response element binding protein, are inhibited, lowering fasting glucose levels [171,172].

Beyond reducing hepatic glucose production, metformin enhances insulin sensitivity by inhibiting lipogenesis, increases peripheral glucose uptake through GLUT4 enhancer factor phosphorylation, and reduces insulin-induced suppression of fatty acid oxidation [173–175]. Additionally, metformin mitigates chronic inflammation through its anti-inflammatory properties and promotes autophagy by inhibiting mTOR phosphorylation via AMPK activation [176]. Individuals with T2DM are at a higher likelihood of experiencing hand or knee OA compared to those without diabetes. Conversely, individuals with OA have an increased risk of developing T2DM compared to age- and sex-matched counterparts without OA.

Metformin, along with weight loss, shows promise as a disease-modifying treatment for knee osteoarthritis in obese patients, potentially reducing cartilage loss and the need for knee replacement surgery [177].

Metformin administration, initiated before or after destabilization of the medial meniscus (DMM) surgery, significantly attenuated cartilage degradation as evidenced by decreased Osteoarthritis Research Society International scores and preserved cartilage areas, associated with upregulated AMPK expression in articular cartilage tissue [178].

Various animal models suggest metformin's potential therapeutic impact on OA, reducing cartilage degradation and modulating pain via AMPK activation [179]. Metformin's chondroprotective effect involves upregulating AMPKα1 expression, demonstrated in genetically modified and DMM-induced OA mice, suggesting therapeutic potential via AMPK/mTOR pathway modulation [180]. Metformin is shown to activate AMPK and SIRT1 pathways, protecting chondrocyte mitochondrial function and potentially preventing OA development clinically [181]. Metformin attenuated IL-1β and TNF-α induced NO and MMP release [182]. Diabetes mellitus, especially type 2, increases skeletal complications and osteoarthritis risk due to hyperglycemia and advanced glycosylation end products, addressed by metformin's bone-protective effects through AMPK [183].

Mesenchymal stem cells (MSCs) possess multilineage differentiation potential and mitigate cartilage degradation through immunomodulatory functions. Metformin-enhanced adipose tissue-derived human MSCs show promising chondroprotective and analgesic effects in osteoarthritis, highlighting their therapeutic potential [182,184]. The study investigated metformin's impact on osteoporotic and normal fracture healing, demonstrating its ability to accelerate healing and promote angiogenesis through HIF-1α upregulation and YAP1/TAZ inhibition, crucial for type H vessel formation [185]. Metformin attenuates IL-1β-induced OA inflammation via SIRT3/PINK1/Parkin signaling, enhancing mitophagy for mitochondrial function [186,187]. The study suggests AMPK and GDF-15 as potential OA therapies, warranting randomized controlled trials for metformin's efficacy [188]. Metformin's pharmacological activity relies on organic cation transporters (OCTs) for tissue penetration and therapeutic efficacy [189–191]. Metformin use showed genetic protection against HER-positive breast cancer, involving testosterone levels [192]. Metformin's efficacy and oral bioavailability depend on transporters [193,194]. Various methods have been explored for improving metformin delivery for musculoskeletal therapies [195–197].

3.3. The Role of GLP-1-Based Therapies in Osteoarthritis: Mechanisms and Potential Benefits

Glucagon-like peptide-1 (GLP-1) and glucose-dependent insulinotropic polypeptide trigger insulin release from pancreatic β cells in response to glucose levels. However, the rapid degradation of native GLP-1 by dipeptidyl peptidase 4 (DPP-4) limits its clinical effectiveness. Consequently, GLP-1 analogues such as liraglutide, exenatide, semaglutide, and lixisenatide, engineered to resist DPP-4 cleavage, are now utilized for managing T2DM [198,199]. GLP-1 agonists are crucial for treating type 2 diabetes and obesity, delaying gastric emptying significantly for glycemic control and weight loss [200]. GLP-1 exerts insulinotropic effects and exhibits anti-inflammatory properties beneficial to the brain, heart, and lungs. GLP-1 receptors are abundant in various tissues, including the pancreas, intestine, and central nervous system [201–203]. Patients on long-acting GLP-1 receptor agonists like semaglutide face aspiration risks during anesthesia [204]. GLP-1 analogues show promise for OA due to their anti-inflammatory effects and presence of GLP-1 receptors in joint tissues [205,206]. GLP-1 receptor agonist therapies, through their potential to induce weight loss, may exert disease-modifying effects on knee OA in individuals with comorbid T2DM [207]. GLP-1's consistent efficacy in reducing food intake and body weight spans across obese individuals, including adolescents and adults. Its mechanism via a single G protein-coupled receptor, coupled with extensive safety data in T2DM patients, supports long-term use for obesity and associated conditions like cardiovascular disease and NASH. Advances suggest GLP-1 therapies may rival bariatric surgery in managing obesity and its complications [208,209].

Drugs that reduce low-grade systemic inflammation might also act locally in the joints [210]. Therefore, incretinomimetics that activate the GLP-1R pathway could be a promising approach for treating OA.

The role of the GLP-1R signaling pathway in chondrocytes has begun to be explored and requires further investigation. Immunohistochemistry detected GLP-1R in normal and OA articular chondrocytes in rat knee sections. GLP-1R signaling is linked to preventing apoptosis, anti-inflammatory activity, and matrix protection [211,212].

Liraglutide protects rat chondrocytes by activating the PI3K/Akt pathway, reducing ER stress-induced apoptosis, increasing Bcl-2, and decreasing cleaved caspase 3 levels. This effect was validated in an ACL rat model [211].

Currently, GLP-1 receptor agonists (GLP-1 RAs) are available in various formulations, including daily injections and a recently approved daily oral preparation of semaglutide, showing efficacy comparable to weekly injections. They share mechanisms such as enhancing insulin secretion, suppressing glucagon release, slowing gastric emptying, reducing post-meal glucose spikes, and promoting weight loss. GLP-1 RAs are recommended as initial injectable therapy for T2DM due to their efficacy in glucose control, weight reduction, and cardiovascular benefits, particularly in high-risk patients with cardiovascular disease. Ongoing research explores their potential in other conditions like type 1 diabetes and neurodegenerative diseases, suggesting a broadening role beyond diabetes management [213].

Activation of GLP-1R inhibits NF-κB, crucial in inflammation and cell regulation [214]. Co-agonist therapies like tirzepatide and amylin combinations show strong clinical promise, enhancing the weight loss potential of GLP-1R agonists like semaglutide [215]. In TNF-activated human chondrocytes and thapsigargin-induced rat chondrocytes, suppressing the NF-κB pathway resulted in decreased release of inflammatory mediators like IL-6, CCL2, and TNF [211]. All GLP-1 RAs improved HbA1c in a 12-week study among Japanese individuals with type 2 diabetes, highlighting varied mechanisms in glucose control and weight loss [216]. In primary mouse chondrocytes, administration of liraglutide decreased the mRNA expression of iNOS, MMP-13, and ADAMTS5, resulting in reduced secretion of inflammatory substances such as nitric oxide, prostaglandin E2, and IL-6 [210]. In the rat model of inflammatory osteoarthritis induced by monoiodoacetate (MIA), activation of GLP-1 receptors initiated the PKA/CREB signaling pathway, leading to a reduction in inflammation within cartilage [217]. Basic scientific studies revealed that GLP-1 analogs exert immunomodulatory effects independent of weight, inhibiting the NF-κB pathway through specific molecular mechanisms in arthritis [218]. GLP-1 analogues demonstrate anti-catabolic effects by decreasing the expression of key enzymes involved in cartilage degradation in response to TNF stimulation. This preservation of extracellular matrix components like aggrecan and type II collagen suggests potential benefits for OA therapy. Additionally, alterations in the phospholipid layer covering the cartilage surface can disrupt joint function and contribute to OA pathogenesis [211,219].

Semaglutide use during total knee arthroplasty reduced sepsis and joint infections but increased myocardial infarction, acute kidney injury, pneumonia, and hypoglycemia risks [220].

GLP-1R expression has been identified in human monocyte-derived macrophages and the murine cell line RAW264.7, but research on GLP-1/GLP-1R signaling in macrophages is limited [221,222]. GLP-1 RAs are approved for diabetes and obesity treatment; they also exhibit anti-inflammatory properties across various tissues and pathways [223].

GLP-1R activation modulates macrophage polarization through PKA/CREB signaling, reducing JNK phosphorylation and enhancing STAT3 phosphorylation, influencing immune responses [221,224,225]. This pathway is critical in murine models for promoting M2 macrophage differentiation, enhancing immune modulation and tissue repair processes [226–228]. Preclinical and clinical studies demonstrate GLP-1 RAs' cardioprotective effects, efficacy in hypertension and dyslipidemia, substantial weight loss in diabetes and obesity, and neuroprotective roles in stroke and neurodegenerative diseases. However, manageable adverse effects include gastrointestinal symptoms, increased heart rate, and potential renal issues [229]. In inflamed synovium, GLP-1R activation in macrophages shifts them from the M1 to the M2 phenotype, decreasing IL-6, TNF-α, and iNOS mRNA expression. This suggests GLP-1 therapies could mitigate inflammation by reducing macrophage infiltration and adhesion molecule expression [62,230]. The study investigates lixisenatide's GLP-1 receptor agonism effects on arthritis pathology in human fibroblast-like synoviocytes, marking the first exploration of this treatment's impact in this context [231]. Studies illustrate liraglutide's role in inhibiting lipid accumulation and oxidative stress triggered by oxidized low-density lipoprotein in macrophages, mediated through GLP-1R pathway activation [232,233].

GLP-1based therapy has emerged as a promising treatment for osteoarthritis, targeting both metabolic and inflammatory pathways involved in the disease's progression. Studies have demonstrated that GLP-1 agonists can reduce inflammation in the synovial membrane and improve cartilage integrity. Additionally, GLP-1 therapy may aid in weight management, thereby alleviating joint stress and further mitigating osteoarthritis symptoms.

4. Conclusions

DM and OA are prevalent chronic conditions associated with significant morbidity and healthcare burden worldwide. Treatment agents for DM have the potential to influence the progression of OA. Insulin, as a key regulator of glucose metabolism, exhibits potential dual roles in OA by influencing cartilage homeostasis and inflammatory responses within joint tissues. Metformin, renowned for its glucose-lowering effects via AMPK activation, also shows promise in mitigating OA progression through its anti-inflammatory properties and potential preservation of cartilage integrity. Additionally, GLP-1-based therapies, which enhance insulin secretion and improve glycemic control in DM, may exert protective effects in osteoarthritis by modulating inflammation, promoting cartilage repair mechanisms, and potentially slowing joint degeneration. Further clinical studies are warranted to elucidate the precise mechanisms and therapeutic efficacy of these agents in OA management, paving the way for integrated treatment strategies targeting both DM and OA comorbidities.

Author Contributions: Conceptualization, I.H., L.B. and O.K. in consultation with co-authors; writing—original draft preparation, I.H., L.B., V.O. and O.K. writing—review and editing, I.H., L.B., V.O. and O.K. All authors have read and agreed to the published version of the manuscript.

Funding: This research received no external funding.

Conflicts of Interest: The authors declare no conflicts of interest.

References

1. Harreiter, J.; Roden, M. Diabetes mellitus: Definition, classification, diagnosis, screening and prevention (Update 2023). *Wien. Klin. Wochenschr.* **2023**, *135* (Suppl. 1), 7–17. [CrossRef] [PubMed]
2. Cloete, L. Diabetes mellitus: An overview of the types, symptoms, complications and management. *Nurs. Stand.* **2022**, *37*, 61–66. [CrossRef] [PubMed]
3. Lovic, D.; Piperidou, A.; Zografou, I.; Grassos, H.; Pittaras, A.; Manolis, A. The Growing Epidemic of Diabetes Mellitus. *Curr. Vasc. Pharmacol.* **2020**, *18*, 104–109. [CrossRef] [PubMed]
4. Li, W.; Huang, E.; Gao, S. Type 1 Diabetes Mellitus and Cognitive Impairments: A Systematic Review. *J. Alzheimer's Dis.* **2017**, *57*, 29–36. [CrossRef] [PubMed]
5. Galicia-Garcia, U.; Benito-Vicente, A.; Jebari, S.; Larrea-Sebal, A.; Siddiqi, H.; Uribe, K.B.; Ostolaza, H.; Martín, C. Pathophysiology of Type 2 Diabetes Mellitus. *Int. J. Mol. Sci.* **2020**, *21*, 6275. [CrossRef]
6. Ruze, R.; Liu, T.; Zou, X.; Song, J.; Chen, Y.; Xu, R.; Yin, X.; Xu, Q. Obesity and type 2 diabetes mellitus: Connections in epidemiology, pathogenesis, and treatments. *Front. Endocrinol.* **2023**, *14*, 1161521. [CrossRef] [PubMed]
7. Santos, M.M.; Santos, A.M.; Nascimento Júnior, J.A.C.; Andrade, T.A.; Rajkumar, G.; Frank, L.A.; Serafini, M.R. The management of osteoarthritis symptomatology through nanotechnology: A patent review. *J. Microencapsul.* **2023**, *40*, 475–490. [CrossRef] [PubMed]
8. Kiełbowski, K.; Herian, M.; Bakinowska, E.; Banach, B.; Sroczyński, T.; Pawlik, A. The Role of Genetics and Epigenetic Regulation in the Pathogenesis of Osteoarthritis. *Int. J. Mol. Sci.* **2023**, *24*, 11655. [CrossRef] [PubMed]
9. Shumnalieva, R.; Kotov, G.; Monov, S. Obesity-Related Knee Osteoarthritis-Current Concepts. *Life* **2023**, *13*, 1650. [CrossRef]
10. Courties, A. Osteoarthritis and diabetes: Is there a true link? *Jt. Bone Spine* **2024**, *91*, 105684. [CrossRef]
11. Veronese, N.; Cooper, C.; Reginster, J.Y.; Hochberg, M.; Branco, J.; Bruyère, O.; Chapurlat, R.; Al-Daghri, N.; Dennison, E.; Herrero-Beaumont, G.; et al. Type 2 diabetes mellitus and osteoarthritis. *Semin. Arthritis Rheum.* **2019**, *49*, 9–19. [CrossRef] [PubMed]
12. Arruda, A.L.; Hartley, A.; Katsoula, G.; Smith, G.D.; Morris, A.P.; Zeggini, E. Genetic underpinning of the comorbidity between type 2 diabetes and osteoarthritis. *Am. J. Hum. Genet.* **2023**, *110*, 1304–1318. [CrossRef]
13. Eitner, A.; Wildemann, B. Diabetes-osteoarthritis and joint pain. *Bone Jt. Res.* **2021**, *10*, 307–309. [CrossRef] [PubMed]
14. Eitner, A.; Culvenor, A.G.; Wirth, W.; Schaible, H.G.; Eckstein, F. Impact of Diabetes Mellitus on Knee Osteoarthritis Pain and Physical and Mental Status: Data From the Osteoarthritis Initiative. *Arthritis Care Res.* **2021**, *73*, 540–548. [CrossRef] [PubMed]
15. Castano Betancourt, M.C.; Morais, C.L.; Vannucci Nunes Lipay, M.; Aragão, J.; de Azevedo, E.S.M.M.; Gomes Machado, E.; Marchi, E. Gender differences in the effect of diabetes mellitus and its treatment on osteoarthritic pain. *BMJ Open Diabetes Res. Care* **2019**, *7*, e000736. [CrossRef]
16. Khor, A.; Ma, C.A.; Hong, C.; Hui, L.L.; Leung, Y.Y. Diabetes mellitus is not a risk factor for osteoarthritis. *RMD Open* **2020**, *6*, 001030. [CrossRef] [PubMed]
17. Rios-Arce, N.D.; Murugesh, D.K.; Hum, N.R.; Sebastian, A.; Jbeily, E.H.; Christiansen, B.A.; Loots, G.G. Preexisting Type 1 Diabetes Mellitus Blunts the Development of Posttraumatic Osteoarthritis. *J. Bone Miner. Res. Plus* **2022**, *6*, e10625. [CrossRef]
18. Dubey, N.K.; Wei, H.J.; Yu, S.H.; Williams, D.F.; Wang, J.R.; Deng, Y.H.; Tsai, F.C.; Wang, P.D.; Deng, W.P. Adipose-derived Stem Cells Attenuates Diabetic Osteoarthritis via Inhibition of Glycation-mediated Inflammatory Cascade. *Aging Dis.* **2019**, *10*, 483–496. [CrossRef]
19. Aiello, F.C.; Trovato, F.M.; Szychlinska, M.A.; Imbesi, R.; Castrogiovanni, P.; Loreto, C.; Musumeci, G. Molecular Links Between Diabetes and Osteoarthritis: The Role of Physical Activity. *Curr. Diabetes Rev.* **2017**, *13*, 50–58. [CrossRef]
20. Knights, A.J.; Redding, S.J.; Maerz, T. Inflammation in osteoarthritis: The latest progress and ongoing challenges. *Curr. Opin. Rheumatol.* **2023**, *35*, 128–134. [CrossRef]
21. Blagov, A.V.; Summerhill, V.I.; Sukhorukov, V.N.; Popov, M.A.; Grechko, A.V.; Orekhov, A.N. Type 1 diabetes mellitus: Inflammation, mitophagy, and mitochondrial function. *Mitochondrion* **2023**, *72*, 11–21. [CrossRef] [PubMed]
22. Klein, S.; Gastaldelli, A.; Yki-Järvinen, H.; Scherer, P.E. Why does obesity cause diabetes? *Cell Metab.* **2022**, *34*, 11–20. [CrossRef] [PubMed]
23. Malone, J.I.; Hansen, B.C. Does obesity cause type 2 diabetes mellitus (T2DM)? Or is it the opposite? *Pediatr. Diabetes* **2019**, *20*, 5–9. [CrossRef] [PubMed]
24. Hoffman, D.J.; Powell, T.L.; Barrett, E.S.; Hardy, D.B. Developmental origins of metabolic diseases. *Physiol. Rev.* **2021**, *101*, 739–795. [CrossRef] [PubMed]
25. Crewe, C.; An, Y.A.; Scherer, P.E. The ominous triad of adipose tissue dysfunction: Inflammation, fibrosis, and impaired angiogenesis. *J. Clin. Investig.* **2017**, *127*, 74–82. [CrossRef] [PubMed]
26. Gugliucci, A. Biomarkers of dysfunctional visceral fat. *Adv. Clin. Chem.* **2022**, *109*, 1–30. [PubMed]
27. Smith, G.I.; Mittendorfer, B.; Klein, S. Metabolically healthy obesity: Facts and fantasies. *J. Clin. Investig.* **2019**, *129*, 3978–3989. [CrossRef] [PubMed]

28. Weisberg, S.P.; McCann, D.; Desai, M.; Rosenbaum, M.; Leibel, R.L.; Ferrante, A.W., Jr. Obesity is associated with macrophage accumulation in adipose tissue. *J. Clin. Investig.* **2003**, *112*, 1796–1808. [CrossRef] [PubMed]
29. Kojta, I.; Chacińska, M.; Błachnio-Zabielska, A. Obesity, Bioactive Lipids, and Adipose Tissue Inflammation in Insulin Resistance. *Nutrients* **2020**, *12*, 1305. [CrossRef]
30. Ying, W.; Fu, W.; Lee, Y.S.; Olefsky, J.M. The role of macrophages in obesity-associated islet inflammation and β-cell abnormalities. *Nat. Rev. Endocrinol.* **2020**, *16*, 81–90. [CrossRef]
31. Fuchs, A.; Samovski, D.; Smith, G.I.; Cifarelli, V.; Farabi, S.S.; Yoshino, J.; Pietka, T.; Chang, S.W.; Ghosh, S.; Myckatyn, T.M.; et al. Associations Among Adipose Tissue Immunology, Inflammation, Exosomes and Insulin Sensitivity in People with Obesity and Nonalcoholic Fatty Liver Disease. *Gastroenterology* **2021**, *161*, 968–981.912. [CrossRef] [PubMed]
32. Smith, G.I.; Polidori, D.C.; Yoshino, M.; Kearney, M.L.; Patterson, B.W.; Mittendorfer, B.; Klein, S. Influence of adiposity, insulin resistance, and intrahepatic triglyceride content on insulin kinetics. *J. Clin. Investig.* **2020**, *130*, 3305–3314. [CrossRef] [PubMed]
33. Smith, G.I.; Shankaran, M.; Yoshino, M.; Schweitzer, G.G.; Chondronikola, M.; Beals, J.W.; Okunade, A.L.; Patterson, B.W.; Nyangau, E.; Field, T.; et al. Insulin resistance drives hepatic de novo lipogenesis in nonalcoholic fatty liver disease. *J. Clin. Investig.* **2020**, *130*, 1453–1460. [CrossRef] [PubMed]
34. Blüher, M. Metabolically Healthy Obesity. *Endocr. Rev.* **2020**, *41*, bnaa004. [CrossRef] [PubMed]
35. Iacobini, C.; Pugliese, G.; Blasetti Fantauzzi, C.; Federici, M.; Menini, S. Metabolically healthy versus metabolically unhealthy obesity. *Metab. Clin. Exp.* **2019**, *92*, 51–60. [CrossRef] [PubMed]
36. Boden, G.; Chen, X.; Iqbal, N. Acute lowering of plasma fatty acids lowers basal insulin secretion in diabetic and nondiabetic subjects. *Diabetes* **1998**, *47*, 1609–1612. [CrossRef] [PubMed]
37. Nedunchezhiyan, U.; Varughese, I.; Sun, A.R.; Wu, X.; Crawford, R.; Prasadam, I. Obesity, Inflammation, and Immune System in Osteoarthritis. *Front. Immunol.* **2022**, *13*, 907750. [CrossRef] [PubMed]
38. Mocciaro, G.; Gastaldelli, A. Obesity-Related Insulin Resistance: The Central Role of Adipose Tissue Dysfunction. *Handb. Exp. Pharmacol.* **2022**, *274*, 145–164. [PubMed]
39. Mittendorfer, B.; Magkos, F.; Fabbrini, E.; Mohammed, B.S.; Klein, S. Relationship between body fat mass and free fatty acid kinetics in men and women. *Obesity* **2009**, *17*, 1872–1877. [CrossRef]
40. Chondronikola, M.; Yoshino, J.; Ramaswamy, R.; Giardina, J.D.; Laforest, R.; Wahl, R.L.; Patterson, B.W.; Mittendorfer, B.; Klein, S. Very-low-density lipoprotein triglyceride and free fatty acid plasma kinetics in women with high or low brown adipose tissue volume and overweight/obesity. *Cell Rep. Med.* **2024**, *5*, 101370. [CrossRef]
41. Hagberg, C.E.; Spalding, K.L. White adipocyte dysfunction and obesity-associated pathologies in humans. *Nat. Rev. Mol. Cell Biol.* **2024**, *25*, 270–289. [CrossRef] [PubMed]
42. Karpe, F.; Dickmann, J.R.; Frayn, K.N. Fatty acids, obesity, and insulin resistance: Time for a reevaluation. *Diabetes* **2011**, *60*, 2441–2449. [CrossRef] [PubMed]
43. Król-Kulikowska, M.; Urbanowicz, I.; Kepinska, M. The Concentrations of Interleukin-6, Insulin, and Glucagon in the Context of Obesity and Type 2 Diabetes and Single Nucleotide Polymorphisms in IL6 and INS Genes. *J. Obes.* **2024**, *2024*, 7529779. [CrossRef] [PubMed]
44. Conte, C.; Fabbrini, E.; Kars, M.; Mittendorfer, B.; Patterson, B.W.; Klein, S. Multiorgan insulin sensitivity in lean and obese subjects. *Diabetes Care* **2012**, *35*, 1316–1321. [CrossRef] [PubMed]
45. Cook, J.R.; Hawkins, M.A.; Pajvani, U.B. Liver insulinization as a driver of triglyceride dysmetabolism. *Nat. Metab.* **2023**, *5*, 1101–1110. [CrossRef] [PubMed]
46. McQuaid, S.E.; Hodson, L.; Neville, M.J.; Dennis, A.L.; Cheeseman, J.; Humphreys, S.M.; Ruge, T.; Gilbert, M.; Fielding, B.A.; Frayn, K.N.; et al. Downregulation of adipose tissue fatty acid trafficking in obesity: A driver for ectopic fat deposition? *Diabetes* **2011**, *60*, 47–55. [CrossRef] [PubMed]
47. Wang, T.; He, C. Pro-inflammatory cytokines: The link between obesity and osteoarthritis. *Cytokine Growth Factor Rev.* **2018**, *44*, 38–50. [CrossRef]
48. Messier, S.P.; Beavers, D.P.; Queen, K.; Mihalko, S.L.; Miller, G.D.; Losina, E.; Katz, J.N.; Loeser, R.F.; DeVita, P.; Hunter, D.J.; et al. Effect of Diet and Exercise on Knee Pain in Patients with Osteoarthritis and Overweight or Obesity: A Randomized Clinical Trial. *Jama* **2022**, *328*, 2242–2251. [CrossRef] [PubMed]
49. Oliveira, M.C.; Vullings, J.; van de Loo, F.A.J. Osteoporosis and osteoarthritis are two sides of the same coin paid for obesity. *Nutrition* **2020**, *70*, 110486. [CrossRef]
50. Godziuk, K.; Hawker, G.A. Obesity and body mass index: Past and future considerations in osteoarthritis research. *Osteoarthr. Cartil.* **2024**, *32*, 452–459. [CrossRef]
51. Williams, M.F.; London, D.A.; Husni, E.M.; Navaneethan, S.; Kashyap, S.R. Type 2 diabetes and osteoarthritis: A systematic review and meta-analysis. *J. Diabetes Complicat.* **2016**, *30*, 944–950. [CrossRef] [PubMed]
52. Yu, H.J.; Ho, M.; Liu, X.; Yang, J.; Chau, P.H.; Fong, D.Y.T. Association of weight status and the risks of diabetes in adults: A systematic review and meta-analysis of prospective cohort studies. *Int. J. Obes.* **2022**, *46*, 1101–1113. [CrossRef] [PubMed]

53. Obotiba, A.D.; Swain, S.; Kaur, J.; Yaseen, K.; Doherty, M.; Zhang, W.; Abhishek, A. Synovitis and bone marrow lesions associate with symptoms and radiographic progression in hand osteoarthritis: A systematic review and meta-analysis of observational studies. *Osteoarthr. Cartil.* **2021**, *29*, 946–955. [CrossRef]
54. Frey, N.; Hügle, T.; Jick, S.S.; Meier, C.R.; Spoendlin, J. Type II diabetes mellitus and incident osteoarthritis of the hand: A population-based case-control analysis. *Osteoarthr. Cartil.* **2016**, *24*, 1535–1540. [CrossRef] [PubMed]
55. Eymard, F.; Parsons, C.; Edwards, M.H.; Petit-Dop, F.; Reginster, J.Y.; Bruyère, O.; Richette, P.; Cooper, C.; Chevalier, X. Diabetes is a risk factor for knee osteoarthritis progression. *Osteoarthr. Cartil.* **2015**, *23*, 851–859. [CrossRef] [PubMed]
56. Mohajer, B.; Moradi, K.; Guermazi, A.; Dolatshahi, M.; Zikria, B.; Najafzadeh, N.; Kalyani, R.R.; Roemer, F.W.; Berenbaum, F.; Demehri, S. Diabetes-associated thigh muscle degeneration mediates knee osteoarthritis-related outcomes: Results from a longitudinal cohort study. *Eur. Radiol.* **2023**, *33*, 595–605. [CrossRef] [PubMed]
57. Magnusson, K.; Hagen, K.B.; Østerås, N.; Nordsletten, L.; Natvig, B.; Haugen, I.K. Diabetes is associated with increased hand pain in erosive hand osteoarthritis: Data from a population-based study. *Arthritis Care Res.* **2015**, *67*, 187–195. [CrossRef] [PubMed]
58. Mulrooney, E.; Neogi, T.; Dagfinrud, H.; Hammer, H.B.; Pettersen, P.S.; Gløersen, M.; Kvien, T.K.; Magnusson, K.; Haugen, I.K. Comorbidities in people with hand OA and their associations with pain severity and sensitization: Data from the longitudinal Nor-Hand study. *Osteoarthr. Cartil. Open* **2023**, *5*, 100367. [CrossRef] [PubMed]
59. Kendzerska, T.; King, L.K.; Lipscombe, L.; Croxford, R.; Stanaitis, I.; Hawker, G.A. The impact of hip and knee osteoarthritis on the subsequent risk of incident diabetes: A population-based cohort study. *Diabetologia* **2018**, *61*, 2290–2299. [CrossRef]
60. Fedorchenko, Y.; Mahmudov, K.; Abenov, Z.; Zimba, O.; Yessirkepov, M. Diabetes mellitus in rheumatic diseases: Clinical characteristics and treatment considerations. *Rheumatol. Int.* **2023**, *43*, 2167–2174. [CrossRef]
61. Puenpatom, R.A.; Victor, T.W. Increased prevalence of metabolic syndrome in individuals with osteoarthritis: An analysis of NHANES III data. *Postgrad. Med.* **2009**, *121*, 9–20. [CrossRef] [PubMed]
62. Lee, D.Y.; Bahar, M.E.; Kim, C.W.; Seo, M.S.; Song, M.G.; Song, S.Y.; Kim, S.Y.; Kim, D.R.; Kim, D.H. Autophagy in Osteoarthritis: A Double-Edged Sword in Cartilage Aging and Mechanical Stress Response: A Systematic Review. *J. Clin. Med.* **2024**, *13*, 3005. [CrossRef] [PubMed]
63. Li, B.; Yang, Z.; Li, Y.; Zhang, J.; Li, C.; Lv, N. Exploration beyond osteoarthritis: The association and mechanism of its related comorbidities. *Front. Endocrinol.* **2024**, *15*, 1352671. [CrossRef] [PubMed]
64. Tomi, A.L.; Sellam, J.; Lacombe, K.; Fellahi, S.; Sebire, M.; Rey-Jouvin, C.; Miquel, A.; Bastard, J.P.; Maheu, E.; Haugen, I.K.; et al. Increased prevalence and severity of radiographic hand osteoarthritis in patients with HIV-1 infection associated with metabolic syndrome: Data from the cross-sectional METAFIB-OA study. *Ann. Rheum. Dis.* **2016**, *75*, 2101–2107. [CrossRef] [PubMed]
65. Mohajer, B.; Kwee, R.M.; Guermazi, A.; Berenbaum, F.; Wan, M.; Zhen, G.; Cao, X.; Haugen, I.K.; Demehri, S. Metabolic Syndrome and Osteoarthritis Distribution in the Hand Joints: A Propensity Score Matching Analysis From the Osteoarthritis Initiative. *J. Rheumatol.* **2021**, *48*, 1608–1615. [CrossRef] [PubMed]
66. Griffin, T.M.; Huebner, J.L.; Kraus, V.B.; Yan, Z.; Guilak, F. Induction of osteoarthritis and metabolic inflammation by a very high-fat diet in mice: Effects of short-term exercise. *Arthritis Rheum.* **2012**, *64*, 443–453. [CrossRef] [PubMed]
67. Batushansky, A.; Zhu, S.; Komaravolu, R.K.; South, S.; Mehta-D'souza, P.; Griffin, T.M. Fundamentals of OA. An initiative of Osteoarthritis and Cartilage. Obesity and metabolic factors in OA. *Osteoarthr. Cartil.* **2022**, *30*, 501–515. [CrossRef] [PubMed]
68. Sun, W.; Yue, J.; Xu, T.; Cui, Y.; Huang, D.; Shi, H.; Xiong, J.; Sun, W.; Yi, Q. Xanthohumol alleviates palmitate-induced inflammation and prevents osteoarthritis progression by attenuating mitochondria dysfunction/NLRP3 inflammasome axis. *Heliyon* **2023**, *9*, e21282. [CrossRef]
69. Rosa, S.C.; Gonçalves, J.; Judas, F.; Mobasheri, A.; Lopes, C.; Mendes, A.F. Impaired glucose transporter-1 degradation and increased glucose transport and oxidative stress in response to high glucose in chondrocytes from osteoarthritic versus normal human cartilage. *Arthritis Res. Ther.* **2009**, *11*, R80. [CrossRef]
70. Goldring, M.B. Update on the biology of the chondrocyte and new approaches to treating cartilage diseases. *Best Pract. Res. Clin. Rheumatol.* **2006**, *20*, 1003–1025. [CrossRef]
71. Anderson, J.R.; Johnson, E.; Jenkins, R.; Jacobsen, S.; Green, D.; Walters, M.; Bundgaard, L.; Hausmans, B.A.C.; van den Akker, G.; Welting, T.J.M.; et al. Multi-Omic Temporal Landscape of Plasma and Synovial Fluid-Derived Extracellular Vesicles Using an Experimental Model of Equine Osteoarthritis. *Int. J. Mol. Sci.* **2023**, *24*, 14888. [CrossRef]
72. Rosa, S.C.; Rufino, A.T.; Judas, F.M.; Tenreiro, C.M.; Lopes, M.C.; Mendes, A.F. Role of glucose as a modulator of anabolic and catabolic gene expression in normal and osteoarthritic human chondrocytes. *J. Cell. Biochem.* **2011**, *112*, 2813–2824. [CrossRef]
73. Seow, S.R.; Mat, S.; Ahmad Azam, A.; Rajab, N.F.; Safinar Ismail, I.; Singh, D.K.A.; Shahar, S.; Tan, M.P.; Berenbaum, F. Impact of diabetes mellitus on osteoarthritis: A scoping review on biomarkers. *Expert Rev. Mol. Med.* **2024**, *26*, e8. [CrossRef]
74. Lentz, T.A.; George, S.Z.; Manickas-Hill, O.; Malay, M.R.; O'Donnell, J.; Jayakumar, P.; Jiranek, W.; Mather, R.C., 3rd. What General and Pain-associated Psychological Distress Phenotypes Exist Among Patients with Hip and Knee Osteoarthritis? *Clin. Orthop. Relat. Res.* **2020**, *478*, 2768–2783. [CrossRef]
75. Davies-Tuck, M.L.; Wang, Y.; Wluka, A.E.; Berry, P.A.; Giles, G.G.; English, D.R.; Cicuttini, F.M. Increased fasting serum glucose concentration is associated with adverse knee structural changes in adults with no knee symptoms and diabetes. *Maturitas* **2012**, *72*, 373–378. [CrossRef]

76. Verzijl, N.; DeGroot, J.; Oldehinkel, E.; Bank, R.A.; Thorpe, S.R.; Baynes, J.W.; Bayliss, M.T.; Bijlsma, J.W.; Lafeber, F.P.; Tekoppele, J.M. Age-related accumulation of Maillard reaction products in human articular cartilage collagen. *Biochem. J.* **2000**, *350 Pt 2*, 381–387. [CrossRef]
77. Steenvoorden, M.M.; Huizinga, T.W.; Verzijl, N.; Bank, R.A.; Ronday, H.K.; Luning, H.A.; Lafeber, F.P.; Toes, R.E.; DeGroot, J. Activation of receptor for advanced glycation end products in osteoarthritis leads to increased stimulation of chondrocytes and synoviocytes. *Arthritis Rheum.* **2006**, *54*, 253–263. [CrossRef]
78. Wei, G.; Lu, K.; Umar, M.; Zhu, Z.; Lu, W.W.; Speakman, J.R.; Chen, Y.; Tong, L.; Chen, D. Risk of metabolic abnormalities in osteoarthritis: A new perspective to understand its pathological mechanisms. *Bone Res.* **2023**, *11*, 63. [CrossRef]
79. Brownlee, M. Biochemistry and molecular cell biology of diabetic complications. *Nature* **2001**, *414*, 813–820. [CrossRef]
80. Ali, S.S.; Ismail, Q.U.A.; Yusuf, A.; Adnan, S.T.A.; Durga, F.; Priyanka, F.; Ghersheen, H.A.; Ahuja, M.; Anwar, A.; Hashmi, A.A. Correlation of Serum Sodium and Potassium with Thiamin Levels in Type 1 and Type 2 Diabetic Patients. *Cureus* **2024**, *16*, e59416. [CrossRef]
81. Rosa, S.C.; Rufino, A.T.; Judas, F.; Tenreiro, C.; Lopes, M.C.; Mendes, A.F. Expression and function of the insulin receptor in normal and osteoarthritic human chondrocytes: Modulation of anabolic gene expression, glucose transport and GLUT-1 content by insulin. *Osteoarthr. Cartil.* **2011**, *19*, 719–727. [CrossRef]
82. Huang, J.; Rozi, R.; Ma, J.; Fu, B.; Lu, Z.; Liu, J.; Ding, Y. Association between higher triglyceride glucose index and increased risk of osteoarthritis: Data from NHANES 2015–2020. *BMC Public Health* **2024**, *24*, 758. [CrossRef]
83. Shi, Y.Y.; Zheng, R.; Cai, J.J.; Qian, S.Z. The association between triglyceride glucose index and depression: Data from NHANES 2005–2018. *BMC Psychiatry* **2021**, *21*, 267. [CrossRef]
84. Griffin, T.M.; Huffman, K.M. Editorial: Insulin Resistance: Releasing the Brakes on Synovial Inflammation and Osteoarthritis? *Arthritis Rheumatol.* **2016**, *68*, 1330–1333. [CrossRef]
85. Liu, Y.; Yao, J.; Xue, X.; Lv, Y.; Guo, S.; Wei, P. Triglyceride-glucose index in the prediction of new-onset arthritis in the general population aged over 45: The first longitudinal evidence from CHARLS. *Lipids Health Dis.* **2024**, *23*, 79. [CrossRef]
86. ElSayed, N.A.; Aleppo, G.; Aroda, V.R.; Bannuru, R.R.; Brown, F.M.; Bruemmer, D.; Collins, B.S.; Hilliard, M.E.; Isaacs, D.; Johnson, E.L.; et al. 2. Classification and Diagnosis of Diabetes: Standards of Care in Diabetes-2023. *Diabetes Care* **2023**, *46*, S19–S40. [CrossRef]
87. Emami, A.; Namdari, H.; Parvizpour, F.; Arabpour, Z. Challenges in osteoarthritis treatment. *Tissue Cell* **2023**, *80*, 101992. [CrossRef]
88. Qiao, L.; Li, Y.; Sun, S. Insulin Exacerbates Inflammation in Fibroblast-Like Synoviocytes. *Inflammation* **2020**, *43*, 916–936. [CrossRef]
89. Liu, S.; Cao, C.; Zhang, Y.; Liu, G.; Ren, W.; Ye, Y.; Sun, T. PI3K/Akt inhibitor partly decreases TNF-α-induced activation of fibroblast-like synoviocytes in osteoarthritis. *J. Orthop. Surg. Res.* **2019**, *14*, 425. [CrossRef]
90. Ribeiro, M.; López de Figueroa, P.; Blanco, F.J.; Mendes, A.F.; Caramés, B. Insulin decreases autophagy and leads to cartilage degradation. *Osteoarthr. Cartil.* **2016**, *24*, 731–739. [CrossRef]
91. Zheng, W.; Feng, Z.; Lou, Y.; Chen, C.; Zhang, C.; Tao, Z.; Li, H.; Cheng, L.; Ying, X. Silibinin protects against osteoarthritis through inhibiting the inflammatory response and cartilage matrix degradation in vitro and in vivo. *Oncotarget* **2017**, *8*, 99649–99665. [CrossRef]
92. Liu, Y.; Lu, T.; Liu, Z.; Ning, W.; Li, S.; Chen, Y.; Ge, X.; Guo, C.; Zheng, Y.; Wei, X.; et al. Six macrophage-associated genes in synovium constitute a novel diagnostic signature for osteoarthritis. *Front. Immunol.* **2022**, *13*, 936606. [CrossRef]
93. Torres, E.S.; Andrade, C.V.; Fonseca, E.C.; Mello, M.A.; Duarte, M.E. Insulin impairs the maturation of chondrocytes in vitro. *Braz. J. Med. Biol. Res.* **2003**, *36*, 1185–1192. [CrossRef]
94. Patil, A.S.; Sable, R.B.; Kothari, R.M. Role of insulin-like growth factors (IGFs), their receptors and genetic regulation in the chondrogenesis and growth of the mandibular condylar cartilage. *J. Cell. Physiol.* **2012**, *227*, 1796–1804. [CrossRef]
95. Kubota, H.; Noguchi, R.; Toyoshima, Y.; Ozaki, Y.; Uda, S.; Watanabe, K.; Ogawa, W.; Kuroda, S. Temporal coding of insulin action through multiplexing of the AKT pathway. *Mol. Cell* **2012**, *46*, 820–832. [CrossRef]
96. Zhou, W.; Li, W.; Wang, S.; Salovska, B.; Hu, Z.; Tao, B.; Di, Y.; Punyamurtula, U.; Turk, B.E.; Sessa, W.C.; et al. An optogenetic-phosphoproteomic study reveals dynamic Akt1 signaling profiles in endothelial cells. *Nat. Commun.* **2023**, *14*, 3803. [CrossRef]
97. Mirdamadi, Y.; Thielitz, A.; Wiede, A.; Goihl, A.; Papakonstantinou, E.; Hartig, R.; Zouboulis, C.C.; Reinhold, D.; Simeoni, L.; Bommhardt, U.; et al. Insulin and insulin-like growth factor-1 can modulate the phosphoinositide-3-kinase/Akt/FoxO1 pathway in SZ95 sebocytes in vitro. *Mol. Cell. Endocrinol.* **2015**, *415*, 32–44. [CrossRef]
98. Kubota, H.; Uda, S.; Matsuzaki, F.; Yamauchi, Y.; Kuroda, S. In Vivo Decoding Mechanisms of the Temporal Patterns of Blood Insulin by the Insulin-AKT Pathway in the Liver. *Cell Syst.* **2018**, *7*, 118–128.e113. [CrossRef]
99. Ho-Palma, A.C.; Toro, P.; Rotondo, F.; Romero, M.D.M.; Alemany, M.; Remesar, X.; Fernández-López, J.A. Insulin Controls Triacylglycerol Synthesis through Control of Glycerol Metabolism and Despite Increased Lipogenesis. *Nutrients* **2019**, *11*, 513. [CrossRef]
100. de Proença, A.R.G.; Pereira, K.D.; Meneguello, L.; Tamborlin, L.; Luchessi, A.D. Insulin action on protein synthesis and its association with eIF5A expression and hypusination. *Mol. Biol. Rep.* **2019**, *46*, 587–596. [CrossRef]

101. Hodonu, A.; Escobar, M.; Beach, L.; Hunt, J.; Rose, J. Glycogen metabolism in mink uterine epithelial cells and its regulation by estradiol, progesterone and insulin. *Theriogenology* **2019**, *130*, 62–70. [CrossRef]
102. De Meyts, P. The Insulin Receptor and Its Signal Transduction Network. In *Endotext*; Feingold, K.R., Anawalt, B., Blackman, M.R., Boyce, A., Chrousos, G., Corpas, E., de Herder, W.W., Dhatariya, K., Dungan, K., Hofland, J., et al., Eds.; MDText.com, Inc.: South Dartmouth, MA, USA, 2000.
103. Dror, E.; Dalmas, E.; Meier, D.T.; Wueest, S.; Thévenet, J.; Thienel, C.; Timper, K.; Nordmann, T.M.; Traub, S.; Schulze, F.; et al. Postprandial macrophage-derived IL-1β stimulates insulin, and both synergistically promote glucose disposal and inflammation. *Nat. Immunol.* **2017**, *18*, 283–292. [CrossRef]
104. Shrestha, S.; Lee, Y.B.; Lee, H.; Choi, Y.K.; Park, B.Y.; Kim, M.J.; Youn, Y.J.; Kim, S.H.; Jung, S.J.; Song, D.K.; et al. Diabetes Primes Neutrophils for Neutrophil Extracellular Trap Formation through Trained Immunity. *Research* **2024**, *7*, 0365. [CrossRef]
105. Yang, P.; Wang, X.; Wang, D.; Shi, Y.; Zhang, M.; Yu, T.; Liu, D.; Gao, M.; Zhang, X.; Liu, Y. Topical insulin application accelerates diabetic wound healing by promoting anti-inflammatory macrophage polarization. *J. Cell Sci.* **2020**, *133*, jcs235838. [CrossRef]
106. Yu, T.; Gao, M.; Yang, P.; Pei, Q.; Liu, D.; Wang, D.; Zhang, X.; Liu, Y. Topical insulin accelerates cutaneous wound healing in insulin-resistant diabetic rats. *Am. J. Transl. Res.* **2017**, *9*, 4682–4693.
107. Sun, Q.; Li, J.; Gao, F. New insights into insulin: The anti-inflammatory effect and its clinical relevance. *World J. Diabetes* **2014**, *5*, 89–96. [CrossRef]
108. Maciver, N.J.; Jacobs, S.R.; Wieman, H.L.; Wofford, J.A.; Coloff, J.L.; Rathmell, J.C. Glucose metabolism in lymphocytes is a regulated process with significant effects on immune cell function and survival. *J. Leukoc. Biol.* **2008**, *84*, 949–957. [CrossRef]
109. Fu, Y.; Chen, Y.; Xie, Z.; Huang, H.; Tan, W.S.; Cai, H. Vitamin combination promotes ex vivo expansion of NK-92 cells by reprogramming glucose metabolism. *Bioresour. Bioprocess.* **2022**, *9*, 87. [CrossRef]
110. Kawahito, S.; Kitahata, H.; Oshita, S. Problems associated with glucose toxicity: Role of hyperglycemia-induced oxidative stress. *World J. Gastroenterol.* **2009**, *15*, 4137–4142. [CrossRef]
111. Robertson, R.P. Antioxidants for Early Treatment of Type 2 Diabetes in Rodents and Humans: Lost in Translation? *Diabetes* **2024**, *73*, 653–658. [CrossRef]
112. Zhang, Z.; Amorosa, L.F.; Coyle, S.M.; Macor, M.A.; Birnbaum, M.J.; Lee, L.Y.; Haimovich, B. Insulin-Dependent Regulation of mTORC2-Akt-FoxO Suppresses TLR4 Signaling in Human Leukocytes: Relevance to Type 2 Diabetes. *Diabetes* **2016**, *65*, 2224–2234. [CrossRef] [PubMed]
113. Tilich, M.; Arora, R.R. Modulation of toll-like receptors by insulin. *Am. J. Ther.* **2011**, *18*, e130–e137. [CrossRef] [PubMed]
114. Chen, W.; Lu, Y.; Zhang, Y.; Wu, J.; McVicar, A.; Chen, Y.; Zhu, S.; Zhu, G.; Lu, Y.; Zhang, J.; et al. Cbfβ regulates Wnt/β-catenin, Hippo/Yap, and Tgfβ signaling pathways in articular cartilage homeostasis and protects from ACLT surgery-induced osteoarthritis. *eLife* **2024**, *13*, e95640. [CrossRef] [PubMed]
115. Bartolome, A.; Guillén, C. Role of the mammalian target of rapamycin (mTOR) complexes in pancreatic β-cell mass regulation. *Vitam. Horm.* **2014**, *95*, 425–469. [PubMed]
116. Ballesteros-Álvarez, J.; Andersen, J.K. mTORC2: The other mTOR in autophagy regulation. *Aging Cell* **2021**, *20*, e13431. [CrossRef] [PubMed]
117. Walrand, S.; Guillet, C.; Boirie, Y.; Vasson, M.P. In vivo evidences that insulin regulates human polymorphonuclear neutrophil functions. *J. Leukoc. Biol.* **2004**, *76*, 1104–1110. [CrossRef] [PubMed]
118. Di Muzio, C.; Cipriani, P.; Ruscitti, P. Rheumatoid Arthritis Treatment Options and Type 2 Diabetes: Unravelling the Association. *BioDrugs* **2022**, *36*, 673–685. [CrossRef]
119. Gerrits, A.J.; Koekman, C.A.; Yildirim, C.; Nieuwland, R.; Akkerman, J.W. Insulin inhibits tissue factor expression in monocytes. *J. Thromb. Haemost.* **2009**, *7*, 198–205. [CrossRef] [PubMed]
120. Tripolino, C.; Ciaffi, J.; Pucino, V.; Ruscitti, P.; van Leeuwen, N.; Borghi, C.; Giacomelli, R.; Meliconi, R.; Ursini, F. Insulin Signaling in Arthritis. *Front. Immunol.* **2021**, *12*, 672519. [CrossRef]
121. Walrand, S.; Guillet, C.; Boirie, Y.; Vasson, M.P. Insulin differentially regulates monocyte and polymorphonuclear neutrophil functions in healthy young and elderly humans. *J. Clin. Endocrinol. Metab.* **2006**, *91*, 2738–2748. [CrossRef]
122. Restrepo, B.I.; Scordo, J.M.; Aguillón-Durán, G.P.; Ayala, D.; Quirino-Cerrillo, A.P.; Loera-Salazar, R.; Cruz-González, A.; Caso, J.A.; Joya-Ayala, M.; García-Oropesa, E.M.; et al. Differential Role of Type 2 Diabetes as a Risk Factor for Tuberculosis in the Elderly versus Younger Adults. *Pathogens* **2022**, *11*, 1551. [CrossRef] [PubMed]
123. Stentz, F.B.; Kitabchi, A.E. Activated T lymphocytes in Type 2 diabetes: Implications from in vitro studies. *Curr. Drug Targets* **2003**, *4*, 493–503. [CrossRef]
124. Biswas, M.; Suvarna, R.; Krishnan, S.V.; Devasia, T.; Shenoy Belle, V.; Prabhu, K. The mechanistic role of neutrophil lymphocyte ratio perturbations in the leading non communicable lifestyle diseases. *F1000Research* **2022**, *11*, 960. [CrossRef] [PubMed]
125. Viardot, A.; Grey, S.T.; Mackay, F.; Chisholm, D. Potential antiinflammatory role of insulin via the preferential polarization of effector T cells toward a T helper 2 phenotype. *Endocrinology* **2007**, *148*, 346–353. [CrossRef] [PubMed]
126. Makhijani, P.; Basso, P.J.; Chan, Y.T.; Chen, N.; Baechle, J.; Khan, S.; Furman, D.; Tsai, S.; Winer, D.A. Regulation of the immune system by the insulin receptor in health and disease. *Front. Endocrinol.* **2023**, *14*, 1128622. [CrossRef] [PubMed]

127. Fischer, H.J.; Sie, C.; Schumann, E.; Witte, A.K.; Dressel, R.; van den Brandt, J.; Reichardt, H.M. The Insulin Receptor Plays a Critical Role in T Cell Function and Adaptive Immunity. *J. Immunol.* **2017**, *198*, 1910–1920. [CrossRef] [PubMed]
128. Shin, J.Y.; Kim, S.Y.; Jeung, M.J.; Eun, S.H.; Woo, C.W.; Yoon, S.Y.; Lee, K.H. Serum adiponectin, C-reactive protein and TNF-alpha levels in obese Korean children. *J. Pediatr. Endocrinol. Metab.* **2008**, *21*, 23–29. [CrossRef]
129. Vernal, R.; Garcia-Sanz, J.A. Th17 and Treg cells, two new lymphocyte subpopulations with a key role in the immune response against infection. *Infect. Disord. Drug Targets* **2008**, *8*, 207–220. [CrossRef] [PubMed]
130. Lee, G.R. The Balance of Th17 versus Treg Cells in Autoimmunity. *Int. J. Mol. Sci.* **2018**, *19*, 730. [CrossRef]
131. Chen, L.; Flies, D.B. Molecular mechanisms of T cell co-stimulation and co-inhibition. *Nat. Rev. Immunol.* **2013**, *13*, 227–242. [CrossRef]
132. Hwang, J.R.; Byeon, Y.; Kim, D.; Park, S.G. Recent insights of T cell receptor-mediated signaling pathways for T cell activation and development. *Exp. Mol. Med.* **2020**, *52*, 750–761. [CrossRef] [PubMed]
133. Zeng, H.; Cohen, S.; Guy, C.; Shrestha, S.; Neale, G.; Brown, S.A.; Cloer, C.; Kishton, R.J.; Gao, X.; Youngblood, B.; et al. mTORC1 and mTORC2 Kinase Signaling and Glucose Metabolism Drive Follicular Helper T Cell Differentiation. *Immunity* **2016**, *45*, 540–554. [CrossRef] [PubMed]
134. Zou, X.; Wang, S.; Zhang, Y.; Wang, X.; Yang, W. The role of follicular T helper cells in the onset and treatment of type 1 diabetes. *Int. Immunopharmacol.* **2020**, *84*, 106499. [CrossRef] [PubMed]
135. Chi, H. Regulation and function of mTOR signalling in T cell fate decisions. *Nat. Rev. Immunol.* **2012**, *12*, 325–338. [CrossRef] [PubMed]
136. Sun, I.H.; Oh, M.H.; Zhao, L.; Patel, C.H.; Arwood, M.L.; Xu, W.; Tam, A.J.; Blosser, R.L.; Wen, J.; Powell, J.D. mTOR Complex 1 Signaling Regulates the Generation and Function of Central and Effector Foxp3$^+$ Regulatory T Cells. *J. Immunol.* **2018**, *201*, 481–492. [CrossRef]
137. Chapman, N.M.; Zeng, H.; Nguyen, T.M.; Wang, Y.; Vogel, P.; Dhungana, Y.; Liu, X.; Neale, G.; Locasale, J.W.; Chi, H. mTOR coordinates transcriptional programs and mitochondrial metabolism of activated T(reg) subsets to protect tissue homeostasis. *Nat. Commun.* **2018**, *9*, 2095. [CrossRef]
138. Mihaylova, M.M.; Shaw, R.J. The AMPK signalling pathway coordinates cell growth, autophagy and metabolism. *Nat. Cell Biol.* **2011**, *13*, 1016–1023. [CrossRef]
139. Tejera-Segura, B.; López-Mejías, R.; Domínguez-Luis, M.J.; de Vera-González, A.M.; González-Delgado, A.; Ubilla, B.; Olmos, J.M.; Hernández, J.L.; González-Gay, M.A.; Ferraz-Amaro, I. Incretins in patients with rheumatoid arthritis. *Arthritis Res. Ther.* **2017**, *19*, 229. [CrossRef] [PubMed]
140. Ristić, G.G.; Subota, V.; Stanisavljević, D.; Vojvodić, D.; Ristić, A.D.; Glišić, B.; Petronijević, M.; Stefanović, D.Z. Impact of disease activity on impaired glucose metabolism in patients with rheumatoid arthritis. *Arthritis Res. Ther.* **2021**, *23*, 95. [CrossRef] [PubMed]
141. Erlandsson, M.C.; Töyrä Silfverswärd, S.; Nadali, M.; Turkkila, M.; Svensson, M.N.D.; Jonsson, I.M.; Andersson, K.M.E.; Bokarewa, M.I. IGF-1R signalling contributes to IL-6 production and T cell dependent inflammation in rheumatoid arthritis. *Biochim. Biophys. Acta Mol. Basis Dis.* **2017**, *1863*, 2158–2170. [CrossRef]
142. Ieronymaki, E.; Daskalaki, M.G.; Lyroni, K.; Tsatsanis, C. Insulin Signaling and Insulin Resistance Facilitate Trained Immunity in Macrophages Through Metabolic and Epigenetic Changes. *Front. Immunol.* **2019**, *10*, 1330. [CrossRef] [PubMed]
143. Klauder, J.; Henkel, J.; Vahrenbrink, M.; Wohlenberg, A.S.; Camargo, R.G.; Püschel, G.P. Direct and indirect modulation of LPS-induced cytokine production by insulin in human macrophages. *Cytokine* **2020**, *136*, 155241. [CrossRef] [PubMed]
144. Pramojanee, S.N.; Phimphilai, M.; Chattipakorn, N.; Chattipakorn, S.C. Possible roles of insulin signaling in osteoblasts. *Endocr. Res.* **2014**, *39*, 144–151. [CrossRef] [PubMed]
145. Guan, J.; Liu, T.; Chen, H.; Yang, K. Association of type 2 Diabetes Mellitus and bone mineral density: A two-sample Mendelian randomization study. *BMC Musculoskelet. Disord.* **2024**, *25*, 130. [CrossRef] [PubMed]
146. Huang, G.; Chen, X.; Chen, Y.; Liu, W.; Chen, C.; Song, W.; Zeng, G. Causal relationship between type 2 diabetes mellitus and bone mineral density: A Mendelian randomization study in an East Asian population. *Osteoporos. Int.* **2023**, *34*, 1719–1727. [CrossRef] [PubMed]
147. Yang, J.; Zhang, X.; Wang, W.; Liu, J. Insulin stimulates osteoblast proliferation and differentiation through ERK and PI3K in MG-63 cells. *Cell Biochem. Funct.* **2010**, *28*, 334–341. [CrossRef] [PubMed]
148. Wikarek, A.; Grabarczyk, M.; Klimek, K.; Janoska-Gawrońska, A.; Suchodolska, M.; Holecki, M. Effect of Drugs Used in Pharmacotherapy of Type 2 Diabetes on Bone Density and Risk of Bone Fractures. *Medicina* **2024**, *60*, 393. [CrossRef] [PubMed]
149. Xian, L.; Wu, X.; Pang, L.; Lou, M.; Rosen, C.J.; Qiu, T.; Crane, J.; Frassica, F.; Zhang, L.; Rodriguez, J.P.; et al. Matrix IGF-1 maintains bone mass by activation of mTOR in mesenchymal stem cells. *Nat. Med.* **2012**, *18*, 1095–1101. [CrossRef] [PubMed]
150. Fitter, S.; Matthews, M.P.; Martin, S.K.; Xie, J.; Ooi, S.S.; Walkley, C.R.; Codrington, J.D.; Ruegg, M.A.; Hall, M.N.; Proud, C.G.; et al. mTORC1 Plays an Important Role in Skeletal Development by Controlling Preosteoblast Differentiation. *Mol. Cell. Biol.* **2017**, *37*, e00668-16. [CrossRef]
151. Oh, J.H.; Lee, N.K. Up-Regulation of RANK Expression via ERK1/2 by Insulin Contributes to the Enhancement of Osteoclast Differentiation. *Mol. Cells* **2017**, *40*, 371–377. [CrossRef]

152. Zhang, Y.; Xu, S.; Li, K.; Tan, K.; Liang, K.; Wang, J.; Shen, J.; Zou, W.; Hu, L.; Cai, D.; et al. mTORC1 Inhibits NF-κB/NFATc1 Signaling and Prevents Osteoclast Precursor Differentiation, In Vitro and In Mice. *J. Bone Miner. Res.* **2017**, *32*, 1829–1840. [CrossRef] [PubMed]
153. Hiraiwa, M.; Ozaki, K.; Yamada, T.; Iezaki, T.; Park, G.; Fukasawa, K.; Horie, T.; Kamada, H.; Tokumura, K.; Motono, M.; et al. mTORC1 Activation in Osteoclasts Prevents Bone Loss in a Mouse Model of Osteoporosis. *Front. Pharmacol.* **2019**, *10*, 684. [CrossRef] [PubMed]
154. Dai, Q.; Xie, F.; Han, Y.; Ma, X.; Zhou, S.; Jiang, L.; Zou, W.; Wang, J. Inactivation of Regulatory-associated Protein of mTOR (Raptor)/Mammalian Target of Rapamycin Complex 1 (mTORC1) Signaling in Osteoclasts Increases Bone Mass by Inhibiting Osteoclast Differentiation in Mice. *J. Biol. Chem.* **2017**, *292*, 196–204. [CrossRef] [PubMed]
155. Courties, A.; Sellam, J.; Berenbaum, F. Metabolic syndrome-associated osteoarthritis. *Curr. Opin. Rheumatol.* **2017**, *29*, 214–222. [CrossRef] [PubMed]
156. Courties, A.; Berenbaum, F.; Sellam, J. The Phenotypic Approach to Osteoarthritis: A Look at Metabolic Syndrome-Associated Osteoarthritis. *Jt. Bone Spine* **2019**, *86*, 725–730. [CrossRef] [PubMed]
157. Bennett, W.L.; Maruthur, N.M.; Singh, S.; Segal, J.B.; Wilson, L.M.; Chatterjee, R.; Marinopoulos, S.S.; Puhan, M.A.; Ranasinghe, P.; Block, L.; et al. Comparative effectiveness and safety of medications for type 2 diabetes: An update including new drugs and 2-drug combinations. *Ann. Intern. Med.* **2011**, *154*, 602–613. [CrossRef] [PubMed]
158. Hu, S.Q.; Zou, Y.P.; Jiang, Y.Q.; Zhang, Q.C.; Cheng, H.X.; Wang, H.R.; Li, X.L. Scutellarin-mediated autophagy activates exosome release of rat nucleus pulposus cells by positively regulating Rab8a via the PI3K/PTEN/Akt pathway. *Cell Biol. Int.* **2022**, *46*, 1588–1603. [CrossRef] [PubMed]
159. Kamyshnyi, O.; Matskevych, V.; Lenchuk, T.; Strilbytska, O.; Storey, K.; Lushchak, O. Metformin to decrease COVID-19 severity and mortality: Molecular mechanisms and therapeutic potential. *Biomed. Pharmacother.* **2021**, *144*, 112230. [CrossRef] [PubMed]
160. Petakh, P.; Kamyshna, I.; Oksenych, V.; Kamyshnyi, O. Metformin Alters mRNA Expression of FOXP3, RORC, and TBX21 and Modulates Gut Microbiota in COVID-19 Patients with Type 2 Diabetes. *Viruses* **2024**, *16*, 281. [CrossRef]
161. Petakh, P.; Griga, V.; Mohammed, I.B.; Loshak, K.; Poliak, I.; Kamyshnyiy, A. Effects of Metformin, Insulin on Hematological Parameters of COVID-19 Patients with Type 2 Diabetes. *Med. Arch.* **2022**, *76*, 329–332. [CrossRef]
162. Petakh, P.; Oksenych, V.; Kamyshnyi, A. The F/B ratio as a biomarker for inflammation in COVID-19 and T2D: Impact of metformin. *Biomed. Pharmacother.* **2023**, *163*, 114892. [CrossRef] [PubMed]
163. Pavlo, P.; Kamyshna, I.; Kamyshnyi, A. Effects of metformin on the gut microbiota: A systematic review. *Mol. Metab.* **2023**, *77*, 101805. [CrossRef] [PubMed]
164. Petakh, P.; Kamyshna, I.; Oksenych, V.; Kainov, D.; Kamyshnyi, A. Metformin Therapy Changes Gut Microbiota Alpha-Diversity in COVID-19 Patients with Type 2 Diabetes: The Role of SARS-CoV-2 Variants and Antibiotic Treatment. *Pharmaceuticals* **2023**, *16*, 904. [CrossRef]
165. Petakh, P.; Kamyshna, I.; Nykyforuk, A.; Yao, R.; Imbery, J.F.; Oksenych, V.; Korda, M.; Kamyshnyi, A. Immunoregulatory Intestinal Microbiota and COVID-19 in Patients with Type Two Diabetes: A Double-Edged Sword. *Viruses* **2022**, *14*, 477. [CrossRef]
166. Petakh, P.; Kamyshna, I.; Kamyshnyi, A. Unveiling the potential pleiotropic effects of metformin in treating COVID-19: A comprehensive review. *Front. Mol. Biosci.* **2023**, *10*, 1260633. [CrossRef]
167. Petakh, P.; Kobyliak, N.; Kamyshnyi, A. Gut microbiota in patients with COVID-19 and type 2 diabetes: A culture-based method. *Front. Cell. Infect. Microbiol.* **2023**, *13*, 1142578. [CrossRef] [PubMed]
168. Yamaguchi, O.; Otsu, K. Role of autophagy in aging. *J. Cardiovasc. Pharmacol.* **2012**, *60*, 242–247. [CrossRef]
169. McBride, H.M.; Neuspiel, M.; Wasiak, S. Mitochondria: More than just a powerhouse. *Curr. Biol.* **2006**, *16*, R551–R560. [CrossRef]
170. Kincaid, J.W.R.; Rimmington, D.; Tadross, J.A.; Cimino, I.; Zvetkova, I.; Kaser, A.; Richards, P.; Patel, S.; O'Rahilly, S.; Coll, A.P. The gastrointestinal tract is a major source of the acute metformin-stimulated rise in GDF15. *Sci. Rep.* **2024**, *14*, 1899. [CrossRef]
171. Rena, G.; Pearson, E.R.; Sakamoto, K. Molecular mechanism of action of metformin: Old or new insights? *Diabetologia* **2013**, *56*, 1898–1906. [CrossRef]
172. Feng, J.; Wang, X.; Ye, X.; Ares, I.; Lopez-Torres, B.; Martínez, M.; Martínez-Larrañaga, M.R.; Wang, X.; Anadón, A.; Martínez, M.A. Mitochondria as an important target of metformin: The mechanism of action, toxic and side effects, and new therapeutic applications. *Pharmacol. Res.* **2022**, *177*, 106114. [CrossRef] [PubMed]
173. Foretz, M.; Hébrard, S.; Leclerc, J.; Zarrinpashneh, E.; Soty, M.; Mithieux, G.; Sakamoto, K.; Andreelli, F.; Viollet, B. Metformin inhibits hepatic gluconeogenesis in mice independently of the LKB1/AMPK pathway via a decrease in hepatic energy state. *J. Clin. Investig.* **2010**, *120*, 2355–2369. [CrossRef] [PubMed]
174. Role of metformin for ovulation induction in infertile patients with polycystic ovary syndrome (PCOS): A guideline. *Fertil. Steril.* **2017**, *108*, 426–441. [CrossRef] [PubMed]
175. Ma, Q.; He, X.; Fu, Z.; Ren, X.; Sun, R.; Zhu, S.; Bian, Y.; Li, X. Clinical observation of laparoscopic sleeve gastrectomy and metformin treatment in obese PCOS patients. *J. Med. Biochem.* **2024**, *43*, 226–233. [CrossRef] [PubMed]
176. Wang, Y.; Xu, W.; Yan, Z.; Zhao, W.; Mi, J.; Li, J.; Yan, H. Metformin induces autophagy and G0/G1 phase cell cycle arrest in myeloma by targeting the AMPK/mTORC1 and mTORC2 pathways. *J. Exp. Clin. Cancer Res.* **2018**, *37*, 63. [CrossRef]
177. Lu, C.H.; Chung, C.H.; Lee, C.H.; Hsieh, C.H.; Hung, Y.J.; Lin, F.H.; Tsao, C.H.; Hsieh, P.S.; Chien, W.C. Combination COX-2 inhibitor and metformin attenuate rate of joint replacement in osteoarthritis with diabetes: A nationwide, retrospective, matched-cohort study in Taiwan. *PLoS ONE* **2018**, *13*, e0191242. [CrossRef] [PubMed]

178. Li, J.; Zhang, B.; Liu, W.X.; Lu, K.; Pan, H.; Wang, T.; Oh, C.D.; Yi, D.; Huang, J.; Zhao, L.; et al. Metformin limits osteoarthritis development and progression through activation of AMPK signalling. *Ann. Rheum. Dis.* **2020**, *79*, 635–645. [CrossRef] [PubMed]
179. Li, H.; Ding, X.; Terkeltaub, R.; Lin, H.; Zhang, Y.; Zhou, B.; He, K.; Li, K.; Liu, Z.; Wei, J.; et al. Exploration of metformin as novel therapy for osteoarthritis: Preventing cartilage degeneration and reducing pain behavior. *Arthritis Res. Ther.* **2020**, *22*, 34. [CrossRef] [PubMed]
180. Feng, X.; Pan, J.; Li, J.; Zeng, C.; Qi, W.; Shao, Y.; Liu, X.; Liu, L.; Xiao, G.; Zhang, H.; et al. Metformin attenuates cartilage degeneration in an experimental osteoarthritis model by regulating AMPK/mTOR. *Aging* **2020**, *12*, 1087–1103. [CrossRef] [PubMed]
181. He, M.; Lu, B.; Opoku, M.; Zhang, L.; Xie, W.; Jin, H.; Chen, S.; Li, Y.; Deng, Z. Metformin Prevents or Delays the Development and Progression of Osteoarthritis: New Insight and Mechanism of Action. *Cells* **2022**, *11*, 3012. [CrossRef]
182. Park, M.J.; Moon, S.J.; Baek, J.A.; Lee, E.J.; Jung, K.A.; Kim, E.K.; Kim, D.S.; Lee, J.H.; Kwok, S.K.; Min, J.K.; et al. Metformin Augments Anti-Inflammatory and Chondroprotective Properties of Mesenchymal Stem Cells in Experimental Osteoarthritis. *J. Immunol.* **2019**, *203*, 127–136. [CrossRef] [PubMed]
183. Bahrambeigi, S.; Yousefi, B.; Rahimi, M.; Shafiei-Irannejad, V. Metformin; an old antidiabetic drug with new potentials in bone disorders. *Biomed. Pharmacother.* **2019**, *109*, 1593–1601. [CrossRef] [PubMed]
184. Lim, Y.Z.; Wang, Y.; Urquhart, D.M.; Estee, M.M.; Wluka, A.E.; Heritier, S.; Cicuttini, F.M. Metformin for knee osteoarthritis with obesity: Study protocol for a randomised, double-blind, placebo-controlled trial. *BMJ Open* **2023**, *13*, e079489. [CrossRef] [PubMed]
185. Ruan, Z.; Yin, H.; Wan, T.F.; Lin, Z.R.; Zhao, S.S.; Long, H.T.; Long, C.; Li, Z.H.; Liu, Y.Q.; Luo, H.; et al. Metformin accelerates bone fracture healing by promoting type H vessel formation through inhibition of YAP1/TAZ expression. *Bone Res.* **2023**, *11*, 45. [CrossRef] [PubMed]
186. Sun, K.; Jing, X.; Guo, J.; Yao, X.; Guo, F. Mitophagy in degenerative joint diseases. *Autophagy* **2021**, *17*, 2082–2092. [CrossRef] [PubMed]
187. Wenting, Z.; Changqing, G.; Mei, D.U.; Yunxuan, M.A.; Yongqi, C.; Xilin, C.; Changqing, G. Acupotomy alleviates knee osteoarthritis in rabbit by regulating chondrocyte mitophagy Pink1-Parkin pathway. *J. Tradit. Chin. Med. = Chung I Tsa Chih Ying Wen Pan* **2024**, *44*, 468–477. [PubMed]
188. Zhang, Y.; Li, D.; Zhu, Z.; Chen, S.; Lu, M.; Cao, P.; Chen, T.; Li, S.; Xue, S.; Zhang, Y.; et al. Evaluating the impact of metformin targets on the risk of osteoarthritis: A mendelian randomization study. *Osteoarthr. Cartil.* **2022**, *30*, 1506–1514. [CrossRef] [PubMed]
189. Pakkir Maideen, N.M.; Jumale, A.; Balasubramaniam, R. Drug Interactions of Metformin Involving Drug Transporter Proteins. *Adv. Pharm. Bull.* **2017**, *7*, 501–505. [CrossRef] [PubMed]
190. Yu, H.; Zhong, X.; Gao, P.; Shi, J.; Wu, Z.; Guo, Z.; Wang, Z.; Song, Y. The Potential Effect of Metformin on Cancer: An Umbrella Review. *Front. Endocrinol.* **2019**, *10*, 617. [CrossRef]
191. Teper, Y.; Ye, L.; Waldron, R.T.; Lugea, A.; Sun, X.; Sinnett-Smith, J.; Hines, O.J.; Pandol, S.J.; Rozengurt, E.; Eibl, G. Low dosage combination treatment with metformin and simvastatin inhibits obesity-promoted pancreatic cancer development in male KrasG12D mice. *Sci. Rep.* **2023**, *13*, 16144. [CrossRef]
192. Chen, Y.; Bai, B.; Ye, S.; Gao, X.; Zheng, X.; Ying, K.; Pan, H.; Xie, B. Genetic effect of metformin use on risk of cancers: Evidence from Mendelian randomization analysis. *Diabetol. Metab. Syndr.* **2023**, *15*, 252. [CrossRef] [PubMed]
193. Cetin, M.; Sahin, S. Microparticulate and nanoparticulate drug delivery systems for metformin hydrochloride. *Drug Deliv.* **2016**, *23*, 2796–2805. [CrossRef] [PubMed]
194. El-Ridy, M.S.; Yehia, S.A.; Elsayed, I.; Younis, M.M.; Abdel-Rahman, R.F.; El-Gamil, M.A. Metformin hydrochloride and wound healing: From nanoformulation to pharmacological evaluation. *J. Liposome Res.* **2019**, *29*, 343–356. [CrossRef] [PubMed]
195. Song, P.; Hwang, J.S.; Park, H.C.; Kim, K.K.; Son, H.J.; Kim, Y.J.; Lee, K.M. Therapeutic Applications of Type 2 Diabetes Mellitus Drug Metformin in Patients with Osteoarthritis. *Pharmaceuticals* **2021**, *14*, 152. [CrossRef] [PubMed]
196. Souto, E.B.; Souto, S.B.; Campos, J.R.; Severino, P.; Pashirova, T.N.; Zakharova, L.Y.; Silva, A.M.; Durazzo, A.; Lucarini, M.; Izzo, A.A.; et al. Nanoparticle Delivery Systems in the Treatment of Diabetes Complications. *Molecules* **2019**, *24*, 4209. [CrossRef] [PubMed]
197. Zhang, S.; Xing, M.; Li, B. Corrigendum to 'Recent advances in musculoskeletal local drug delivery' [Acta Biomaterialia 2019, 93, 135–151]. *Acta Biomater.* **2020**, *105*, 336. [CrossRef] [PubMed]
198. Hunter, D.J. Pharmacologic therapy for osteoarthritis--the era of disease modification. *Nat. Rev. Rheumatol.* **2011**, *7*, 13–22. [CrossRef]
199. Zhang, Y.; Chen, H.; Wu, J.; McVicar, A.; Chen, Y.; Su, J.; Li, Y.P.; Chen, W. Deficiency of Cbfβ in articular cartilage leads to osteoarthritis-like phenotype through Hippo/Yap, TGFβ, and Wnt/β-catenin signaling pathways. *Int. J. Biol. Sci.* **2024**, *20*, 1965–1977. [CrossRef] [PubMed]
200. Willson, C.M.; Patel, L.; Middleton, P.; Desai, M. Glucagon-Like Peptide-1 Agonists and General Anesthesia: Perioperative Considerations and the Utility of Gastric Ultrasound. *Cureus* **2024**, *16*, e58042. [CrossRef]
201. Yoon, G.; Kim, Y.K.; Song, J. Glucagon-like peptide-1 suppresses neuroinflammation and improves neural structure. *Pharmacol. Res.* **2020**, *152*, 104615. [CrossRef]

202. Kim, S.; Jeong, J.; Jung, H.S.; Kim, B.; Kim, Y.E.; Lim, D.S.; Kim, S.D.; Song, Y.S. Anti-inflammatory Effect of Glucagon Like Peptide-1 Receptor Agonist, Exendin-4, through Modulation of IB1/JIP1 Expression and JNK Signaling in Stroke. *Exp. Neurobiol.* **2017**, *26*, 227–239. [CrossRef]
203. Mehdi, S.F.; Pusapati, S.; Anwar, M.S.; Lohana, D.; Kumar, P.; Nandula, S.A.; Nawaz, F.K.; Tracey, K.; Yang, H.; LeRoith, D.; et al. Glucagon-like peptide-1: A multi-faceted anti-inflammatory agent. *Front. Immunol.* **2023**, *14*, 1148209. [CrossRef] [PubMed]
204. Gulak, M.A.; Murphy, P. Regurgitation under anesthesia in a fasted patient prescribed semaglutide for weight loss: A case report. *Can. J. Anaesth. J. Can. D'anesthesie* **2023**, *70*, 1397–1400. [CrossRef] [PubMed]
205. Nauck, M. Incretin therapies: Highlighting common features and differences in the modes of action of glucagon-like peptide-1 receptor agonists and dipeptidyl peptidase-4 inhibitors. *Diabetes Obes. Metab.* **2016**, *18*, 203–216. [CrossRef] [PubMed]
206. Son, J.W.; Lim, S. Glucagon-Like Peptide-1 Based Therapies: A New Horizon in Obesity Management. *Endocrinol. Metab.* **2024**, *39*, 206–221. [CrossRef] [PubMed]
207. Zhu, H.; Zhou, L.; Wang, Q.; Cai, Q.; Yang, F.; Jin, H.; Chen, Y.; Song, Y.; Zhang, C. Glucagon-like peptide-1 receptor agonists as a disease-modifying therapy for knee osteoarthritis mediated by weight loss: Findings from the Shanghai Osteoarthritis Cohort. *Ann. Rheum. Dis.* **2023**, *82*, 1218–1226. [CrossRef] [PubMed]
208. Drucker, D.J. GLP-1 physiology informs the pharmacotherapy of obesity. *Mol. Metab.* **2022**, *57*, 101351. [CrossRef] [PubMed]
209. Abdelmalek, M.F.; Harrison, S.A.; Sanyal, A.J. The role of glucagon-like peptide-1 receptor agonists in metabolic dysfunction-associated steatohepatitis. *Diabetes Obes. Metab.* **2024**, *26*, 2001–2016. [CrossRef] [PubMed]
210. Meurot, C.; Martin, C.; Sudre, L.; Breton, J.; Bougault, C.; Rattenbach, R.; Bismuth, K.; Jacques, C.; Berenbaum, F. Liraglutide, a glucagon-like peptide 1 receptor agonist, exerts analgesic, anti-inflammatory and anti-degradative actions in osteoarthritis. *Sci. Rep.* **2022**, *12*, 1567. [CrossRef]
211. Chen, J.; Xie, J.J.; Shi, K.S.; Gu, Y.T.; Wu, C.C.; Xuan, J.; Ren, Y.; Chen, L.; Wu, Y.S.; Zhang, X.L.; et al. Glucagon-like peptide-1 receptor regulates endoplasmic reticulum stress-induced apoptosis and the associated inflammatory response in chondrocytes and the progression of osteoarthritis in rat. *Cell Death Dis.* **2018**, *9*, 212. [CrossRef]
212. Wen, Z.Q.; Lin, J.; Xie, W.Q.; Shan, Y.H.; Zhen, G.H.; Li, Y.S. Insights into the underlying pathogenesis and therapeutic potential of endoplasmic reticulum stress in degenerative musculoskeletal diseases. *Mil. Med. Res.* **2023**, *10*, 54. [CrossRef]
213. Nauck, M.A.; Quast, D.R.; Wefers, J.; Meier, J.J. GLP-1 receptor agonists in the treatment of type 2 diabetes—state-of-the-art. *Mol. Metab.* **2021**, *46*, 101102. [CrossRef]
214. Mei, J.; Sun, J.; Wu, J.; Zheng, X. Liraglutide suppresses TNF-α-induced degradation of extracellular matrix in human chondrocytes: A therapeutic implication in osteoarthritis. *Am. J. Transl. Res.* **2019**, *11*, 4800–4808. [PubMed]
215. Baggio, L.L.; Drucker, D.J. Glucagon-like peptide-1 receptor co-agonists for treating metabolic disease. *Mol. Metab.* **2021**, *46*, 101090. [CrossRef] [PubMed]
216. Kuwata, H.; Yabe, D.; Murotani, K.; Fujiwara, Y.; Haraguchi, T.; Kubota, S.; Kubota-Okamoto, S.; Usui, R.; Ishitobi, M.; Yamazaki, Y.; et al. Effects of glucagon-like peptide-1 receptor agonists on secretions of insulin and glucagon and gastric emptying in Japanese individuals with type 2 diabetes: A prospective, observational study. *J. Diabetes Investig.* **2021**, *12*, 2162–2171. [CrossRef]
217. Que, Q.; Guo, X.; Zhan, L.; Chen, S.; Zhang, Z.; Ni, X.; Ye, B.; Wan, S. The GLP-1 agonist, liraglutide, ameliorates inflammation through the activation of the PKA/CREB pathway in a rat model of knee osteoarthritis. *J. Inflamm.* **2019**, *16*, 13. [CrossRef] [PubMed]
218. Karacabeyli, D.; Lacaille, D. Glucagon-Like Peptide 1 Receptor Agonists in Patients with Inflammatory Arthritis or Psoriasis: A Scoping Review. *J. Clin. Rheumatol.* **2024**, *30*, 26–31. [CrossRef]
219. Kosinska, M.K.; Ludwig, T.E.; Liebisch, G.; Zhang, R.; Siebert, H.C.; Wilhelm, J.; Kaesser, U.; Dettmeyer, R.B.; Klein, H.; Ishaque, B.; et al. Articular Joint Lubricants during Osteoarthritis and Rheumatoid Arthritis Display Altered Levels and Molecular Species. *PLoS ONE* **2015**, *10*, e0125192. [CrossRef]
220. Magruder, M.L.; Yao, V.J.H.; Rodriguez, A.N.; Ng, M.K.; Sasson, V.; Erez, O. Does Semaglutide Use Decrease Complications and Costs Following Total Knee Arthroplasty? *J. Arthroplast.* **2023**, *38*, 2311–2315.e2311. [CrossRef]
221. Shiraishi, D.; Fujiwara, Y.; Komohara, Y.; Mizuta, H.; Takeya, M. Glucagon-like peptide-1 (GLP-1) induces M2 polarization of human macrophages via STAT3 activation. *Biochem. Biophys. Res. Commun.* **2012**, *425*, 304–308. [CrossRef]
222. Chrysavgis, L.G.; Kazanas, S.; Bafa, K.; Rozani, S.; Koloutsou, M.E.; Cholongitas, E. Glucagon-like Peptide 1, Glucose-Dependent Insulinotropic Polypeptide, and Glucagon Receptor Agonists in Metabolic Dysfunction-Associated Steatotic Liver Disease: Novel Medication in New Liver Disease Nomenclature. *Int. J. Mol. Sci.* **2024**, *25*, 3832. [CrossRef] [PubMed]
223. Bendotti, G.; Montefusco, L.; Lunati, M.E.; Usuelli, V.; Pastore, I.; Lazzaroni, E.; Assi, E.; Seelam, A.J.; El Essawy, B.; Jang, J.; et al. The anti-inflammatory and immunological properties of GLP-1 Receptor Agonists. *Pharmacol. Res.* **2022**, *182*, 106320. [CrossRef]
224. Noguchi, T.; Katoh, H.; Nomura, S.; Okada, K.; Watanabe, M. The GLP-1 receptor agonist exenatide improves recovery from spinal cord injury by inducing macrophage polarization toward the M2 phenotype. *Front. Neurosci.* **2024**, *18*, 1342944. [CrossRef]
225. Wan, S.; Sun, H. Glucagon-like peptide-1 modulates RAW264.7 macrophage polarization by interfering with the JNK/STAT3 signaling pathway. *Exp. Ther. Med.* **2019**, *17*, 3573–3579. [CrossRef]
226. Porcheray, F.; Viaud, S.; Rimaniol, A.C.; Léone, C.; Samah, B.; Dereuddre-Bosquet, N.; Dormont, D.; Gras, G. Macrophage activation switching: An asset for the resolution of inflammation. *Clin. Exp. Immunol.* **2005**, *142*, 481–489. [CrossRef]
227. Matsukawa, A.; Takeda, K.; Kudo, S.; Maeda, T.; Kagayama, M.; Akira, S. Aberrant inflammation and lethality to septic peritonitis in mice lacking STAT3 in macrophages and neutrophils. *J. Immunol.* **2003**, *171*, 6198–6205. [CrossRef]

228. Millrine, D.; Cardus Figueras, A.; Uceda Fernandez, J.; Andrews, R.; Szomolay, B.; Cossins, B.C.; Rice, C.M.; Li, J.; Tyrrell, V.J.; McLeod, L.; et al. Th1 Cells Alter the Inflammatory Signature of IL-6 by Channeling STAT Transcription Factors to Alu-like Retroelements. *J. Immunol.* **2023**, *211*, 274–286. [CrossRef] [PubMed]
229. Seufert, J.; Gallwitz, B. The extra-pancreatic effects of GLP-1 receptor agonists: A focus on the cardiovascular, gastrointestinal and central nervous systems. *Diabetes Obes. Metab.* **2014**, *16*, 673–688. [CrossRef] [PubMed]
230. Lee, Y.S.; Jun, H.S. Anti-Inflammatory Effects of GLP-1-Based Therapies beyond Glucose Control. *Mediat. Inflamm.* **2016**, *2016*, 3094642. [CrossRef]
231. Du, X.; Zhang, H.; Zhang, W.; Wang, Q.; Wang, W.; Ge, G.; Bai, J.; Guo, X.; Zhang, Y.; Jiang, X.; et al. The protective effects of lixisenatide against inflammatory response in human rheumatoid arthritis fibroblast-like synoviocytes. *Int. Immunopharmacol.* **2019**, *75*, 105732. [CrossRef]
232. Wang, Y.G.; Yang, T.L. Liraglutide reduces oxidized LDL-induced oxidative stress and fatty degeneration in Raw 264.7 cells involving the AMPK/SREBP1 pathway. *J. Geriatr. Cardiol.* **2015**, *12*, 410–416. [PubMed]
233. Bu, T.; Sun, Z.; Pan, Y.; Deng, X.; Yuan, G. Glucagon-Like Peptide-1: New Regulator in Lipid Metabolism. *Diabetes Metab. J.* **2024**, *48*, 354–372. [CrossRef] [PubMed]

biomedicines

MDPI

Review

What Is the Role of Basal Weekly Insulin in Clinical Practice? The State of the Art

Christiano Argano [1,*], Laura Priola [1], Francesco Manno [1] and Salvatore Corrao [1,2]

[1] Department of Internal Medicine, National Relevance and High Specialization Hospital Trust ARNAS Civico, Di Cristina, Benfratelli, 90127 Palermo, Italy; laura.priola@libero.it (L.P.); francescomanno0@gmail.com (F.M.); s.corrao@tiscali.it (S.C.)

[2] Department of Health Promotion Sciences, Maternal and Infant Care, Internal Medicine and Medical Specialties (PROMISE), University of Palermo, 90127 Palermo, Italy

* Correspondence: christiano.argano@arnascivico.it; Tel.: +39-091-655-2065; Fax: +39-091-666-3167

Abstract: Despite the advent of innovative therapies in the treatment of diabetes, ever-increasing awareness is still directed to the role of insulin since it has continued to be at the centre of diabetes therapy for decades, as a therapeutic integration of innovative agents in type 2 diabetes mellitus (T2DM), as the only replacement therapy in type 1 diabetes mellitus (T1DM) and also in gestational diabetes. In this context, the study of molecules such as weekly basal insulins, both for their technological and pharmacodynamic innovation and their manageability and undoubted benefits in compliance with drug therapy, can only be a turning point in diabetes and for all its phenotypes. This review aims to provide insight into the knowledge of basal weekly insulins and their use in type 1 and 2 diabetes mellitus by examining their safety, efficacy, manageability and increased therapeutic compliance.

Keywords: weekly insulin; icodec; LY3209590 basal insulin Fc (BIF); type 1 diabetes mellitus; type 2 diabetes mellitus

1. Introduction

Globally, diabetes represents a considerable burden to healthcare systems with an increasing prevalence, primarily due to a rise in obesity [1]. In 2021, the global age-standardized total prevalence was 6.1% (5.8–6.5) [1], resulting in health expenditures of U.S. $966 billion that are expected to rise, reaching more than $1054 billion by 2045 [2]. According to the Global Burden of Diseases, Injuries, and Risk Factors Study (GBD) 2019, diabetes was the eighth cause of death and disability globally [3]. Furthermore, the global burden of diabetes is predicted to increase among elderly patients due to reduced physical activity relating to T2DM mellitus, unhealthy diets, rising incidences of T1DM and the aging of the world population, determining a further surge in the hospitalization of subjects with diabetes and comorbidities, which are essential determinants of diabetes burden in terms of their considerable impact on a patient's quality of life, health status and outcomes [4,5]. In 2021, approximately 530 million adults worldwide were affected by diabetes [2], and 11.6% of the U.S. population (38.4 million people of all ages) had diabetes. In particular, 14.7% of all U.S. adults (38.1 million adults million adults aged 18 years or older) had diabetes. A total of 35 per 10,000 children and adolescents younger than age 20 years (352,000) had been diagnosed with diabetes. This datum includes 304,000 with type 1 diabetes [1,6]. In Europe, the prevalence of diabetes is 9.2%, and the number of people with diabetes (61 million) will increase to 13% by 2045 [7]. Nowadays, insulin continues to be an agent of ordinary and necessary use in the pharmacological treatment of diabetes, firstly in T1DM and in gestational diabetes, where insulin is the only pharmacological option and the only considerable replacement therapy. Secondly, the treatment of T2DM also takes into account the cardiovascular risk, often as an add-on to other molecules, in order to achieve the pre-established glycemic objectives despite the various pharmacological alternatives.

According to the National Statistics Report of the Centers for Disease Control and Prevention, 5.7% of all U.S. adults (1.7 million adults aged 20 years or older) with diagnosed diabetes use insulin. A total of 12.3% (3.6 million adults aged 20 years or older) of all U.S. adults with diagnosed diabetes started using insulin within a year of their diagnosis [6].

Although the currently available basal insulin formulations are effective and have a reduced hypoglycemic risk compared to past formulations, their therapeutic introduction could be more timely, mainly due to clinical inertia, patient concerns and poor compliance and education by medical personnel [8,9]. Poor adherence to daily dosing is widespread and associated with poor glycemic control [10,11]. Further problems relate to titration based on glycemic compensation and daily needs [12]. In addition, insulin non-adherence was associated with several injection-related factors, such as number of injections, dose calculation and injection technique, interference with daily activities and embarrassment [13,14]. In this sense, to overcome these problems, the research has moved towards developing basal insulin with longer than twenty-four hours of action and a flatter insulin profile [15].

Once-weekly basal insulin administration would reduce clinical inertia, increase treatment adherence and improve patients' quality of life, provided the risk of hypoglycemia remains low. Comparisons of once-weekly Glucagon-like peptide-1 receptor agonists (GLP-1 RAs) with once-daily GLP-1 RAs come to our aid [16–19].

Recent studies have showed that once-weekly insulin treatment had glucose-lowering efficacy and a safety profile [20,21]. Given this background, this review explored current knowledge about basal weekly insulins and their use in type 1 and 2 diabetes.

2. Methods

An extensive search of SCOPUS, PubMed and CENTRAL was performed using the following string: "(once-weekly insulin) AND ((("Clinical Trial, Phase III" [Publication Type]) OR ("Clinical Trial, Phase II" [Publication Type]) OR "Clinical Trial, Phase IV" [Publication Type]) OR "Randomized Controlled Trial" [Publication Type])" [22–24]. The search string retrieved 167 manuscripts. Hand-searching for principal generalist, human nutrition and basic research journals was also carried out. Two authors (L.P. and F.M.) independently reviewed the retrieved articles' titles, abstracts and full texts to determine their potential inclusion. Any disagreements were resolved via discussion with other authors (S.C and C.A.). Manuscripts regarding the role of weekly insulin in type 1 and 2 diabetes were extracted for this review.

3. Basal Weekly Insulin

Over the last 100 years, insulin therapy has evolved in parallel with advances in biochemistry and biotechnology [25]. Despite numerous milestones over the last 100 years, insulin is still in constant technological development to facilitate compliance [26]. The first insulins were crude preparations from bovine or porcine pancreas. These were associated with side effects such as lipodystrophy and allergic reactions [27,28] and were administered several times a day given their short duration of action. Basal insulin is essential to insulin therapy in T1DM and rapid insulin. In some cases, insulin is necessary to regulate blood sugar levels during fasting at night and after meals in people with T2DM. This is particularly important during episodes of acute glycometabolic decompensation and for individuals who cannot tolerate newer treatments [29].

Problems related to therapeutic adherence, quality of life, hypoglycemic risk and secondary disability or the expected compensation often arise [30].

Basal insulin is the most common insulin therapy in type 1 and T2DM. It is required for multiple injection therapy in T1DM and can be used as an adjunctive drug in T2DM, along with other drugs usually administered in the decompensation phase. Subsequently, there has been a shift from basal insulin with a duration of action of 5–7 h to once-daily dosing and now to once-weekly dosing with an extended half-life.

New weekly insulins have been developed, including Fc-fusion proteins of native single-chain insulin and a panel of recombinant native single-chain insulin molecules. In a pre-clinical study [31], these insulins led to a significant decrease in blood glucose levels for five days in db/db mice after a single dose, by more than 50% compared to the controls ($p < 0.05$). Another molecule was PEGylated insulin AB101, which demonstrated activity over seven days in a phase 1 trial. However, its variability in time to onset and drug concentration could be more robust, so it is no longer in development [32]. Another two molecules, the Fc-fusion insulins HM12460A and HM12470, were presented in 2016. Unfortunately, there have been no reports on their progress for several years [33–35]. Insumera insulin (PE0139) was analyzed in a randomized controlled phase 2 trial study completed in 2016 (NCT02581657). However, the results have not been published, and it is unknown whether Insumera is still in active development [36]. Currently, two alternative molecules have been further developed: Basal insulin Fc (BIF, LY3209590) and Insulin Icodec.

4. Basal Insulin Fc (BIF, LY3209590)

The LY3209590 basal insulin Fc (BIF) is a fusion protein that combines a single-chain insulin variant with a human immunoglobulin G fragment crystallizable domain. It is a selective agonist for insulin receptors and provides full agonism [37]. BIF comprises a human insulin receptor (IR) agonist fused to a human immunoglobulin G2 (IgG2) fragment crystallizable (Fc) domain and has a molecular weight of 64.1 kDa. Each homodimer monomer comprises a single-chain variant of insulin, an interdomain linker and the Fc domain from IgG2. In vitro, the data exhibited a reduced IR-binding affinity, yet with full agonism, selectivity against the insulin-like growth factor-1 receptor and functional properties similar to native human insulin, so it is a selective agonist for insulin receptors and provides full agonism [38] (Figure 1).

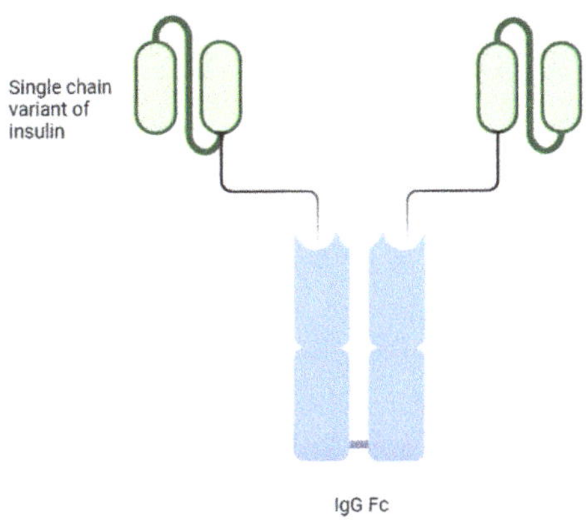

Figure 1. Schematic structure of basal weekly insulin Fc (BIF).

It was designed for once-weekly subcutaneous administration in treating patients with T2DM or T1DM. Phase 1 studies indicated that BIF has a low weekly peak-to-trough ratio (1.14, or <15% variation in insulin concentration) and a half-life of 17 days [38] (Figure 2).

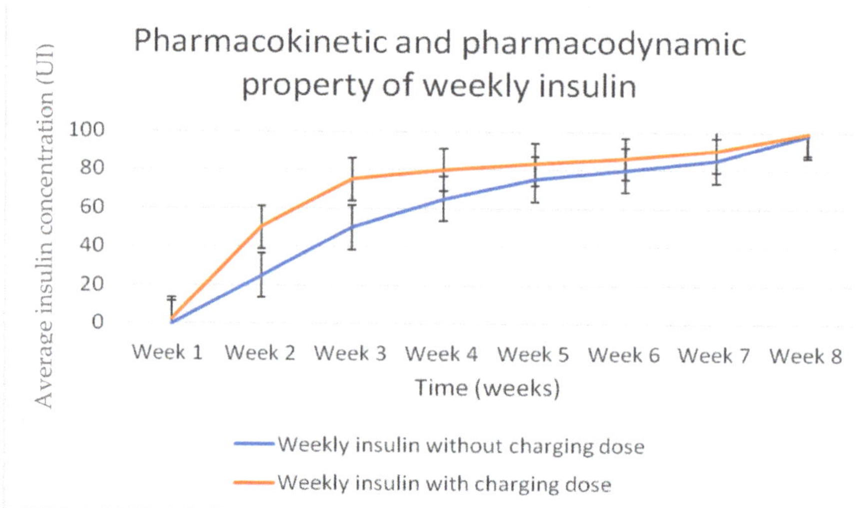

Figure 2. Basal weekly insulin Fc (BIF) pharmacokinetic profile.

5. Insulin Icodec

Icodec insulin is one of two ultra-slow, weekly-acting analogues currently being studied to treat diabetes [39]. In particular, icodec insulin is an acylated analogue (due to the addition of icosanedioic acid, hence the name). It owes its long duration of action to the pharmacodynamic effect that this modification entails, together with the replacement of three amino acids, ensuring a stronger bond with albumin and more remarkable persistence in the bloodstream [40] (Figure 3). By introducing a solid but reversible bond with albumin, icodec guarantees circulating deposition of the drug bound to albumin, which is inactive (through the addition of a side chain containing C20 fatty acid), and three amino acid substitutions (A14E, B16H and B25H), which provides molecular stability with which icodec insulin can activate slowly and steadily, thereby ensuring a prolonged half-life adequate for weekly administration. [40] A clinical pharmacology study demonstrated that icodec has an estimated half-life of 196 h and a uniform hypoglycemic effect throughout the week [40,41] (Figure 4). In vitro cytology studies have demonstrated that icodec activates the same dose-dependent IR-mediated signaling and metabolic responses as endogenous human insulin [41]. Furthermore, the in vitro mitogenic effect of icodec insulin in various human cells was low compared to other types [40,42].

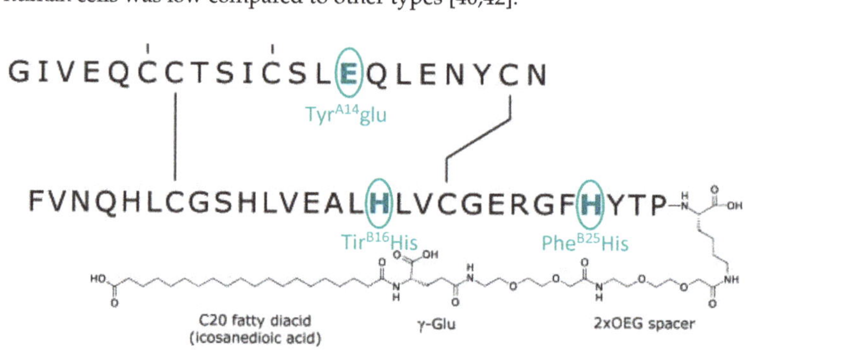

Figure 3. Schematic description and biological properties of basal weekly insulin icodec. The insulin icodec structure shows changes to the human insulin amino acid sequence and chemical modification attached to the lysine in position B29 of insulin.

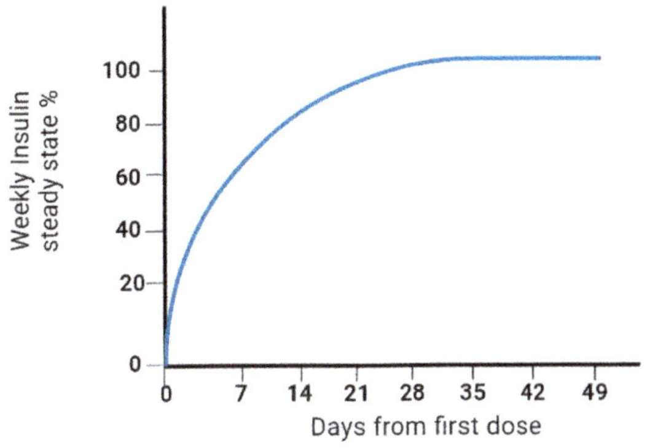

Figure 4. Pharmacokinetic properties (steady state) of weekly insulin.

To date, the two most advanced clinical development programs are basal insulin Fc (BIF, LY3209590) (Table 1) and the basal insulin icodec ONWARDS program (Table 2).

Table 1. Synthesis of randomized trials regarding insulin Fc (phase 2 trials).

	Insulin Fc vs. Degludec in DMt2 Patients Previously Treated with Basal Insulin [40]	Insulin Fc vs. Degludec in DMt2 Patients Insulino-Naïve [43]	Insulin Fc vs. Degludec in DMt1 Patients [44]
Study design	- Multicenter (44 sites) - Randomized, 1:1, open-label - Phase 2 trial - Non-inferiority study vs. basal insulin for efficacy and safety - Basal insulin and up to three oral antidiabetic medicines	- Multicenter (61 sites) - Randomized, 1:1, open-label - Phase 2 trial - Non-inferiority study vs. degludec in DMt2 insulin-naïve patients - Insulin-naïve DMt2 patients previously treated with metformin alone or in combination with dipeptidyl peptidase 4 and/or sodium-glucose cotransporter 2 for at least 3 months prior to screening	- Multicenter (49 sites) - Randomized, 1:1, open-label - Phase 2 trial - Non-inferiority study vs. Degludec in DMt2 insulin-naive patients - Patients with T1D treated with multiple daily basal injections of glargine (U-100 or U-300), detemir, degludec (U-100 or U-200) as basal insulin and as boluses of insulin lispro, aspart, FiAsp or glulisine
Period	November 2018–February 2020	5 March 2021–19 July 2023	6 June 2020–22 January 2021
Endpoint I	HbA1c reduction at 32 weeks	HbA1c reduction at 26 weeks	HbA1c reduction at 26 weeks
Endpoint II	- ΔFPG vs. baseline - Average insulin dose: at weeks 50–52 and 76–78 - Δweight vs. baseline - No. level 2, 3 and combined hypoglycemia vs. baseline - ΔTIR 70–180 mg/dL between groups at weeks 48–52	- Δweight vs. baseline - ΔFPG from baseline to week 26 - No. level 2, 3 and combined hypoglycemia vs. baseline	- Δ percent time in range (TIR) (70–180 mg/dL) on continuous glucose monitoring (CGM) fasting glucose (FG) level - Rate of hypoglycemia
Titration protocol	The loading and initial weekly doses were based on their previous daily basal insulin dose and their glycemic control according to baseline HbA1c (using a threshold of 8.5. BIF dosing in the Phase 2 program used mg increments and not insulin international units (IU))	Initial dose 10 IU/day (70 IU/week for icodec) Weekly titration on average FPG of the last 3 days Target: FPG 80–130 mg/dL	Titration was based on mean fasting blood glucose levels using CGM measurements on at least 3 days of the week using a paper-based algorithm. BIF was titrated weekly for weeks 1–12 and then every 4 weeks until the end of the treatment period

Table 1. *Cont.*

	Insulin Fc vs. Degludec in DMt2 Patients Previously Treated with Basal Insulin [40]	Insulin Fc vs. Degludec in DMt2 Patients Insulino-Naïve [43]	Insulin Fc vs. Degludec in DMt1 Patients [44]
Numbers of patients	- Enrolled (at least 1 dose): 399 - Completed trials: 351	- Enrolled (at least 1 dose): 278 - Completed trials: 241	- Enrolled (at least 1 dose): 238 - Completed trials: 190
Population	- DT2 (average duration 15 years) - Average age 60.2 years - 51% female - Average BMI 30 kg/m^2 (<32.2 kg/m^2) - Baseline HbA1c 8.1% (7–11%) - Mean daily basal insulin dose at randomization (39 IU)	- DT2 (average duration 10 years) - Average age 58 years - 45% female - Average BMI 30 kg/m^2 (<32.2 kg/m^2) - Baseline HbA1c 8% (7–9.5%) - Mean daily basal insulin dose at randomization (39 IU)	- DT1 (average duration 22 years) - Average age 46 years - 38% female - Average BMI 27.5 kg/m^2 (<32.2 kg/m^2) - Baseline HbA1c 7.5% (7–9.5%)
Results	- HbA1c reduction −0.1% (CI Δ 0.4–0.03%), $p < 0.001$ - Increase in patients at target (HbA1c < 7%) without significant hypoglycemia: +10% - ΔFPG not significant - Average insulin dose at 52 weeks: 31 IU/day icodec vs. 32 IU/day glargine; on average 0.35 IU/kg/day - Δweight not significant (+2 kg both groups) - TIR increase +4.3% (CI 1.9–6.6%) $p < 0.001$	- At week 26, icodec demonstrated non-inferiority and superiority to degludec in reducing mean HbA1c from baseline. Rates of clinically significant hypoglycemia were not significantly different between treatment groups at week 26.	- At week 26, a non-inferior reduction in HbA1c from baseline was observed compared to patients treated with degludec, with a statistically significant difference of 0.17% ($p = 0.07$) - Time in range (TIR) was similar for patients in the BIF (56.1%) and degludec (58.9%; $p = 0.112$) groups at week 26
Hypoglycemic events	The event rates of all documented hypoglycemia were about 25% lower in the Fc groups, and those for nocturnal hypoglycemia were at least 33% lower from baseline to week 32 compared with insulin degludec	The rate of severe hypoglycemic events was not significant between treatment groups (p 0.64)	Hypoglycemia occurrence over 24 h was similar for BIF and degludec for level 1 ($p = 0.960$) or level 2 ($p = 0.517$) hypoglycemia during treatment. The occurrence of serious adverse events was similar between the BIF and degludec groups.
Adverse events	Mostly mild/moderate events and not associated with treatment Deaths: 3 (2%) in degludec, 1 (1%) in glargine No reactions at the injection site or critical issues related to medication errors described	Mostly mild/moderate events and not associated with treatment: Fc 5.6% (n = 143) Degludec 3% (n = 135) Deaths: 2 (1%) in Fc, 3 (1.5%) in degludec	Mostly mild/moderate events and not associated with treatment. The occurrence of serious adverse events was similar between the BIF and degludec groups.

Table 2. Synthesis of randomized trials regarding icodec: the ONWARDS program.

	ONWARDS 1 Icodec vs. Glargine U100 in DT2 Insulino-Naïve [45]	**ONWARDS 2 Icodec vs. Degludec U100 in Basal Bolus [46]**	**ONWARDS 3 Icodec vs. Degludec in DT2 Insulino-Naïve [47]**	**ONWARDS 4 Icodec vs. Glargine U100 in DT2 in Basal Bolus [48]**	**ONWARDS 5 Icodec vs. Once-Daily Insulin in DT2 Insulino-Naïve with Dosing Guide App [49]**	**ONWARDS 6 Icodec vs. Degludec in T1D [50]**
Study design	- Multicenter (147 sites) - Randomized, 1:1, open-label - Non-inferiority study vs. glargine U100 for efficacy and safety - Basal insulin in addition to any hypoglycemic agent, except S.U. and glinides	- Multicenter (71 sites) - Randomized, 1:1, open-label - Non-inferiority study vs. degludec for efficacy and safety - Basal insulin in insulin-naïve patients, in addition to any hypoglycemic agent, including S.U. and glinides; double-blinded CGM	- Multicenter (92 sites) - Randomized 1:1, double blind - Non-inferiority study vs. degludec for efficacy and safety - Basal insulin in addition to any hypoglycemic agent, including S.U. and glinides	- Multicenter (80 sites) - Randomized, 1:1, open-label - Non-inferiority study vs. glargine U100 for efficacy and safety in patients previously in basal bolus treatment - Basal insulin in addition to any hypoglycemic agent, except S.U. and glinides	- Multicenter (176 sites) - Randomized, 1:1, open-label, parallel group with real-world elements - Non-inferiority study versus once-daily basal insulin analogues (O.D. analogues) dosed per standard practice using a dose-checking app	- Multicenter (99 sites) - Randomized, 1:1, open label - Non-inferiority study vs. degludec for efficacy and safety - Basal insulin in addition to insulin aspart for active group and control group
Period	November 2020–May 2023	5 March 2021–19 July 2023	March 2021–June 2022	March 2021–October 2021	1 March 2021–12 August 2022	30 April 2021–15 October 2021
Endpoint I	HbA1c reduction at 52 weeks	HbA1c reduction at 26 weeks	HbA1c reduction at 26 weeks	HbA1c reduction at 26 weeks	HbA1c reduction at 52 weeks	HbA1c reduction at 26 weeks
Endpoint II	- ΔFPG vs. baseline - Average insulin dose: at weeks 50–52 and 76–78 - Δweight vs. baseline - No. level 2, 3 and combined hypoglycemia vs. baseline - ΔTIR 70–180 mg/dL between groups at weeks 48–52	- Δweight vs. baseline - ΔFPG from baseline to week 26 - No. level 2, 3 and combined hypoglycemia vs. baseline	- ΔFPG vs. baseline - Average insulin dose: at weeks 24–26 - Δweight vs. baseline - No. Level 2, 3 and combined hypoglycemia vs. baseline	- ΔFPG from baseline to week 26 - Δweight vs. baseline - No. level 2, 3 and combined hypoglycemia vs. baseline	- Time from baseline to treatment discontinuation or intensification - No. level 2, 3 and combined hypoglycemia vs. baseline	- HbA1c from baseline to week 52 - ΔFPG from baseline to week 26 - Percentage of time in range (TIR; 3.9–10.0 mmol/L [70–180 mg/dL]) during weeks 22–26 - Δweight vs. baseline - Average insulin dose: at weeks 24–26 and at weeks 50–52 - No. level 2, 3 and combined hypoglycemia vs. baseline
Titration protocol	Initial dose of 10 IU/day (70 IU/week for icodec) Weekly titration on average FPG of the last 3 days Target: FPG 80–130 mg/dL	Initial dose of 10 IU/day (70 IU/week for icodec) Weekly titration on average FPG of the last 3 days Target: FPG 80–130 mg/dL	Initial dose of 10 IU/day (70 IU/week for icodec) Weekly titration on average FPG of the last 3 days Target: FPG 80–130 mg/dL Increments of 3 IU/day (20 IU/week for icodec)	Initial dose of 10 IU/day (70 IU/week for icodec) Weekly titration on average FPG of the last 3 days Target: FPG 80–130 mg/dL	Icodec titrated with a dosing guide app (icodec with app)	Initial dose of 10 IU/day (70 IU/week for icodec) Weekly titration on average FPG of the last 3 days Target: FPG 80–130 mg/dL Increments of 3 IU/day (20 IU/week for icodec)

Table 2. *Cont.*

	ONWARDS 1 Icodec vs. Glargine U100 in DT2 Insulino-Naïve [45]	ONWARDS 2 Icodec vs. Degludec U100 in Basal Bolus [46]	ONWARDS 3 Icodec vs. Degludec in DT2 Insulino-Naïve [47]	ONWARDS 4 Icodec vs. Glargine U100 in DT2 in Basal Bolus [48]	ONWARDS 5 Icodec vs. Once-Daily Insulin in DT2 Insulino-Naïve with Dosing Guide App [49]	ONWARDS 6 Icodec vs. Degludec in T1D [50]
Numbers of patients	- Enrolled (at least 1 dose): 984 - Completed trials: 954	- Enrolled (at least 1 dose): 526 - Completed trials: 510	- Enrolled (at least 1 dose): 588 - Completed trials: 564	- Enrolled (at least 1 dose): 582 - Completed trials: 582	- Enrolled (at least 1 dose): 1085 - Completed trials: 1008	- Enrolled (at least 1 dose): 582 - Completed trials: 540
Population	- DT2 (average duration 11.5 years) - Average age: 59 years - 40% female - Average BMI: 30 kg/m^2 (<40 kg/m^2) - Baseline HbA1c: 8.5% (7–11%)	- DT2 (average duration 10.5 years) - Average age: ≥18 years - HbA1c: 7.0–10.0%	- DT2 (average duration 10.5 years) - Average age: 58 years - 37% female - Average BMI: 29.5 kg/m^2 (<40 kg/m^2) - Baseline HbA1c: 8.5% (7–11%) - Layering for S.U./glinide use	- DT2 (average duration 10.5 years) - Average age: 44.9 years - 41% female - Average BMI: 26.5 kg/m^2 (<40 kg/m^2) - Baseline HbA1c: 7.51% (7–10%)	- DT2 (average duration 10.5 years) - Average age: ≥18 years - HbA1c: 7.0–10.0%, insulin-naïve	- TD1 (average duration 19.5 years) - Average age: 44.2 years - 42% female - Average BMI: 26.5 kg/m^2 (<40 kg/m^2) - Baseline HbA1c: 7.61% (7–11%)
Results	- HbA1c reduction: −0.2% (CI Δ 0.4–0.03%), p <0.001 - Increase in patients at target (HbA1c < 7%) without significant hypoglycemia: +10% - ΔFPG not significant - Average insulin dose at 52 weeks: 31 IU/day icodec vs. 32 IU/day glargine; on average 0.35 IU/kg/day - Δweight not significant (+2 kg both groups) - TIR increase +4.3% (CI 1.9–6.6%) p < 0.001	- At week 26, icodec demonstrated non-inferiority and superiority to degludec in reducing HbA1c from baseline. Clinically significant hypoglycemia rates were not significant between the two groups at week 31	- HbA1c reduction −0.2% (CI Δ 0.3–0.1%), p < 0.001 - Increase in patients at target (HbA1c < 7%) without significant hypoglycemia: +15% - ΔFPG not significant - Average insulin dose at 26 weeks: 29 IU/day icodec vs. 27 IU/day degludec; on average 0.3 IU/kg/day - Δweight not significant (+2.5 kg both groups)	At week 26, the mean change in HbA1c was −1.16 percentage points in the icodec group (baseline 8.29%) and −1.18 percentage points in the glargine U100 group (baseline 8.31%). Combined level 2 and level 3 hypoglycemia rates were similar between treatment groups.	At week 52, insulin icodec used in conjunction with the dosing guide app demonstrated non-inferiority and superiority versus the basal insulin analogues in reducing the estimated mean HbA1c from baseline	- HbA1c reduction: −0.47% (p < 0.0001) - Increase in patients at target (HbA1c <7%) without significant hypoglycemia: +9.5% - ΔFPG (icodec −15.08 mg/dL—degludec −33.66 mg/dL ETD 18.58 (8.58 to 28.58), p = 0.0003 - Estimated mean weekly total insulin dose, U/week (U/day) at 26 weeks icodec 311 (~44) vs. degludec 323 (~46) ETR 0.96 (0.90 to 1.03), p = 0.27 - Δweight icodec 1.29 vs. degludec 1.01 ETD 0.28 (−0.37 to 0.92), p = 0.41

Table 2. *Cont.*

	ONWARDS 1 Icodec vs. Glargine U100 in DT2 Insulino-Naïve [45]	ONWARDS 2 Icodec vs. Degludec U100 in Basal Bolus [46]	ONWARDS 3 Icodec vs. Degludec in DT2 Insulino-Naïve [47]	ONWARDS 4 Icodec vs. Glargine U100 in DT2 in Basal Bolus [48]	ONWARDS 5 Icodec vs. Once-Daily Insulin in DT2 Insulino-Naïve with Dosing Guide App [49]	ONWARDS 6 Icodec vs. Degludec in T1D [50]
Hypoglycemic events	Icodecs: - 226 episodes in 61 pcs (12.4%) - 1 episode of severe hypoglycemia Glargine: - 114 episodes in 66 pcs (13.4%) - 7 episodes of severe hypoglycemia	Clinically significant hypoglycemia rates were not significant between the two groups at week 31	Icodecs: - 53 episodes in 26 pcs (9%) - 0 episodes of severe hypoglycemia Degludec: - 23 episodes in 17 pieces (6%) - 2 episodes of severe hypoglycemia	Icodecs: - 35 serious adverse events were reported in 22 (8%) of 291 participants Degludec U100: - 33 serious adverse events were reported in 25 (9%) of 291 participants	Clinically significant or severe hypoglycemia rates were not significantly different between the treatment groups at week 57	Icodecs: - 2789 episodes in 246 pcs (19.60%) - 47 episodes of severe hypoglycemia (0.33%) Degludec: - 1478 episodes in 223 pieces (10.26%) - 17 episodes of severe hypoglycemia (0.12%)
Adverse events	Mostly mild/moderate events and not associated with treatment Deaths: 5 in icodec, 4 in glargine No reactions at the injection site or critical issues related to medication errors described	Mostly mild/moderate events and not associated with treatment Deaths: 5 in icodec, 4 in glargine No reactions at the injection site or critical issues related to medication errors described	Mostly mild/moderate events and not associated with treatment Deaths: 2 in icodec, 1 in degludec 8.5 vs. 4.4% injection site reactions for icodec vs. degludec Usage errors <5%	Mostly mild/moderate events and not associated with treatment No reactions at the injection site or critical issues related to medication errors described	Mostly mild/moderate events and not associated with treatment No reactions at the injection site or critical issues related to medication errors described	Mostly mild/moderate events and not associated with treatment Deaths: 1 in icodec, 0 in degludec 0.07% vs. 0.06% injection site reactions for icodec vs. degludec

6. Type 2 Diabetes Mellitus and Weekly Insulin

Even if many new drugs are available now, some patients need to be treated with insulin therapy to achieve personalized glycemic control [51,52]. According to the guidelines, basal insulin needs to be used in a patient with T2DM and severe hyperglycemia (generally blood glucose $\geq$ 300 mg/dL [$\geq$16.7 mmol/L] or glycated hemoglobin [HbA1c] > 10%) or symptomatic hyperglycemia or if the patient has signs of catabolism (hypertriglyceridemia, weight loss or ketosis) [20]. It is worth outlining that a glycemia level greater than 250 mg/dL [$\geq$13.89 mmol/L] represents a strong predictor of in-hospital mortality in older people hospitalized in internal medicine wards [53]. If a glucagon-like peptide-1 receptor agonist (GLP-1RA) is not suitable, if a more robust approach is needed or if it is a personal preference, insulin therapy is recommended [54,55]. Poor adherence to insulin therapy is a common problem and is responsible for poor outcomes and high healthcare costs. One of the most common causes of reduced adherence is the frequency of injection. This problem could be solved by once-weekly insulin injections, improving patients' quality of life and leading to better outcomes. This statement is even more pertinent in patients receiving multiple glucose-lowering agents who need injection assistance or are intolerant to other treatments [56]. The rates and reasons for discontinuations vary by study [10,45–47,57], but injection frequency is always one important contributing factor. In this sense, the ONWARDS program [39] has been developed to evaluate the safety and efficacy of insulin icodec in T2DM. Six trials are part of it. Five of these trials enrolled T2DM subjects. Going into the specifics of the icodec trial, in the ONWARDS 1 study [48], with head-to-head comparison between icodec and glargine 100 conducted with a large sample of patients in the two groups (492 patients) and with homologous basic characteristics in the two groups, the mean reduction in glycated hemoglobin at 52 weeks and the percentage of TIR (time in range) were evaluated, demonstrating the non-inferiority and superiority of icodec compared to glargine 100. The two groups' rates of combined clinically significant events or severe hypoglycemia were similar, concluding that once-weekly insulin icodec achieves better glycemic control than once-daily insulin glargine U100.

The ONWARDS 2 [49] study aimed to evaluate the safety and efficacy of once-weekly icodec compared to once-daily insulin degludec in treating T2DM patients already on basal insulin treatment. The study found that once-weekly icodec was better than once-daily degludec in reducing HbA1c levels without causing significant adverse effects.

Similarly, in the ONWARDS 3 [43] study, which focused on insulin-naïve T2DM patients, once-weekly icodec was more effective in reducing HbA1c levels than once-daily degludec after 26 weeks of treatment. The study found no significant difference in secondary outcomes such as weight change and level 2 or 3 hypoglycemic events.

In the clinical trial ONWARDS 4 [58], researchers studied individuals with long-standing T2DM who were on a basal bolus insulin regimen. The study aimed to compare the efficacy of once-weekly insulin icodec to once-daily insulin glargine U100. The results indicated that weekly icodec resulted in better glycemic control with fewer basal insulin injections and lower bolus insulin doses, without increasing the risk of hypoglycemia, in comparison to daily glargine U100.

ONWARDS 5 [59], with attention to technology, is a trial regarding once-weekly insulin codec vs. once-daily basal insulin analogues in people who have T2DM and have not received insulin treatment before with a dosing guide app. Once-weekly icodec resulted in similar improvements in glycemic control compared to once-daily glargine, with fewer basal insulin injections, a lower bolus insulin dose and no increase in hypoglycemic rates compared to glargine U100. Icodec used in conjunction with a dosing guide app demonstrated non-inferiority and superiority versus basal insulin analogues in reducing the estimated mean HbA1c from baseline. A superior time in range was achieved for once-weekly insulin icodec compared with insulin glargine, while the clinically significant or severe hypoglycemia rates were not significantly different between the treatment groups. Weekly BIF was tested in patients with T2DM, achieving a similar efficacy to degludec despite higher fasting glucose targets in the BIF groups for basal insulin Fc. The higher fasting glucose targets and lower glucose variability might have contributed to its lower BIF hypoglycemia rates than degludec [51]. After 26 weeks of treatment once weekly, BIF achieved excellent glycemic control, similar to degludec, with no concerning hypoglycemia in subjects with T2DM [44]. A very recent systematic review [50] demonstrated superior glycometabolic compensation was achieved in patients with T2DM with icodec insulin compared to once-weekly Fc insulin, with no clinically significant differences in major hypoglycemic events.

7. Type 1 Diabetes Mellitus and Weekly Insulin

Basal insulin treatment is indispensable for patients with T1DM since it is a replacement therapy. Once-weekly insulin use is more complex in T1DM than in T2DM, but adherence can significantly improve, especially in people prone to missing doses, like teenagers, with better stability and lower episodes of diabetic ketoacidosis. [56,60] Once-weekly BIF demonstrated non-inferior glycemic control to once-daily degludec and no difference in hypoglycemia or other safety findings in patients with T1DM [61].

In ONWARDS 6 [62], the only phase 3 trial regarding the use of once-weekly insulin icodec vs. once-daily insulin degludec in combination with insulin aspart in people with T1DM, insulin icodec was non-inferior to insulin degludec in terms of HbA1c reduction, but severe hypoglycemia episodes occurred in the insulin icodec group.

Nevertheless, patients with diabetes have a positive attitude toward once-weekly injections [26], and a lower frequency of injections is a valuable attribute for injectable therapies [63].

8. Discussion

From a therapeutic point of view, considering the burden of the pathology, insulin continues to be an agent of ordinary and necessary use in the pharmacological treatment of diabetes, especially in T1DM and despite the various pharmacological alternatives for the treatment of T2DM [GLP1-RA, sodium-glucose co-transporter-2 inhibitors (SGLT2i), Dipeptidyl peptidase 4 (DPP4)], often as an add-on to other molecules, in order to achieve the pre-established glycemic objectives [11,57,60]. Although glucose regulation often becomes inadequate with these options as the disease progresses, there is some degree of "clinical inertia" due to the complexity and fear of insulin therapy, both from the perspectives of healthcare providers and people with diabetes. Nevertheless, there are cases of insulinopenic phenotypes where insulin becomes of fundamental use; think of patients with diabetes secondary to pancreaticoduodenectomy, patients with LADA and low c-peptide levels, patients with severe sarcopenia or with side effects and contraindications to GLP1RA or SGLT2i. The challenge in achieving reasonable glycemic control with insulin therapy can be attributed to the complexity of matching the dose and timing of daily insulin injections to the actual physiological requirements.

In this sense, real-world data from an extensive U.S. electronic medical records database, including 6597 subjects, suggested that among patients with T2DM who initiated basal insulin after oral antidiabetic drugs, the likelihood of reaching glycemic control diminished over time and remained low from 12 months onwards [64]. Another real-world observational study showed that the median time to treatment intensification in patients with elevated HbA1c following basal insulin initiation was 4.3 years [65].

The difficulty of integrating insulin use into daily lifestyle due to regimen complexity, reducing the frequency of daily injections and medical affordability are the most common reasons for basal insulin discontinuation [66].

For patients with T1DM, there are currently no therapeutic options available other than insulin therapy using multiple daily insulin injections or micro-infusion pumps. However, despite the advent of innovative therapies for the treatment of patients with T2DM, in many cases, as expressed above, insulin remains a valid option. In this regard, it is delaying the start of insulin therapy in T2DM that results in poor glycometabolic control. Long-acting basal insulin that can exert a hypoglycemic effect in an effective, safe and long-lasting way with just one injection per week should reduce the treatment burden, ensuring better compliance and glycemic control. Clearly, for once-weekly basal insulin to be clinically relevant, it must be comparable to or superior to conventional once-daily insulin treatment in the absence of an increased risk of hypoglycemic events. It remains crucial that both healthcare personnel and patients must learn to switch from conventional insulin therapy, titrate weekly insulin and manage concomitant preprandial insulin if as a basal bolus. At the start of the therapeutic switch, patients switching from once-daily to once-weekly basal insulin may be predisposed to worse initial glycometabolic compensation before reaching a new steady state. However, this can be addressed with a higher initial loading dose and subsequent titration to lower doses, as recently shown with insulin icodec and Fc [38,42,61]. Consistent insulin titration for new users is critical to achieving timely glycemic control [67] and well evidenced, but straightforward titration regimens will be essential to provide confidence in using once-weekly insulins.

The molecular modifications introduced into insulin icodec and insulin Fc provide novel basal insulin with biological and pharmacokinetic/pharmacodynamic properties suitable for once-weekly dosing. Weekly analogues promise a better quality of life and better therapeutic adherence, reducing the number of injections required from patients.

A clinical phase 3 trial in people with type 1 and 2 diabetes showed that insulin icodec was well tolerated and had pharmacokinetic/pharmacodynamic properties suited for once-weekly dosing. The same is valid for the phase 2 clinical trial of insulin Fc. These once-weekly preparations have demonstrated similar glycemic control to long-acting once-daily insulin analogues, with their hypoglycemic episode rates similar to those of the usual basal insulin preparations. In this sense, a recent meta-analysis showed that insulin icodec was associated with significantly decreased HbA1C, an increased time with glucose in range and similar hypoglycemic and severe adverse effects compared with long-acting insulin in people with T2DM [68]. The possibility of employing basal weekly insulin, beyond its proven safety and efficacy, makes the long duration of action and the reduced need for daily injections noteworthy, as shown by Bajaj and colleagues [69]. All this is undoubtedly associated with better compliance, effectiveness, safety and, consequently, quality of life, which are always to be considered in the management of patients during follow-up. Insulin is a growth factor, and the possibility of reducing the daily dosage per kilogram could, in the long term, reduce the risks linked to its mitotic effect on cells and anabolic effects on tissues, reducing the activation of the insulin receptor and the post-receptor pathways, which may have a stronger mitogenic potency on cancer cells [70]. This argument is a future "open question" for scientific research.

We can, however, consider the use of weekly basal insulin in other rare forms of diabetes that are independent of T1DM or 2 T2DM and which, over time, will be of increasingly more significant scientific interest since there is no solid evidence in place in the literature on the subject. These forms include T2DM patients in the decompensation phase due to steroid therapy, purely "meta steroid" diabetes or patients with LADA. Further application may occur in forms of diabetes secondary to endocrine and exocrine deficiency of the pancreas, such as in chronic pancreatitis or in patients undergoing major pancreatic surgery or severe sarcopenia. Another example, indeed more frequent from an epidemiological point of view, is gestational diabetes, which could be a valid, safe and effective option. Since, a bit like in T1DM, insulin therapy is practically the only valid weapon in gestational diabetes, another open issue remains for gestational diabetes, in which it could be a valid, safe and effective option, reducing the frequency of daily injections; more solid and future clinical data are needed in this regard. These clinical settings represent "open issues" for which there is no current literature but will undoubtedly be of particular scientific interest later on.

9. Conclusions

In conclusion, basal weekly long-acting insulin shows similar and better glycemic efficacy than daily basal insulin in T1DM and T2DM due to its association with less hypoglycemia, a reduction in the number of injections and its proven effectiveness. In particular, nowadays, icodec insulin is a candidate to become the primary basal weekly insulin, increasing patient compliance because of its tolerability and encouraging safety results related to hypoglycemia [71]. Consequently, once-weekly insulin could lower the polypharmacy burden among patients with T2DM, primarily comorbid and elderly [4,72], and at the same time, favor their acceptance of insulin therapy.

Although many questions remain unanswered, the future of once-weekly insulin preparations appears bright, and the data regarding some of the clinical issues are encouraging.

Author Contributions: Conceptualization, C.A. and S.C.; methodology, C.A. and S.C.; software, C.A. and S.C.; validation, C.A. and S.C.; formal analysis, L.P. and F.M.; investigation, L.P. and F.M.; resources, L.P. and F.M.; data curation L.P. and F.M.; writing—original draft preparation, C.A.; writing—review and editing, C.A, L.P., F.M. and S.C.; visualization, L.P. and F.M; supervision, S.C.; project administration, C.A. All authors have read and agreed to the published version of the manuscript.

Funding: This research received no external funding.

Conflicts of Interest: The authors declare no conflict of interest.

References

1. Ong, K.L.; Stafford, L.K.; McLaughlin, S.A.; Boyko, E.J.; Vollset, S.E.; Smith, A.E.; Dalton, B.E.; Duprey, J.; Cruz, J.A.; Hagins, H.; et al. Global, Regional, and National Burden of Diabetes from 1990 to 2021, with Projections of Prevalence to 2050: A Systematic Analysis for the Global Burden of Disease Study 2021. *Lancet* **2023**, *402*, 203–234. [CrossRef] [PubMed]
2. IDF Diabetes Atlas 2021 | IDF Diabetes Atlas. Available online: https://diabetesatlas.org/atlas/tenth-edition/ (accessed on 13 February 2024).
3. Vos, T.; Lim, S.S.; Abbafati, C.; Abbas, K.M.; Abbasi, M.; Abbasifard, M.; Abbasi-Kangevari, M.; Abbastabar, H.; Abd-Allah, F.; Abdelalim, A.; et al. Global Burden of 369 Diseases and Injuries in 204 Countries and Territories, 1990–2019: A Systematic Analysis for the Global Burden of Disease Study 2019. *Lancet* **2020**, *396*, 1204–1222. [CrossRef] [PubMed]
4. Argano, C.; Natoli, G.; Mularo, S.; Nobili, A.; Monaco, M.L.; Mannucci, P.M.; Perticone, F.; Pietrangelo, A.; Corrao, S. Impact of Diabetes Mellitus and Its Comorbidities on Elderly Patients Hospitalized in Internal Medicine Wards: Data from the RePoSi Registry. *Healthcare* **2022**, *10*, 86. [CrossRef] [PubMed]
5. Corrao, S.; Natoli, G.; Nobili, A.; Mannucci, P.M.; Perticone, F.; Arcoraci, V.; Argano, C. The "Diabetes Comorbidome": A Different Way for Health Professionals to Approach the Comorbidity Burden of Diabetes. *Healthcare* **2022**, *10*, 1459. [CrossRef] [PubMed]
6. National Diabetes Statistics Report | Diabetes | CDC. Available online: https://www.cdc.gov/diabetes/data/statistics-report/index.html (accessed on 10 February 2024).
7. Europe Diabetes Report 2000–2045. Available online: https://www.diabetesatlas.org/data/ (accessed on 10 February 2024).
8. Russell-Jones, D.; Pouwer, F.; Khunti, K. Identification of Barriers to Insulin Therapy and Approaches to Overcoming Them. *Diabetes Obes. Metab.* **2018**, *20*, 488–496. [CrossRef]
9. Khunti, K.; Gomes, M.B.; Pocock, S.; Shestakova, M.V.; Pintat, S.; Fenici, P.; Hammar, N.; Medina, J. Therapeutic Inertia in the Treatment of Hyperglycaemia in Patients with Type 2 Diabetes: A Systematic Review. *Diabetes Obes. Metab.* **2018**, *20*, 427–437. [CrossRef] [PubMed]
10. Boye, K.S.; Curtis, S.E.; Lage, M.J.; Garcia-Perez, L.-E. Associations between Adherence and Outcomes among Older, Type 2 Diabetes Patients: Evidence from a Medicare Supplemental Database. *Patient Prefer. Adherence* **2016**, *10*, 1573–1581. [CrossRef] [PubMed]
11. Donnelly, L.A.; Morris, A.D.; Evans, J.M.M.; DARTS/MEMO Collaboration. Adherence to Insulin and Its Association with Glycaemic Control in Patients with Type 2 Diabetes. *J. Assoc. Physicians* **2007**, *100*, 345–350. [CrossRef] [PubMed]
12. Kuritzky, L.; Reid, T.S.; Wysham, C.H. Practical Guidance on Effective Basal Insulin Titration for Primary Care Providers. *Clin. Diabetes* **2019**, *37*, 368–376. [CrossRef] [PubMed]
13. Peyrot, M.; Rubin, R.R.; Kruger, D.F.; Travis, L.B. Correlates of Insulin Injection Omission. *Diabetes Care* **2010**, *33*, 240–245. [CrossRef]
14. Peyrot, M.; Barnett, A.H.; Meneghini, L.F.; Schumm-Draeger, P.-M. Factors Associated with Injection Omission/Non-Adherence in the Global Attitudes of Patients and Physicians in Insulin Therapy Study. *Diabetes Obes. Metab.* **2012**, *14*, 1081–1087. [CrossRef] [PubMed]
15. Sugumar, V.; Ang, K.P.; Alshanon, A.F.; Sethi, G.; Yong, P.V.C.; Looi, C.Y.; Wong, W.F. A Comprehensive Review of the Evolution of Insulin Development and Its Delivery Method. *Pharmaceutics* **2022**, *14*, 1406. [CrossRef]
16. Qiao, Q.; Ouwens, M.J.; Grandy, S.; Johnsson, K.; Kostev, K. Adherence to GLP-1 Receptor Agonist Therapy Administered by Once-Daily or Once-Weekly Injection in Patients with Type 2 Diabetes in Germany. *Diabetes Metab. Syndr. Obes.* **2016**, *9*, 201–205. [CrossRef] [PubMed]

17. Qin, L.; Chen, S.; Flood, E.; Shaunik, A.; Romero, B.; de la Cruz, M.; Alvarez, C.; Grandy, S. Glucagon-Like Peptide-1 Receptor Agonist Treatment Attributes Important to Injection-Experienced Patients with Type 2 Diabetes Mellitus: A Preference Study in Germany and the United Kingdom. *Diabetes Ther.* **2017**, *8*, 335–353. [CrossRef] [PubMed]
18. Weeda, E.R.; Muraoka, A.K.; Brock, M.D.; Cannon, J.M. Medication Adherence to Injectable Glucagon-like Peptide-1 (GLP-1) Receptor Agonists Dosed Once Weekly vs Once Daily in Patients with Type 2 Diabetes: A Meta-Analysis. *Int. J. Clin. Pract.* **2021**, *75*, e14060. [CrossRef] [PubMed]
19. Weiss, T.; Carr, R.D.; Pal, S.; Yang, L.; Sawhney, B.; Boggs, R.; Rajpathak, S.; Iglay, K. Real-World Adherence and Discontinuation of Glucagon-Like Peptide-1 Receptor Agonists Therapy in Type 2 Diabetes Mellitus Patients in the United States. *Patient Prefer. Adherence* **2020**, *14*, 2337–2345. [CrossRef] [PubMed]
20. Rosenstock, J.; Bajaj, H.S.; Janež, A.; Silver, R.; Begtrup, K.; Hansen, M.V.; Jia, T.; Goldenberg, R.; NN1436-4383 Investigators. Once-Weekly Insulin for Type 2 Diabetes without Previous Insulin Treatment. *N. Engl. J. Med.* **2020**, *383*, 2107–2116. [CrossRef] [PubMed]
21. Skyler, J.S. Weekly Insulin Becoming a Reality. *Diabetes Care* **2021**, *44*, 1459–1461. [CrossRef] [PubMed]
22. Corrao, S.; Colomba, D.; Arnone, S.; Argano, C.; Di Chiara, T.; Scaglione, R.; Licata, G. Improving Efficacy of PubMed Clinical Queries for Retrieving Scientifically Strong Studies on Treatment. *J. Am. Med. Inf. Assoc.* **2006**, *13*, 485–487. [CrossRef] [PubMed]
23. Corrao, S.; Colomba, D.; Argano, C.; Calvo, L.; Scaglione, R.; Licata, G. Optimized Search Strategy for Detecting Scientifically Strong Studies on Treatment through PubMed. *Intern. Emerg. Med.* **2012**, *7*, 283–287. [CrossRef] [PubMed]
24. Haynes, R.B.; McKibbon, K.A.; Wilczynski, N.L.; Walter, S.D.; Werre, S.R.; Hedges Team. Optimal Search Strategies for Retrieving Scientifically Strong Studies of Treatment from Medline: Analytical Survey. *BMJ* **2005**, *330*, 1179. [CrossRef] [PubMed]
25. Rubino, A.; McQuay, L.J.; Gough, S.C.; Kvasz, M.; Tennis, P. Delayed Initiation of Subcutaneous Insulin Therapy after Failure of Oral Glucose-Lowering Agents in Patients with Type 2 Diabetes: A Population-Based Analysis in the UK. *Diabet. Med.* **2007**, *24*, 1412–1418. [CrossRef] [PubMed]
26. Polonsky, W.H.; Fisher, L.; Hessler, D.; Bruhn, D.; Best, J.H. Patient Perspectives on Once-Weekly Medications for Diabetes. *Diabetes Obes. Metab.* **2011**, *13*, 144–149. [CrossRef]
27. Paley, R.G.; Scott, M.H. Severe Insulin Lipodystrophy as a Possible Cause of Instability in Diabetics. *Br. Med. J.* **1958**, *2*, 1331–1334. [CrossRef] [PubMed]
28. Watson, E.M. Non-Hypoglycaemic (Allergic) Insulin Reactions. *Can. Med. Assoc. J.* **1942**, *47*, 336–339. [PubMed]
29. American Diabetes Association 9. Pharmacologic Approaches to Glycemic Treatment: Standards of Medical Care in Diabetes-2020. *Diabetes Care* **2020**, *43*, S98–S110. [CrossRef] [PubMed]
30. Polonsky, W.H.; Henry, R.R. Poor Medication Adherence in Type 2 Diabetes: Recognizing the Scope of the Problem and Its Key Contributors. *Patient Prefer. Adherence* **2016**, *10*, 1299–1307. [CrossRef]
31. Howard, V.; Church, C.; Oldham, S.; Hornigold, D.; Trevaskis, J.; Baker, D.; Rhodes, C.; Rossi, A.; Naylor, J.; Dhillon, J.; et al. 1086-P: Preclinical Development of an Ultralong-Acting Insulin for Once-Weekly Dosing. *Diabetes* **2019**, *68*, 1086-P. [CrossRef]
32. Rezolute, Inc. Announces Top-Line Results from Phase 1 Trial Evaluating AB101 in Patients with Diabetes. Available online: https://www.biospace.com/article/rezolute-inc-announces-top-line-results-from-phase-1-trial-evaluating-ab101-in-patients-with-diabetes-/ (accessed on 17 February 2024).
33. Insulin Long-Acting (HM 12470)—Hanmi Pharmaceutical—AdisInsight. Available online: https://adisinsight.springer.com/drugs/800040862 (accessed on 17 February 2024).
34. Hanmi | Hanmi Pharmaceutical's Official Site. Available online: https://www.hanmipharm.com/main.hm (accessed on 17 February 2024).
35. Kurtzhals, P.; Nishimura, E.; Haahr, H.; Høeg-Jensen, T.; Johansson, E.; Madsen, P.; Sturis, J.; Kjeldsen, T. Commemorating Insulin's Centennial: Engineering Insulin Pharmacology towards Physiology. *Trends Pharmacol. Sci.* **2021**, *42*, 620–639. [CrossRef] [PubMed]
36. Marquez, F.; Brazg, R.; Christiansen, M.; Free, A.; Matson, M.; Jones, S.; Georgopoulos, L.; Malatesta, J.; Arnold, S.; Kramer, W.; et al. PE0139, the First Recombinant Fully Human Monomeric Super-Long-Acting Basal Insulin to Display a Sustained Nearly Peakless Insulin Profile Following a Single Subcutaneous Dose in Subjects with T2DM Supporting Weekly Dosing. In Proceedings of the 75th Scientific Sessions of the American Diabetes Association, Boston, MA, USA, 5–9 June 2014; p. A26.
37. Moyers, J.S.; Hansen, R.J.; Day, J.W.; Dickinson, C.D.; Zhang, C.; Ruan, X.; Ding, L.; Brown, R.M.; Baker, H.E.; Beals, J.M. Preclinical Characterization of LY3209590, a Novel Weekly Basal Insulin Fc-Fusion Protein. *J. Pharmacol. Exp. Ther.* **2022**, *382*, 346–355. [CrossRef] [PubMed]
38. Heise, T.; Chien, J.; Beals, J.M.; Benson, C.; Klein, O.; Moyers, J.S.; Haupt, A.; Pratt, E.J. Pharmacokinetic and Pharmacodynamic Properties of the Novel Basal Insulin Fc (Insulin Efsitora Alfa), an Insulin Fusion Protein in Development for Once-Weekly Dosing for the Treatment of Patients with Diabetes. *Diabetes Obes. Metab.* **2023**, *25*, 1080–1090. [CrossRef] [PubMed]
39. Philis-Tsimikas, A.; Bajaj, H.S.; Begtrup, K.; Cailleteau, R.; Gowda, A.; Lingvay, I.; Mathieu, C.; Russell-Jones, D.; Rosenstock, J. Rationale and Design of the Phase 3a Development Programme (ONWARDS 1-6 Trials) Investigating Once-Weekly Insulin Icodec in Diabetes. *Diabetes Obes. Metab.* **2023**, *25*, 331–341. [CrossRef] [PubMed]
40. Nishimura, E.; Pridal, L.; Glendorf, T.; Hansen, B.F.; Hubálek, F.; Kjeldsen, T.; Kristensen, N.R.; Lützen, A.; Lyby, K.; Madsen, P.; et al. Molecular and Pharmacological Characterization of Insulin Icodec: A New Basal Insulin Analog Designed for Once-Weekly Dosing. *BMJ Open Diabetes Res. Care* **2021**, *9*, e002301. [CrossRef] [PubMed]

41. Danne, T.; Heinemann, L.; Pieber, T.R. New Insulins, Biosimilars, and Insulin Therapy. *Diabetes Technol. Ther.* **2023**, *25*, S44–S69. [CrossRef] [PubMed]
42. Belal, H.; Gandhi, G.Y. In T2DM Uncontrolled with Noninsulin Glucose-Lowering Agents, Weekly Icodec Reduced HbA1c vs. Daily Degludec at 26 Wk. *Ann. Intern. Med.* **2023**, *176*, JC112. [CrossRef] [PubMed]
43. Lingvay, I.; Asong, M.; Desouza, C.; Gourdy, P.; Kar, S.; Vianna, A.; Vilsbøll, T.; Vinther, S.; Mu, Y. Once-Weekly Insulin Icodec vs Once-Daily Insulin Degludec in Adults with Insulin-Naive Type 2 Diabetes: The ONWARDS 3 Randomized Clinical Trial. *JAMA* **2023**, *330*, 228–237. [CrossRef] [PubMed]
44. Bue-Valleskey, J.M.; Kazda, C.M.; Ma, C.; Chien, J.; Zhang, Q.; Chigutsa, E.; Landschulz, W.; Haupt, A.; Frias, J.P. Once-Weekly Basal Insulin Fc Demonstrated Similar Glycemic Control to Once-Daily Insulin Degludec in Insulin-Naive Patients with Type 2 Diabetes: A Phase 2 Randomized Control Trial. *Diabetes Care* **2023**, *46*, 1060–1067. [CrossRef]
45. Roussel, R.; Charbonnel, B.; Behar, M.; Gourmelen, J.; Emery, C.; Detournay, B. Persistence with Insulin Therapy in Patients with Type 2 Diabetes in France: An Insurance Claims Study. *Diabetes Ther.* **2016**, *7*, 537–549. [CrossRef] [PubMed]
46. Yavuz, D.G.; Ozcan, S.; Deyneli, O. Adherence to Insulin Treatment in Insulin-Naïve Type 2 Diabetic Patients Initiated on Different Insulin Regimens. *Patient Prefer. Adherence* **2015**, *9*, 1225–1231. [CrossRef] [PubMed]
47. Wu, J.; Morrison, F.; Zhao, Z.; Haynes, G.; He, X.; Ali, A.K.; Shubina, M.; Malmasi, S.; Ge, W.; Peng, X.; et al. Reasons for Discontinuing Insulin and Factors Associated with Insulin Discontinuation in Patients with Type 2 Diabetes Mellitus: A Real-World Evidence Study. *Clin. Diabetes Endocrinol.* **2021**, *7*, 1. [CrossRef] [PubMed]
48. Rosenstock, J.; Bain, S.C.; Gowda, A.; Jódar, E.; Liang, B.; Lingvay, I.; Nishida, T.; Trevisan, R.; Mosenzon, O.; ONWARDS 1 Trial Investigators. Weekly Icodec versus Daily Glargine U100 in Type 2 Diabetes without Previous Insulin. *N. Engl. J. Med.* **2023**, *389*, 297–308. [CrossRef] [PubMed]
49. Philis-Tsimikas, A.; Asong, M.; Franek, E.; Jia, T.; Rosenstock, J.; Stachlewska, K.; Watada, H.; Kellerer, M. Switching to Once-Weekly Insulin Icodec versus Once-Daily Insulin Degludec in Individuals with Basal Insulin-Treated Type 2 Diabetes (ONWARDS 2): A Phase 3a, Randomised, Open Label, Multicentre, Treat-to-Target Trial. *Lancet Diabetes Endocrinol.* **2023**, *11*, 414–425. [CrossRef] [PubMed]
50. Wang, P.; Zhang, Y.; Xu, W.; He, J.; Peng, L.; Feng, Y.; Xu, P.; Chong, W.; Hai, Y.; Jia, L.; et al. Efficacy and Safety of Once-Weekly Insulin Regimes on Glycemic Control for Type 2 Diabetes: A Systematic Review and Network Meta-Analysis. *Diabetol. Metab. Syndr.* **2024**, *16*, 3. [CrossRef] [PubMed]
51. Frias, J.; Chien, J.; Zhang, Q.; Chigutsa, E.; Landschulz, W.; Syring, K.; Wullenweber, P.; Haupt, A.; Kazda, C. Safety and Efficacy of Once-Weekly Basal Insulin Fc in People with Type 2 Diabetes Previously Treated with Basal Insulin: A Multicentre, Open-Label, Randomised, Phase 2 Study. *Lancet Diabetes Endocrinol.* **2023**, *11*, 158–168. [CrossRef] [PubMed]
52. Lingvay, I.; Buse, J.B.; Franek, E.; Hansen, M.V.; Koefoed, M.M.; Mathieu, C.; Pettus, J.; Stachlewska, K.; Rosenstock, J. A Randomized, Open-Label Comparison of Once-Weekly Insulin Icodec Titration Strategies Versus Once-Daily Insulin Glargine U100. *Diabetes Care* **2021**, *44*, 1595–1603. [CrossRef] [PubMed]
53. Corrao, S.; Nobili, A.; Natoli, G.; Mannucci, P.M.; Perticone, F.; Pietrangelo, A.; Argano, C.; REPOSI Investigators. Hyperglycemia at admission, comorbidities, and in-hospital mortality in elderly patients hospitalized in internal medicine wards: Data from the RePoSI Registry. *Acta Diabetol.* **2021**, *58*, 1225–1236, Correction in *Acta Diabetol.* **2021**, *58*, 1237. [CrossRef]
54. Candido, R.; Nicolucci, A.; Larosa, M.; Rossi, M.C.; Napoli, R.; Gabellieri, E.; Tortato, E.; Rabini, R.A.; Crazzolara, D.; Lucibelli, L.; et al. Treatment Intensification Following Glucagon-like Peptide-1 Receptor Agonist Treatment in Type 2 Diabetes: The RESTORE-G Real-World Study. *Nutr. Metab. Cardiovasc. Dis.* **2023**, *33*, 2294–2305. [CrossRef]
55. Guerci, B.; Chanan, N.; Kaur, S.; Jasso-Mosqueda, J.G.; Lew, E. Lack of Treatment Persistence and Treatment Nonadherence as Barriers to Glycaemic Control in Patients with Type 2 Diabetes. *Diabetes Ther.* **2019**, *10*, 437–449. [CrossRef] [PubMed]
56. Rosenstock, J.; Del Prato, S. Basal Weekly Insulins: The Way of the Future! *Metabolism* **2022**, *126*, 154924. [CrossRef] [PubMed]
57. Baser, O.; Tangirala, K.; Wei, W.; Xie, L. Real-World Outcomes of Initiating Insulin Glargine-Based Treatment versus Premixed Analog Insulins among US Patients with Type 2 Diabetes Failing Oral Antidiabetic Drugs. *Clin. Outcomes Res.* **2013**, *5*, 497–505. [CrossRef] [PubMed]
58. Mathieu, C.; Ásbjörnsdóttir, B.; Bajaj, H.S.; Lane, W.; Matos, A.L.S.A.; Murthy, S.; Stachlewska, K.; Rosenstock, J. Switching to Once-Weekly Insulin Icodec versus Once-Daily Insulin Glargine U100 in Individuals with Basal-Bolus Insulin-Treated Type 2 Diabetes (ONWARDS 4): A Phase 3a, Randomised, Open-Label, Multicentre, Treat-to-Target, Non-Inferiority Trial. *Lancet* **2023**, *401*, 1929–1940. [CrossRef] [PubMed]
59. Bajaj, H.S.; Aberle, J.; Davies, M.; Donatsky, A.M.; Frederiksen, M.; Yavuz, D.G.; Gowda, A.; Lingvay, I.; Bode, B. Once-Weekly Insulin Icodec with Dosing Guide App versus Once-Daily Basal Insulin Analogues in Insulin-Naive Type 2 Diabetes (ONWARDS 5): A Randomized Trial. *Ann. Intern. Med.* **2023**, *176*, 1476–1485. [CrossRef] [PubMed]
60. Lockhart, M.J.; Dinneen, S.F. In Type 2 Diabetes, Weekly Basal Insulin Fc Was Noninferior to Daily Insulin Degludec for HbA1c at 26 Wk. *Ann. Intern. Med.* **2023**, *176*, JC81. [CrossRef] [PubMed]
61. Kazda, C.M.; Bue-Valleskey, J.M.; Chien, J.; Zhang, Q.; Chigutsa, E.; Landschulz, W.; Wullenweber, P.; Haupt, A.; Dahl, D. Novel Once-Weekly Basal Insulin Fc Achieved Similar Glycemic Control with a Safety Profile Comparable to Insulin Degludec in Patients with Type 1 Diabetes. *Diabetes Care* **2023**, *46*, 1052–1059. [CrossRef] [PubMed]

62. Russell-Jones, D.; Babazono, T.; Cailleteau, R.; Engberg, S.; Irace, C.; Kjaersgaard, M.I.S.; Mathieu, C.; Rosenstock, J.; Woo, V.; Klonoff, D.C. Once-Weekly Insulin Icodec versus Once-Daily Insulin Degludec as Part of a Basal-Bolus Regimen in Individuals with Type 1 Diabetes (ONWARDS 6): A Phase 3a, Randomised, Open-Label, Treat-to-Target Trial. *Lancet* **2023**, *402*, 1636–1647. [CrossRef] [PubMed]
63. Fifer, S.; Rose, J.; Hamrosi, K.K.; Swain, D. Valuing Injection Frequency and Other Attributes of Type 2 Diabetes Treatments in Australia: A Discrete Choice Experiment. *BMC Health Serv. Res.* **2018**, *18*, 675. [CrossRef] [PubMed]
64. Blonde, L.; Meneghini, L.; Peng, X.V.; Boss, A.; Rhee, K.; Shaunik, A.; Kumar, S.; Balodi, S.; Brulle-Wohlhueter, C.; McCrimmon, R.J. Probability of Achieving Glycemic Control with Basal Insulin in Patients with Type 2 Diabetes in Real-World Practice in the USA. *Diabetes Ther.* **2018**, *9*, 1347–1358. [CrossRef] [PubMed]
65. Khunti, K.; Nikolajsen, A.; Thorsted, B.L.; Andersen, M.; Davies, M.J.; Paul, S.K. Clinical Inertia with Regard to Intensifying Therapy in People with Type 2 Diabetes Treated with Basal Insulin. *Diabetes Obes. Metab.* **2016**, *18*, 401. [CrossRef] [PubMed]
66. Zhang, P.; Zhang, H.; Li, X.; Chen, M.; Wang, D.; Ji, L. Factors and Outcomes Associated with Discontinuation of Basal Insulin Therapy in Patients with Type 2 Diabetes Mellitus. *Endocrinol. Diabetes Metab.* **2020**, *3*, e00122. [CrossRef] [PubMed]
67. Khunti, K.; Giorgino, F.; Berard, L.; Mauricio, D.; Harris, S.B. The Importance of the Initial Period of Basal Insulin Titration in People with Diabetes. *Diabetes Obes. Metab.* **2020**, *22*, 722–733. [CrossRef] [PubMed]
68. Abuelazm, M.; Ibrahim, A.A.; Khlidj, Y.; Badr, A.; Amin, A.M.; Elzeftawy, M.A.; Gowaily, I.; Elsaeidy, A.S.; Abdelazeem, B. Once-weekly Insulin Icodec versus Once-daily Long-acting Insulin for Type II Diabetes: A Meta-analysis of Randomized Controlled Trials. *J. Endocr. Soc.* **2023**, *8*, bvad177. [CrossRef] [PubMed]
69. Bajaj, H.S.; Bergenstal, R.M.; Christoffersen, A.; Davies, M.J.; Gowda, A.; Isendahl, J.; Lingvay, I.; Senior, P.A.; Silver, R.J.; Trevisan, R.; et al. Switching to Once-Weekly Insulin Icodec versus Once-Daily Insulin Glargine U100 in Type 2 Diabetes Inadequately Controlled on Daily Basal Insulin: A Phase 2 Randomized Controlled Trial. *Diabetes Care* **2021**, *44*, 1586–1594. [CrossRef] [PubMed]
70. Sciacca, L.; Vella, V.; Frittitta, L.; Tumminia, A.; Manzella, L.; Squatrito, S.; Belfiore, A.; Vigneri, R. Long-actinginsulinanalogs and cancer. *Nutr. Metab. Cardiovasc. Dis.* **2018**, *28*, 436–443. [CrossRef] [PubMed]
71. Aktas, G.; Taslamacioglu Duman, T. Current usage of long-acting insulin analogs in patients with type 2 diabetes mellitus. *Expert Rev. Endocrinol. Metab.* **2024**, *19*, 155–161. [CrossRef] [PubMed]
72. Corrao, S.; Argano, C.; Natoli, G.; Nobili, A.; Corazza, G.R.; Mannucci, P.M.; Perticone, F.; REPOSI Investigators. Sex-Differences in the Pattern of Comorbidities, Functional Independence, and Mortality in Elderly Inpatients: Evidence from the RePoSI Register. *J. Clin. Med.* **2019**, *8*, 81. [CrossRef] [PubMed]

biomedicines
MDPI

Review

100 Years since the Discovery of Insulin, from Its Discovery to the Insulins of the Future

Carmen Lambert [1,2,*] and Elias Delgado [1,3,4,5,*]

1 Endocrinology, Nutrition, Diabetes and Obesity Group, Health Research Institute of the Principality of Asturias (ISPA), 33011 Oviedo, Asturias, Spain
2 Faculty of Educational Sciences, University of Oviedo, 33005 Oviedo, Asturias, Spain
3 Asturias Central University Hospital, 33011 Oviedo, Asturias, Spain
4 Faculty of Medicine, University of Oviedo, 33006 Oviedo, Asturias, Spain
5 Centre for Biomedical Network Research on Rare Diseases (CIBERER), Institute of Health Carlos III, 28222 Madrid, Spain
* Correspondence: carmen.lambert@ispasturias.es (C.L.); delgadoelias@uniovi.es (E.D.)

Abstract: The term diabetes first emerged in the 3rd century BC, in a reference by Demetrius of Apamea, who described the disease as a dropsy in which any liquid ingested is eliminated in the form of urine. However, the great discovery that revolutionized this field came from the Canadian doctor Frederick Banting, who together with his student and assistant Charles Best, managed to isolate insulin and treat a patient with diabetes on 23 January 1922. This patient was Leonard Thompson, and the results obtained from him were surprising. His glycosuria and ketonuria disappeared and his blood glucose returned to normal. He received daily injections and lived 13 more years. Advances in the treatment of diabetes have been numerous in the 100 years since its discovery. In this review, we recapitulate the most important events that have occurred, and where research is progressing today.

Keywords: insulin; diabetes; Frederick Banting

1. History of Diabetes

The first references to diabetes date back to the Egyptians in 1500 BC who described it in "*The Ebers Papyrus*", a new disease characterized by weight lost, continuous hunger, abundant urination, and an enormous thirst [1]. Many other ancient cultures also described this disease, including the Hindus, ancient Chinese, Greeks, and Romans, among others [2]. In fact, it was the Greek doctor Demetrius of Apamea (3rd century BC), who described the disease as a dropsy in which any fluid that is drunk is discharged as urine, and named it for the first time as Diabetes [3].

Many discoveries were made in the 19th century. In 1815, Michel-Eugene Chevreul identified glucose in urine; a few years later, in 1869, Paul Langerhans described nests of cells in the pancreas; these were later named the "Islets of Langerhans" by Gustave-Edouard Laguesse in 1983 (Figure 1). Twenty years later, in 1889, Von Mering and Minkowsky, two physiologists from the University of Strasbourg, removed a pancreas to test it in a living organism (dog) and observed that its absence induced an excess of sugar in the urine, and subsequently, they found that the pancreas secreted something that reduced the levels of sugar [4,5]. A few years later, in 1891, Eugène Gley confirmed this discovery and revealed that the atrophy of the acinar pancreas did not result in experimental diabetes, and looked for pancreatic extracts which reduced glucosuria; however, Gley did not publish his results [5]. Instead, it was Georg Ludwig Zuelzer who was the first to publish the use of pancreatic extracts, which he called "Acomatol", on diabetic dogs. He also tried to use Acomatol to treat eight diabetic patients, observing variable reductions in glycosuria and ketonuria, but this also resulted in very severe side effects [6].

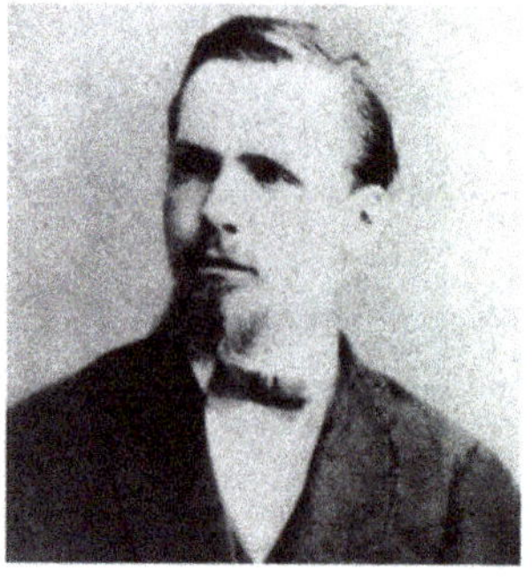

(a)

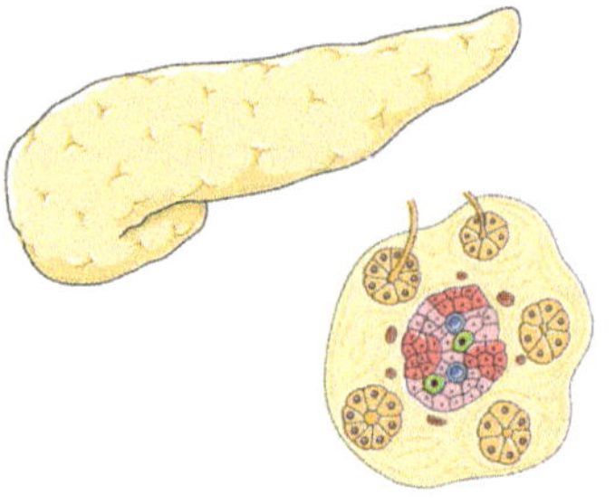

(b)

Figure 1. The islets of Langerhans. (**a**) Photograph of Paul Langerhans, discoverer of the islets [7]. (**b**) Drawing of pancreatic islets.

During the first half of the 20th century, many physiologists focused their attention on the field of diabetes, one of which was Nicolas Paulesco, who carried out several experiments on pancreatectomized dogs and in 1916 isolated an aqueous pancreatic extract, showing the disappearance of diabetes in pancreatectomized dogs when injected with said extract. Paulesco called this substance "pancreine" and obtained a Romanian patent on the 12 April 1922. However, despite attempts to purify it, pancreine was too toxic to be used in humans [8].

2. The Discovery of Insulin

Frederick Banting was born on 14 November 1891 in Alliston, Ontario. He graduated from the school of medicine in 1916 and after completing his specialization in Orthopedics at the Hospital for Sick Children in Toronto, he moved to London, Ontario, and opened a general medicine clinic. Simultaneously, he accepted a part-time position as a professor of surgery and physiology at London's Western University [2,9]. On November 1st he had to give a course on carbohydrate metabolism. The day before, he was preparing his talk and went to bed after reading the article "The relation of the islets of Langerhans with special reference to cases of pancreatic lithiasis" by pathologist Moses Barron [2,10], a clinical professor of Medicine at the University of Minnesota, published in the latest issue of the journal Surgery, Gynecology and Obstetrics, where he reviewed the pathology of the pancreas and the effects of Wirsung duct ligation on diabetic patients suffering from the obstruction of the pancreatic ducts by stones, and recalled the gradual atrophy of the acini in contrast to the islets of Langerhans. Fascinated by this article, he woke up with an idea at 2.00 a.m. on 31 October 1920 and wrote: "*Diabetus. Ligate pancreatic ducts of dog. Keep dogs alive till acini degenerate leaving islets. Try to isolate the internal secretion of these to relieve glycosurea*" [11,12]. With no proper research training, Banting moved to the University of Toronto for a summer internship, where he worked with Prof. John Macleod who provided Banting with laboratory space, equipment, dogs and a student assistant, Charles Best.

On 17 May 1921, Banting and Best began their experiments with erratic results. Then, Banting began to believe that the islets were formed before the exocrine, and used fetal pancreases as a source for extractions. The first positive results were obtained on 18 November, when the pancreatectomized dog No. 33, called Majorie, was intravenously treated with 10 cc of fetal calf pancreas extract. Her urine became sugar-free within an hour, and she lived for 70 days [8,13]. Their objective was then to produce sufficient stable quantities of pancreatic extract, for which they had the help of the biochemist Dr. James Collip. In order to extract the insulin before it was digested by pancreatic enzymes, they used an extraction method based on the use of varying concentrations of alcohol, which were slightly acidic and kept at a low temperature, and they managed to inactivate the pancreatic enzymes [2,8,13,14]. In this way, Banting and Collip succeeded in producing a pancreatic extract with sufficient potency and purity for human consumption (Figure 2).

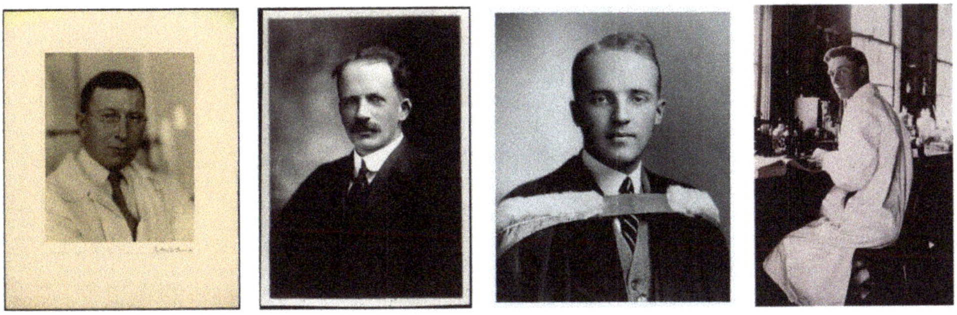

(a) (b) (c) (d)

Figure 2. The faces of insulin discovery [7]. (**a**) Frederick Banting, the principal investigator; (**b**) John Macleod, Banting's supervisor; (**c**) Charles Best, Banting's assistant and (**d**) James Collip, the individual responsible for developing a method to purify a safe and stable insulin extract.

After the first failed attempts in humans, on 23 January 1922, the new extract purified by Collip was administered subcutaneously to Leonard Thompson, and the results were spectacular; glycosuria and ketonuria had disappeared, and the blood glucose became normalized. Daily injections of this new extract enabled Leonard to live 13 more years (Figure 3) [15]. However, they did not record the steps they had taken, so it was not until the spring of 1922 that the team was able to successfully produce insulin again. Although they were capable of synthesizing insulin, large-scale production was not feasible for the Toronto group. It was then that Collip and Banting shared their methodology with George H. A. Clowes of Eli Lilly and Company, which had the infrastructure to produce larger quantities of insulin. But it was not until autumn when, using isoelectric precipitation, they were finally able to produce purified insulin on a large scale [16]. Banting, Best and Collip patented the discovery and gave it to the University of Toronto for USD 1, as they wanted everyone who needed it to have access to insulin. As Banting famously said: "Insulin does not belong to me, it belongs to the world".

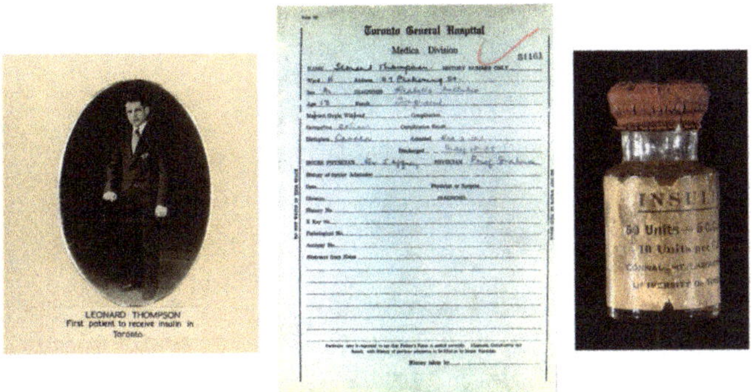

(a) (b) (c)

Figure 3. The first successful insulin administration [7]. (**a**) Photography by Leonard Thompson. (**b**) Extract from the patient's medical record at the Toronto hospital after insulin administration. (**c**) Insulin vial.

On 25 October 1923, the Nobel Prize jury granted the award to Banting and Macleod. Then, Banting, angry after seeing Macleod awarded, decided to share his prize with Best, as did Macleod with Collip soon after. For the first time in the history of the Nobel Prizes, none of the winners attended the award ceremony, which took place on 10 December 1923.

Insulin Arrives in Europe

In the fall of 1922, August Krogh, a professor at the University of Copenhagen, and his wife, Marie, a physician, came to the United States at the invitation of Yale University to give a series of lectures across the country on their medical research after receiving the Nobel Prize in Physiology in 1920 [17]. During this trip, they heard daily reports of people with diabetes being treated with insulin, and Marie Krogh, who had type 2 diabetes, took a special interest in the treatment. In Boston, Dr. Elliot P. Joslin (the first American diabetes doctor) treated Marie with insulin, and the couple decided to contact Professor Macleod to request permission to manufacture and sell insulin in Scandinavia. August Krogh founded the company Nordisk Insulinlaboratorium with his Danish partner, Dr. Hans Christian Hagedorn, and with funding from the Danish pharmacist August Kongsted [17,18].

In 1925, after a heated argument with Hagendorn, the brothers Harald and Thorvald Pedersen, former Nordisk employees, founded their own company: Novo Terapeutisk Laboratorium. Novo and Nordisk became the world's leading insulin manufacturers and competed with each other for almost 65 years, until they finally merged in 1989 to form today's Novo Nordisk s.a. [18].

3. The Evolution of the Treatment of Diabetes

3.1. The Evolution of Insulin Therapy

Since the discovery of insulin in 1922, there have been numerous advances in the treatment of diabetes, with the common goal of trying to bring the blood glucose and insulin levels of people with diabetes into line with those of healthy people.

Specifically, we know that, in people without diabetes, the maximum peak of insulin secretion occurs 1 h after ingestion and returns to normal levels after another 2 h. However, to achieve a normal insulin profile for 24 h and avoid nocturnal hypoglycemia in diabetic patients, it is necessary to use other insulin formulations that prolong the duration of action.

In this way, we have different types of insulin, with different release times, which allow the patient to better control their disease. Among the different types of insulin, two stand out: rapid-acting insulins, whose action is practically immediate after administration and is short-lived; and long-acting insulins, whose effect takes longer to occur, but lasts longer (Figure 4) [19].

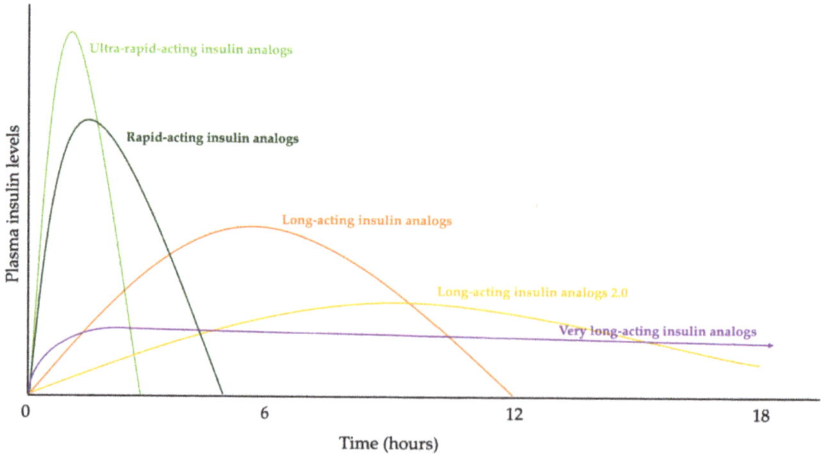

Figure 4. Graph that shows the action time of insulin and its plasma levels according to the type of insulin administered.

At first, after its discovery, the insulin used was the so-called "amorphous or regular insulin", but it was an insulin that was not very stable and had many impurities. In 1926, John Jacob Abel, professor of pharmacology at the Johns Hopkins School of Medicine, managed to crystallize amorphous insulin for the first time by adding acetic acid pyridine and zinc, which caused crystals to form, and gave it greater stability, with a slightly later onset of action and producing fewer allergic reactions. This new crystallized insulin quickly displaced amorphous insulin [20]. However, although effective, both insulins required a large number of daily injections. It was then that, in 1936, the first long-acting insulin, the protamine insulin, appeared. Hans Christian Hagedorn, Birger Norman Jensen, Ingrid Wodstrup-Nielsen and Niels B. Krarup published their work, wherein they demonstrated that insulin, together with protamine (a protein from the histone group, obtained from the semen of river trout), increased its action time to almost twenty-four hours. They made the presumption that the greater the insolubility that protamine gave it, the more useful it would be in treatment [21]. The problem was that the solution had to be buffered just before injecting it, making its administration more complicated. Despite this, protamine–insulin boosted the search for new methods to increase the action time of insulin. The next step was the use of metals that would help stabilize the molecule, with nickel and cobalt being the first to appear; however, they did not seem valid. The solution was obtained by Canadians Albert Madden Fisher and David Alymer Scott in 1935, using the most abundant metal in the pancreas, zinc [22]; 10 years later, in 1946, Nordisk was able to form crystals of protamine and insulin using zinc insulin (PZI), and marketed it in 1950 as NPH insulin. NPH insulin had the advantage that it could be mixed with regular insulin directly in the same syringe and had a faster and longer-lasting action than its predecessor [23].

In 1965, Novo (Novo Industri A/S, Bagsværd, Denmark) once again focused its attention on rapid insulins, a field without any progress for around 30 years, and introduced two new insulins: the rapid-acting insulin Actrapid® and the intermediate-acting insulin Crystal II [24]. Researchers already knew that, for many patients, crystalline or regular insulin took too long to act, and a more immediate-acting insulin was needed. Actrapid®, also called neutral soluble insulin, was prepared from recrystallized porcine insulin and had a pH of 7.0, at which porcine insulin crystals are soluble. Therefore, it had a faster action than acidic soluble insulin, which had to go from pH 3.0 to a neutral pH before achieving its biological activity [25]. As for Crystal II, insulin came from recrystallized bovine insulin, whose crystals were less soluble and therefore their action was slower [24]. This is when combined insulin treatments appeared, which alternated the use of slow insulins and rapid-acting insulins during the day.

Until that moment, all insulins that had been produced were of animal origin, requiring approximately 50 pigs to cover the annual insulin needs of a patient. This meant that insulin treatment was only available to a few. That changed in 1953, when the British biochemist Frederick Sanger finally determined, after 10 years of work, the amino acid sequence of bovine insulin. Sanger determined that it had two chains, which he called A and B [26]. Chain A had 21 amino acids and chain B, 30 amino acids (Figure 5a,b). They were joined by two disulfide bridges and there was another of these bridges between the amino acids of chain A. Years later, in 1969, it was Dr. Dorothy Crowfoot Hodgkin who would finally describe the three-dimensional structure of the molecule (Figure 5c,d) [27]. Both received the Nobel Prize in Chemistry in 1958 and 1964, respectively, and their discoveries were the beginning of the race to achieve the synthesis of the insulin molecule [12,13].

Porcine insulin differs from human insulin by one amino acid, and from bovine insulin by three. This small difference was enough for some patients to develop an allergy and forced them to abandon treatment. To solve this problem, in 1980 Hoechst, applying a chemical process called transpeptidization, managed to replace the different amino acid in porcine insulin (an alanine) with the amino acid of the human sequence (a threonine). However, despite having achieved its synthesis, insulin was still very expensive.

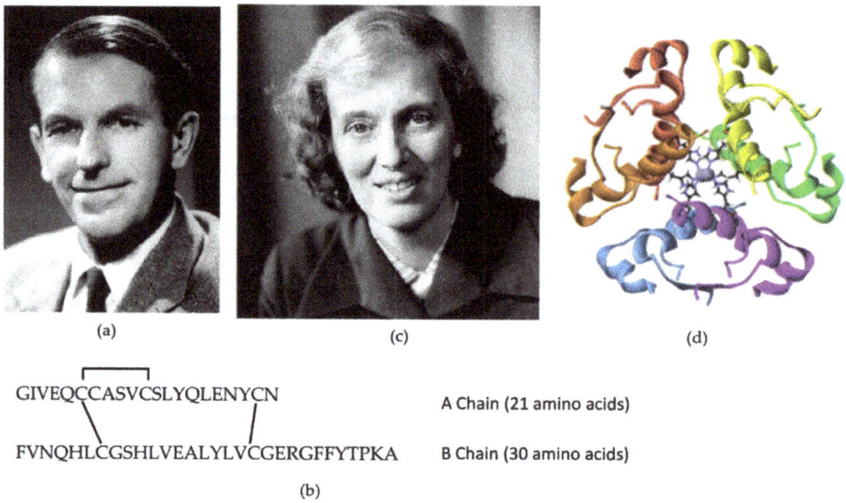

Figure 5. Insulin structure. (**a**) Frederick Sanger, awarded the Nobel Prize in 1958 for the discovery of the amino acid sequence of bovine insulin. (**b**) Amino acid sequence of insulin, made up of two chains, A and B. (**c**) Dr. Dorothy Crowfoot Hodgkin, awarded the Nobel Prize in 1964 for the discovery of the (**d**) three-dimensional structure of insulin.

In 1973, Cohen and Boyer created the first transgenic bacteria that were capable of expressing a foreign gene, and everything seemed to indicate that this technique could be used for the production of proteins or peptides of medical interest [28]. However, it was still necessary to identify the gene encoding insulin in the human genome, which was achieved in 1977 by W. Gilbert and Lydia Villa-Komaroff [29]. However, another problem still had to be solved: insulin is produced from a single chain that is cut in several places until it becomes two chains joined by disulfide bonds, and while bacteria or yeast could synthesize the precursor, they could not process it, so the result would be useless. To solve this problem, the parallel synthesis of the two molecules separately was proposed, which would later be joined by chemical methods. The first to achieve it were Riggs, Itaura and Boyer in 1977. The first clinical trial was carried out on 17 volunteers in July 1980 at Guy's Hospital in London, and the process was commercialized by Eli Lilly in consortium with Boyer himself and Genetech in 1982 under the trade name Humulin. That new insulin was cheaper to produce, powerful and safe, since it did not show the problems that animal counterparts produced. It began to be distributed in the early 1980s as a treatment for diabetes, being (once again) the first recombinant protein approved as a medicine [30].

Nowadays, practically all diabetics are treated with some type of recombinant insulin, as numerous analogues have been developed, each with different qualities (delayed effect, more powerful, etc.).

The advantage of genetic engineering is that we are not limited to mere copying, but can improve according to the patient's needs (insulin with immediate effect during a hyperglycemic shock, for example, or persistent over time) [31]. Thus, in 1996, the first rapid insulin analogue, Humalog®, was produced; a form of insulin that, by changing the position of two amino acids, managed to increase the speed of the effect. Soon after, in 2000, the first long-acting insulin analogue, insulin Glargine (Lantus®), was marketed by Sanofi-Aventis Germany Ltd. (Frankfurt, Germany) throughout the European Union. This new long-acting insulin evolved into a three-times more concentrated formulation of glargine (Glarginia U300), marketed as Toujeo®, and was launched following FDA approval in 2015. Additionally, in 2016, the first second-generation long-acting insulin analogue appeared, insulin degludec, marketed by Novo Nordisk as Tresiba®; it had a half-life of 25.4 h, reaching its steady state after 3 days [30–34]. New advances have also appeared in rapid insulins, such as the ultra-rapid insulin Faster Aspart (FiAsp®), marketed by Novo Nordisk (Bagsværd, Denmark), which was approved in 2017 both in Europe and the USA. This new insulin is formulated with two excipients: vitamin B3 (niacinamide), which increases local blood flow, accelerating the absorption of insulin at that level, and L-arginine, which acts as a stabilizer, achieving a faster onset of action (4.9 min vs. 11.2 min) and a 35% reduction in the time it takes to reach 50% of the maximum concentration [35] (Figure 6).

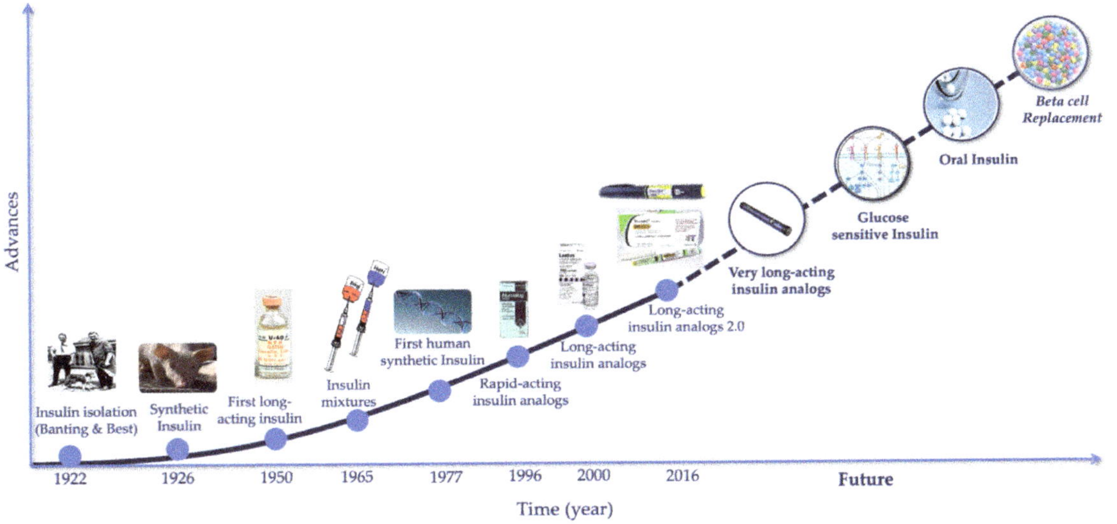

Figure 6. Past and future advances in insulin development.

Additionally, to investigate insulin's time of action, combinations of insulin treatment with other hypoglicemiant drugs were also researched. In this line, the American Diabetes Association has recommended, since 2019, the administration of a combination of GLP-1RA (glucagon-like peptide 1 receptor agonist) with basal insulin in type 2 diabetes when GLP-1RA is not enough to achieve an optimum glucose control, and injectable therapy is needed [36]. Basal insulin provides a constant level of insulin throughout the day, helping to control fasting blood sugar levels, while GLP-1RAs act to stimulate insulin secretion, inhibit glucagon release, slow gastric emptying and promote satiety, which leads to better blood sugar control, as well as possible weight loss. Due to the different ways in which both medications act, their combination in a fixed-dose injectable formulation offers several advantages. First, it simplifies the treatment regimen for patients by reducing the number of injections needed each day. Second, it addresses multiple aspects of diabetes pathology, focusing on both fasting and postprandial hyperglycemia, as well as providing potential benefits for weight management. Additionally, the combination of these two classes of medications may have synergistic effects, leading to better glycemic control compared to either therapy alone [36–38].

3.2. The Evolution of Insulin Therapy, More Than Insulin Analogues

After all the advances that took place in the development of new insulins, the efforts began to focus on administration methods as well as the development of equipment capable of measuring blood glucose levels in a rapid, precise and non-invasive way (Figure 7) [39].

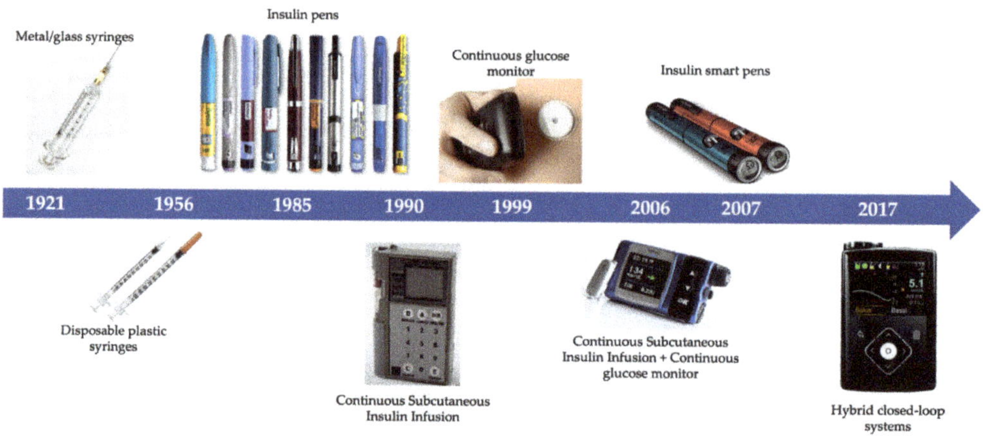

Figure 7. The evolution of insulin administration and glucose monitoring systems.

3.2.1. Syringes

The administration of insulin in diabetic patients is carried out subcutaneously. Thus, not only have advances in insulin analogues been important during these 100 years, but so too has the progress in methods of insulin administration. Initially, insulin was administered using reusable metal or glass syringes. These hypodermic syringes were sterilized after each use, yet cases of disease transmission have been documented, including hepatitis, malaria, polio and tuberculosis [40].

It was the New Zealand veterinarian and pharmacist Colin Murdoch who, in 1956, developed the first model of disposable syringe, trying to improve on those used to vaccinate animals [41]. He designed a single-use model that would be sold already loaded with the vaccine. When he presented his idea to the New Zealand Department of Health it was considered too futuristic, and the idea did not progress until years later, when it was sold around the world thanks to the Australian company Tasman Vaccine Ltd. Empty disposable plastic syringes did not came onto the market until 1964, pioneered by the leading American medical instrument company Becton Dickinson, which nowadays continues to manufacture about 5 million syringes a day [39].

3.2.2. Insulin Pens

Despite the great advantages, both in terms of safety and comfort for the patient, that the introduction of disposable syringes offered, advances continued towards their disappearance, with the first insulin prefilled pens appearing in 1985—NovoPen from the company Novo Nordisk. Those pens comprised three parts: a single-click-per-unit dosage system, a cartridge for insulin and a disposable needle. That device allowed the patient greater discretion and freedom and better long-term profitability, translating into better adherence to treatment. In 1989, NovoLet was launched, based on the same technology as the previous NovoPen prefilled pens, but in this case, it was disposable and biodegradable [42].

In the year 2007, Next-Generation Insulin pens, also known as "smart pens", arrived on the market. These devices contain a multidose memory function that records the date, time and dose of previous administrations, which helps better control the insulin doses administered, helping with the better monitoring of the treatment by the doctor. Furthermore, it is important to highlight that the new models on the market allow the administration of insulin in increments of 0.1 units, starting from a minimum dose of half a unit, helping to better adjust the insulin dose needed at all times.

3.2.3. Continuous Subcutaneous Insulin Infusion-CSII

The first commercially used insulin pump was the "Autosyringe" model in 1978, also known as the "Big Blue Brick" [43]. Despite the great enthusiasm of the medical community for this new instrument, they were large devices with very limited reliability. Therefore, it was not until the 1990s when CSII models could finally be introduced into the treatment routine of patients with type 1 diabetes, thanks to the reduction in pump size, increased safety and greater reliability in the administrations. These systems are capable of simulating the physiological secretion of insulin by islet cells more accurately than is performed with multiple daily injections [39,43].

These insulin infusion systems have been evolving over the past few years, allowing the prior programming of doses, as well as adjustments by the patient to special insulin needs such as exercise, illness, hormonal changes, or other circumstances that are out of the ordinary. These changes can be made precisely in increments as small as 0.05–0.25 units per hour. Different clinical trials have demonstrated that the use of CSII improves the glycemic state, and reduces the insulin dosage as well as the glycemic variability of type 1 diabetes patients [40].

Another important advance in the treatment of diabetes was the appearance of continuous glucose monitors, which allow the glucose in the interstitial fluid to be continuously monitored using a sensor inserted into the subcutaneous tissue. Since the beginning of the 2000s, these systems have been capable of integration with an CSII, combining the benefits of both technologies, so that the administration of insulin by the pump is adjusted with the measurements of the continuous glucose monitor, enabling one able to identify trends of increase or decrease in glucose, thus anticipating the necessary dose of insulin [44].

The latest advances in this field occurred in 2017, with the appearance of hybrid closed-loop systems or automated insulin infusion systems, which integrate three components: a real-time continuous glucose monitor, which measures interstitial glucose at regular intervals; a control algorithm, which can be integrated into the insulin pump; an external device or a mobile application; and finally, an insulin pump that allows its continuous release, increasing significantly the time required of patients and reducing HbA1c levels, as well as the number of sever hypo- and hyperglycemia. Since the implementation of the closed-loop systems, their use has increased exponentially, and, currently, 60% of patients with type 1 diabetes in the US use them [45–47].

4. The Future of Insulin Therapy

Multiple different insulin formulations have been marketed since its discovery in 1922. Currently, according to the FDA [48], we can find three types of approved and marketed insulin: basal insulins, prandial insulins, and insulin mixtures (Table 1). However, research into new formulations and ways of administration of insulin continues, with the near future holing once-weekly basal insulin analogues, glucose-sensitive insulins (also known as smart insulins), and non-injectable insulins.

Table 1. Different types of insulin approved by FDA.

	Type of Insulin	Brand Name	Other Names
PRANDIAL	Rapid-Acting	Admelog	insulin lispro injection
		Afrezza (inhalation powder)	regular human insulin
		Apidra	insulin glulisine
		Fiasp	insulin aspart
		Humalog	insulin lispro
		Novolog	insulin aspart

Table 1. *Cont.*

	Type of Insulin	Brand Name	Other Names
BASAL	Intermediate-Acting	Humulin N	NPH human insulin
		Novolin N	
	Short-Acting	Humulin R	regular human insulin
		Novolin R	
	Long-Acting	Basaglar KwikPen	insulin glargine
		Lantus	
		Toujeo	
		Levemir	insulin detemir
		Tresiba FlexTouch	insulin degludec
MIXTURES	Intermediate- and Rapid-Acting	Humalog Mix 75/25	75% insulin lispro protamine suspension
			25% insulin lispro injection
		Humalog 70/30	70% human insulin isophane suspension
			30% human insulin injection
		Humalog Mix 50/50	50% insulin lispro protamine suspension
			50% insulin lispro injection
		NovoLog Mix 70/30	70% insulin aspart protamine suspension
			30% insulin aspart injection
	Long- and Rapid-Acting	Ryzodeg 70/30 FlexTouch	70% insulin degludec
			30% insulin aspart
	Intermediate- and Short-Acting	Humulin 70/30	70% NPH human insulin
			30% regular human insulin injection
		Novolin 70/30	70% NPH Human Insulin
			30% Regular Human Insulin Injection

NPH: neutral protamine Hagedorn.

4.1. Once-Weekly Basal Insulin Analogue

One of the main lines of research that is currently being carried out is the search for very long-acting basal insulins, which allow the elimination of daily basal insulin injections, thus requiring only rapid insulin boluses. This is how insulin icodec was developed, developed by Novo Nordisk and whose effectiveness is currently being studied. Icodec has achieved, through structural modifications and binding to C20 fatty diacids, greater molecular stability, less enzymatic degradation and reduced receptor-mediated clearance, allowing less degradation and increasing its lifetime to 196 h [49,50].

4.2. Glucose Sensitivity

Also known as smart insulins, the objective of glucose-sensitive insulins is to act in case of hyperglycemia and cease their action after reaching normoglycemia, thus promoting optimal glucose levels in the body. The first studies on these insulins date back to the 1970s; specifically, in 1979, a modified insulin molecule appeared, linked to a lectin, called concavalin A. This molecule would bind to carbohydrates such as glucose and produce a greater release of insulin from this complex; but its final effect was not the desired one [51,52]. Over the years, other studies have been carried out using different types of insulin encapsulations or polymers intended for subcutaneous deposits, among other options. However, none of these products have been translated into therapeutic practice, mainly due to their slow reaction to increases in glucose, meaning that, today, only two molecules have been tested in humans. The main characteristics that a glucose-sensitive insulin must show in order to be transferred to clinical practice are the selective detection of glycemia, no toxicity or side effects, responsiveness to physiological glycemic ranges, and a quick and efficient reaction, reversible in the case of glucose changes [51,53]. Although to date there has been no molecule found that is capable of meeting all these characteristics, there are several pharmaceutical laboratories that are committed to this line of research.

4.3. Non-Injectable Insulins

Another line of research that is currently blooming in different pharmaceutical laboratories is the search for non-invasive routes of insulin administration, among which inhaled, intranasal, oral, buccal, and transdermal formulations stand out.

The first non-injectable insulin administration method to hit the market was inhaled insulin, marketed in 2006 by Pfizer under the name Exubera; however, it was quickly withdrawn from the market due to its adverse effects, mainly coughing and alterations of lung function [53,54]. Over the years, new formulations have come to the market, and although none have yet been able to replace injectable insulin, several inhaled insulins are in the clinical trial phase, and seek to establish themselves as a real alternative to injectable insulin in clinical practice.

Possibly the most promising non-invasive route of insulin administration is the oral route, due to its easy administration, which is why there are multiple pharmaceutical laboratories working in this line. Among the main challenges faced by these laboratories are the poor permeability of the epithelial cell due to its high molecular weight, and the enzymatic degradation of oral insulin by gastrointestinal peptidases, so increasing the bioavailability of oral insulin is considered one of the main challenges [55,56].

We can also highlight the long-acting basal insulin analogue 338 (I338), an insulin modified to be less susceptible to proteolytic degradation in the gastrointestinal tract. Its principle is based on a strong and reversible binding to albumin that gives it a long life, with an average plasma concentration of about 70 h [57]. In relation to oral insulins, a capsule-shaped device has been developed, the self-orienting millimeter-scale applicator, SOMA, which after being ingested adheres to the intestinal mucosa to release insulin, and whose objective is to increase the bioavailability of oral insulin [58]. Although preclinical studies are very promising, further research is needed in this field.

5. Conclusions

The idea that woke up Frederick Banting in the early morning of 31 October 1920 marked a paradigm shift, not only in the world of diabetes, but in the field of medicine in general, highlighting the importance of collaboration between clinicians, researchers and pharmaceutical companies seeking to improve the lives of people with diabetes. On the other hand, the refusal of the discoverers to conduct business with its discovery allowed significant progress from the first years, as opposed to new developers who have decided to patent the new insulin formulas.

Despite a century having passed since the discovery of insulin, with consequent advances in diabetes research, we are still very far from being able to achieve a real cure for type 1 diabetes that prevents the autoimmune destruction of pancreatic beta cells, although the lives of these patients improve year after year with the new discoveries in this field.

Author Contributions: Both authors researched data for the article and wrote the manuscript. All authors have read and agreed to the published version of the manuscript.

Funding: CL is the recipient of a Sara Borrel postdoctoral grant from the Carlos III Institute of Health, Spain (Grant number: CD23/00037).

Conflicts of Interest: The authors declare no conflicts of interest.

References

1. King, K.M.; Rubin, G. A History of Diabetes- from Antiquity to Discovering Insulin. *Br. J. Nurs.* **2003**, *12*, 1091–1095. [CrossRef]

2. Karamanou, M.; Protogerou, A.; Tsoucalas, G.; Androutsos, G.; Poulakou-Rebelakou, E. Milestones in the History of Diabetes Mellitus: The Main Contributors. *World J. Diabetes* **2016**, *7*, 1. [CrossRef] [PubMed]
3. Gemmill, C.L. The Greek Concept of Diabetes. *Bull. N. Y. Acad. Med.* **1972**, *48*, 1033.
4. Chevreul, M.E. Note Sur Le Sucre Du Diabète. *Ann. Chem.* **1815**, *95*, 319–320.
5. De Leiva-Hidalgo, A.; De Leiva-Pérez, A. I-European Research, the Cradle of the Discovery of the Antidiabetic Hormone: The Pioneer Roles and the Relevance of Oskar Minkowski and Eugène Gley. *Acta Diabetol.* **1976**, *59*, 1635–1651. [CrossRef] [PubMed]
6. De Leiva-Hidalgo, A.; De Leiva-Pérez, A. Pancreatic Extracts for the Treatment of Diabetes (1889–1914): Acomatol. *Am. J. Ther.* **2020**, *27*, E1–E12. [CrossRef] [PubMed]
7. The Discovery and Early Development of Insulin. Available online: https://insulin.library.utoronto.ca/ (accessed on 30 January 2024).
8. Karamitsos, D.T. The Story of Insulin Discovery. *Diabetes Res. Clin. Pract.* **2011**, *93* (Suppl. S1), S2–S8. [CrossRef] [PubMed]
9. Bliss, M. *Banting: A Biography*; University of Toronto Press: Toronto, ON, Canada, 1993; ISBN 9780802073860.
10. Barron, M. The Relation of the Islets of Langerhans with Special Reference to Cases of Pancreatic Lithiasis. *Surg. Gynecol. Obs.* **1920**, *31*, 437–448.
11. Tan, S.Y.; Merchant, J. Frederick Banting (1891–1941): Discoverer of Insulin. *Singap. Med. J.* **2017**, *58*, 2–3. [CrossRef]
12. Hegele, R.A.; Maltman, G.M. Insulin's Centenary: The Birth of an Idea. *Lancet Diabetes Endocrinol.* **2020**, *8*, 971–977. [CrossRef]
13. Marshall, S.M. Celebrating 100 Years of Insulin. *Diabetologia* **2021**, *64*, 944–946. [CrossRef] [PubMed]
14. Collip, J.B. The Original Method as Used for the Isolation of Insulin in Semipure Form for the Treatment of the First Clinical Cases. *J. Biol. Chem.* **1923**, *55*, 40–41.
15. Banting, F.G.; Barron, M.; Best, C.H. The Internal Secretion of the Pancreas. *J. Lab. Clin. Med.* **1922**, *7*, 465–480.
16. Macleod, J.J.R. Insulin and the Steps Taken to Secure an Effective Preparation. *Can. Med. Assoc. J.* **1922**, *12*, 899–900.
17. Poole, D.C.; Pittman, R.N.; Musch, T.I.; Østergaard, L. August Krogh: Physiology Genius and Compassionate Humanitarian. *J. Physiol.* **2020**, *598*, 4423–4424. [CrossRef]
18. Poulsen, J.E. The Impact of August Krogh on the Insulin Treatment of Diabetes and Our Present Status. *Acta Med. Scand. Suppl.* **1975**, *578*, 7–14. [CrossRef]
19. Ahmad, K. Insulin Sources and Types: A Review of Insulin in Terms of Its Mode on Diabetes Mellitus. *J. Tradit. Chin. Med.* **2014**, *34*, 234–237. [CrossRef]
20. John Jacob Abel (1875–1938). Available online: https://www.historiadelamedicina.org/abel.html (accessed on 3 January 2024).
21. Hagedorn, H.C.; Jensen, B.N.; Krarup, N.B.; Wodstrup, I. Protamine Insulinate. *J. Am. Med. Assoc.* **1936**, *106*, 177–180. [CrossRef]
22. Fisher, A.M.; Scott, D.A. Zinc Content of Bovine Pancreas. *Biochem. J.* **1935**, *29*, 1055–1058. [CrossRef] [PubMed]
23. Jamieson, M.; Lacey, A.H.; Fisher, A.M. NPH Insulin. *Can. Med. Assoc. J.* **1951**, *65*, 20–23. [PubMed]
24. Clarki, B.F.; Munro, J.F.; Duncan, L.J.P. Time-Action Studies and Clinical Trial of Actrapid and Crystal II Novo Insulins. *Br. Med. J.* **1965**, *2*, 265–267. [CrossRef]
25. Schlichtkrull, J.; Munck, O.; Jersild, M. Insulin Rapitard and Insulin Actrapid. *Acta Med. Scand.* **1965**, *177*, 103–113. [CrossRef]
26. SANGER, F.; THOMPSON, E.O. The Amino-Acid Sequence in the Glycyl Chain of Insulin. II. The Investigation of Peptides from Enzymic Hydrolysates. *Biochem. J.* **1953**, *53*, 366–374. [CrossRef]
27. Glusker, J.P. Dorothy Crowfoot Hodgkin (1910–1994). *Protein Sci.* **1994**, *3*, 2465–2469. [CrossRef] [PubMed]
28. Cohen, S.N.; Chang, A.C.Y.; Boyer, H.W.; Helling, R.B. Construction of Biologically Functional Bacterial Plasmids In Vitro. *Proc. Natl. Acad. Sci. USA* **1973**, *70*, 3240–3244. [CrossRef] [PubMed]
29. Villa-Komaroff, L.; Efstratiadis, A.; Broome, S.; Lomedico, P.; Tizard, R.; Naber, S.P.; Chick, W.L.; Gilbert, W. A Bacterial Clone Synthesizing Proinsulin. *Proc. Natl. Acad. Sci. USA* **1978**, *75*, 3727–3731. [CrossRef] [PubMed]
30. Borgoño, C.A.; Zinman, B. Insulins: Past, Present, and Future. *Endocrinol. Metab. Clin. N. Am.* **2012**, *41*, 1–24. [CrossRef] [PubMed]
31. Baghban Taraghdari, Z.; Imani, R.; Mohabatpour, F. A Review on Bioengineering Approaches to Insulin Delivery: A Pharmaceutical and Engineering Perspective. *Macromol. Biosci.* **2019**, *19*, e1800458. [CrossRef] [PubMed]
32. Bolli, G.B.; Cheng, A.Y.Y.; Owens, D.R. Insulin: Evolution of Insulin Formulations and Their Application in Clinical Practice over 100 Years. *Acta Diabetol.* **2022**, *59*, 1129–1144. [CrossRef]
33. Home, P. The Evolution of Insulin Therapy. *Diabetes Res. Clin. Pract.* **2021**, *175*, 108816. [CrossRef]
34. Danne, T.; Bolinder, J. New Insulins and Insulin Therapy. *Int. J. Clin. Pract. Suppl.* **2011**, *65*, 26–30. [CrossRef]
35. Wilson, L.M.; Castle, J.R. Recent Advances in Insulin Therapy. *Diabetes Technol. Ther.* **2020**, *22*, 929–936. [CrossRef]
36. Jung, H.N.; Cho, Y.K.; Min, S.H.; Kim, H.S.; Kim, Y.J.; Park, J.Y.; Lee, W.J.; Jung, C.H. Free versus Fixed-Ratio Combination of Basal Insulin and GLP-1 Receptor Agonists in Type 2 Diabetes Uncontrolled with GLP-1 Receptor Agonists: A Systematic Review and Indirect Treatment Comparison. *Front. Endocrinol.* **2022**, *13*, 870722. [CrossRef] [PubMed]
37. Anderson, S.L.; Trujillo, J.M. Basal Insulin Use With GLP-1 Receptor Agonists. *Diabetes Spectr.* **2016**, *29*, 152–160. [CrossRef] [PubMed]
38. GLP-1 Receptor Agonist and Basal Insulin Co-Therapy in Type 2 Diabetes: Clinical Evidence and Practicalities of Use—PCDS. Available online: https://www.pcdsociety.org/resources/details/glp-1-receptor-agonist-and-basal-insulin-co-therapy-in-type-2-diabetes-clinical-evidence-and-practicalities-of-use (accessed on 15 February 2024).
39. Kesavadev, J.; Saboo, B.; Krishna, M.B.; Krishnan, G. Evolution of Insulin Delivery Devices: From Syringes, Pens, and Pumps to DIY Artificial Pancreas. *Diabetes Ther.* **2020**, *11*, 1251–1269. [CrossRef]

40. Shah, R.B.; Patel, M.; Maahs, D.M.; Shah, V.N. Insulin Delivery Methods: Past, Present and Future. *Int. J. Pharm. Investig.* **2016**, *6*, 1. [CrossRef]
41. Pincock, S. Colin Murdoch. *Lancet* **2008**, *371*, 1994. [CrossRef]

Rai, I.; Wanjari, A.; Acharya, S. Recent Advances in Insulin Delivery Devices and Modes of Insulin Therapy. *J. Pharm. Res. Int.* **2021**, *33*, 358–367. [CrossRef]

. Alsaleh, F.M.; Smith, F.J.; Keady, S.; Taylor, K.M.G. Insulin Pumps: From Inception to the Present and toward the Future. *J. Clin. Pharm. Ther.* **2010**, *35*, 127–138. [CrossRef] [PubMed]

44. Ontario, H.Q. Continuous Monitoring of Glucose for Type 1 Diabetes: A Health Technology Assessment. *Ont. Health Technol. Assess. Ser.* **2018**, *18*, 1.
45. Beck, R.W.; Bergenstal, R.M.; Laffel, L.M.; Pickup, J.C. Advances in Technology for Management of Type 1 Diabetes. *Lancet* **2019**, *394*, 1265–1273. [CrossRef]
46. Warshauer, J.T.; Bluestone, J.A.; Anderson, M.S. New Frontiers in the Treatment of Type 1 Diabetes. *Cell Metab.* **2020**, *31*, 46–61. [CrossRef] [PubMed]
47. Faulds, E.R.; Zappe, J.; Dungan, K.M. Real-World Implications of Hybrid Close Loop (HCl) Insulin Delivery System. *Endocr. Pract.* **2019**, *25*, 477–484. [CrossRef] [PubMed]
48. Insulin | FDA. Available online: https://www.fda.gov/consumers/free-publications-women/insulin (accessed on 15 February 2024).
49. Rosenstock, J.; Bain, S.C.; Gowda, A.; Jódar, E.; Liang, B.; Lingvay, I.; Nishida, T.; Trevisan, R.; Mosenzon, O. Weekly Icodec versus Daily Glargine U100 in Type 2 Diabetes without Previous Insulin. *N. Engl. J. Med.* **2023**, *389*, 297–308. [CrossRef] [PubMed]
50. Rosenstock, J.; Bajaj, H.S.; Janež, A.; Silver, R.; Begtrup, K.; Hansen, M.V.; Jia, T.; Goldenberg, R. Once-Weekly Insulin for Type 2 Diabetes without Previous Insulin Treatment. *N. Engl. J. Med.* **2020**, *383*, 2107–2116. [CrossRef]
51. Hoeg-Jensen, T. Review: Glucose-Sensitive Insulin. *Mol. Metab.* **2021**, *46*, 101107. [CrossRef]
52. Brownlee, M.; Cerami, A. A Glucose-Controlled Insulin-Delivery System: Semisynthetic Insulin Bound to Lectin. *Science* **1979**, *206*, 1190–1191. [CrossRef]
53. Nkonge, K.M.; Nkonge, D.K.; Nkonge, T.N. Insulin Therapy for the Management of Diabetes Mellitus: A Narrative Review of Innovative Treatment Strategies. *Diabetes Ther.* **2023**, *14*, 1801–1831. [CrossRef]
54. Mohanty, R.R.; Das, S. Inhaled Insulin—Current Direction of Insulin Research. *J. Clin. Diagn. Res.* **2017**, *11*, OE01–OE02. [CrossRef] [PubMed]
55. Wong, C.Y.; Al-Salami, H.; Dass, C.R. Recent Advancements in Oral Administration of Insulin-Loaded Liposomal Drug Delivery Systems for Diabetes Mellitus. *Int. J. Pharm.* **2018**, *549*, 201–217. [CrossRef]
56. Wong, C.Y.; Al-Salami, H.; Dass, C.R. Microparticles, Microcapsules and Microspheres: A Review of Recent Developments and Prospects for Oral Delivery of Insulin. *Int. J. Pharm.* **2018**, *537*, 223–244. [CrossRef] [PubMed]
57. Halberg, I.B.; Lyby, K.; Wassermann, K.; Heise, T.; Zijlstra, E.; Plum-Mörschel, L. Efficacy and Safety of Oral Basal Insulin versus Subcutaneous Insulin Glargine in Type 2 Diabetes: A Randomised, Double-Blind, Phase 2 Trial. *Lancet Diabetes Endocrinol.* **2019**, *7*, 179–188. [CrossRef] [PubMed]
58. Abramson, A.; Caffarel-Salvador, E.; Khang, M.; Dellal, D.; Silverstein, D.; Gao, Y.; Frederiksen, M.R.; Vegge, A.; Hubálek, F.; Water, J.J.; et al. An Ingestible Self-Orienting System for Oral Delivery of Macromolecules. *Science* **2019**, *363*, 611–615. [CrossRef] [PubMed]

biomedicines

Systematic Review

Once-Weekly Insulin Icodec in Diabetes Mellitus: A Systematic Review and Meta-Analysis of Randomized Clinical Trials (ONWARDS Clinical Program)

Giuseppe Lisco [1], Anna De Tullio [1], Vincenzo De Geronimo [2], Vito Angelo Giagulli [1], Edoardo Guastamacchia [1], Giuseppina Piazzolla [1], Olga Eugenia Disoteo [3,*] and Vincenzo Triggiani [1]

1 Interdisciplinary Department of Medicine, School of Medicine, University of Bari "Aldo Moro", Piazza Giulio Cesare 11, 70124 Bari, Italy; giuseppe.lisco@uniba.it (G.L.); annadetullio16@gmail.com (A.D.T.); vitogiagulli58@gmail.com (V.A.G.); edoardo.guastamacchia@uniba.it (E.G.); giuseppina.piazzolla@uniba.it (G.P.); vincenzo.triggiani@uniba.it (V.T.)

2 Unit of Endocrinology, Policlinico Morgagni CCD, 95125 Catania, Italy; vdg@iol.it

3 Unit of Endocrinology, Diabetology, Dietetics and Clinical Nutrition, Sant Anna Hospital, San Fermo della Battaglia, 22020 Como, Italy

* Correspondence: olgaeugenia.disoteo.amediabete@gmail.com

Abstract: Background. One hundred years have passed since the discovery of insulin, which is one of the most relevant events of the 20th century. This period resulted in extraordinary progress in the development of novel molecules to improve glucose control, simplify the insulin regimen, and ameliorate the quality of life. In late March 2024, the first once-weekly basal analog Icodec was approved for diabetes mellitus, generating high expectations. Our aim was to systematically review and meta-analyze the efficacy and safety of Icodec compared to once-daily insulin analogs in type 1 (T1D) and type 2 diabetes (T2D). Methods. PubMed/MEDLINE, Cochrane Library, and ClinicalTrials.gov were searched for randomized clinical trials (RCTs). Studies were included for the synthesis according to the following prespecified inclusion criteria: uncontrolled T1D or T2D, age $\geq$ 18 years, insulin Icodec vs. active comparators (Degludec U100, Glargine U100, Glargine U300, and Detemir), phase 3, multicenter, double-blind or open-label RCTs, and a study duration $\geq$ 24 weeks. Results. The systematic review included 4347 patients with T1D and T2D inadequately controlled (2172 randomized to Icodec vs. 2175 randomized to once-daily basal analogs). Icodec, compared to once-daily basal analogs, slightly reduced the levels of glycated hemoglobin (HbA1c) with an estimated treatment difference (ETD) of −0.14% [95%CI −0.25; −0.03], p = 0.01, and I^2 68%. Patients randomized to Icodec compared to those on once-daily basal analogs had a greater probability to achieve HbA1c < 7% without clinically relevant or severe hypoglycemic events in 12 weeks from randomization with an estimated risk ratio (ERR) of 1.17, [95%CI 1.01, 1.36], p = 0.03, and I^2 66%. We did not find a difference in fasting glucose levels, time in range, and time above range between Icodec and comparators. Icodec, compared to once-daily basal analogs, resulted in a slight but statistically significant weight gain of 0.62 kg [95%CI 0.25; 0.99], p = 0.001, and I^2 25%. The frequency of hypoglycemic events (ERR 1.16 [95%CI 0.95; 1.41]), adverse events (ERR 1.04 [95%CI 1.00; 1.08]), injection-site reactions (ERR 1.08 [95%CI 0.62; 1.90]), and the discontinuation of treatments were similar between the two groups. Icodec was found to work better when used in a basal-only than basal-bolus regimen with an ETD in HbA1c of −0.22%, a probability of achieving glucose control of +33%, a probability of achieving glucose control without clinically relevant or severe hypoglycemia of +28%, more time spent in target (+4.55%) and less time spent in hyperglycemia (−5.14%). The risk of clinically relevant or severe hypoglycemic events was significantly higher when background glinides and sulfonylureas were added to basal analogs (ERR 1.42 [95%CI 1.05; 1.93]). Conclusion. Insulin Icodec is substantially non-inferior to once-daily insulin analogs in T2D, either insulin-naïve or insulin-treated. However, Icodec works slightly better than competitors when used in a basal-only rather than basal-bolus regimen. Weight gain and hypoglycemic risk are substantially low but not negligible. Patients' education, adequate lifestyle and pharmacological interventions, and appropriate therapy adjustments are essential to minimize risks. This systematic review is registered as PROSPERO CRD42024568680.

Keywords: Icodec; once-weekly basal insulin; type 1 diabetes; type 2 diabetes; ONWARDS; randomized clinical trials; meta-analysis

1. Background

The discovery of insulin represents one of the most valuable scientific events of the 20th century, as it significantly contributed to the comprehension of diabetes mellitus pathophysiology and had relevant fallouts from a therapeutic viewpoint [1].

After the first identification of pancreatic islets by Paul Langerhans in 1869, more than 50 years passed until insulin was isolated for the first time by Sir Frederick Banting and Charles Best under the direction of John James Richard MacLeod at Toronto University (1921) [2]. Leonard Thompson was the first patient with type 1 diabetes (T1D) to receive the first insulin dose to control glucose levels, marking an extremely important event that would dramatically change the prognosis of future patients with insulinopenic diabetes. Banting and MacLeod's discovery was then honored with the Nobel Prize in Physiology or Medicine in 1923.

Subsequent decades were characterized by the fervid development of the pharmaceutical industry and biotechnologies with the aim of (1) expanding the production and distribution of insulin worldwide, given the progressively growing demand for the hormone in North America and Europe; (2) improving insulin safety and tolerability; and (3) developing novel insulin analogs with a long half-life to overcome the need for multiple administrations of short-acting insulin [3].

Frederick Sanger in 1958 and Dorothy Hodgkin in 1969 isolated the primary sequence and quaternary structure of human insulin, respectively [4,5], opening the gate to the future development of synthetic and completely humanized insulin analog, which took place in 1978 by David Goeddel with recombinant DNA technology (and amplification in *Escherichia coli*) [6].

Over the last 45 years, we have observed significant progress in the fields of Diabetology, Biotechnology, and Pharmacology after the development and approval of several insulin analogs with a rapid, ultra-rapid, and ultra-slow length of action and pre-filled pens that simplified the handling of insulin regimens significantly, especially for patients treated with multiple daily injections (MDI). At the same time, we observed a growing contribution of technology with glucometers, insulin pumps, glucose sensors, bolus calculators, and integrated systems, allowing increasingly more comfortable and tailored insulin delivery and better glucose control (Figure 1).

A recent investigation focused on the development of modern agents with different routes of administration (e.g., oral, transdermal, or inhalation), extremely long half-life (i.e., once weekly insulins), and analogs conjugated with glucose sensors and conveyed by specific platforms (smart insulins), which can act in a glucose-dependent manner [7–9].

Nowadays, the prevalence of diabetes is around 10% of the adult population worldwide, with estimations indicating that 635 million people will have established diabetes by 2030 and 783 million (+46%) by 2045 [10]. Type 2 diabetes (T2D) is the most common cause of diabetes, representing 90% of all cases, while T1D is less common (8–10%). Trends in insulin prescriptions in diabetes indicate a relevant increase in the number of insulin users among T2D patients, with around 17.4% and 52% of them, respectively, on basal-only and basal-bolus regimens [11]. Despite the novel agents currently available for T2D, the percentage of patients who are candidates for insulin treatment is expected to increase over the following decades due to the extension of life expectancy and the absolute increase in the number of patients living with T2D. As another issue, only 1 in 4 insulin users with T2D achieve their glucose targets, making frequent therapy adjustments compulsory, including a switch to other basal analogs, to improve glucose control [12]. The lack of adherence to insulin regimens, especially for patients on MDI, with the suboptimal frequency of glucose checks and therapeutic inertia of prompt insulin titration, represent the most common causes of insulin failure [13]. Overcoming these barriers can result in better glucose management in patients with diabetes.

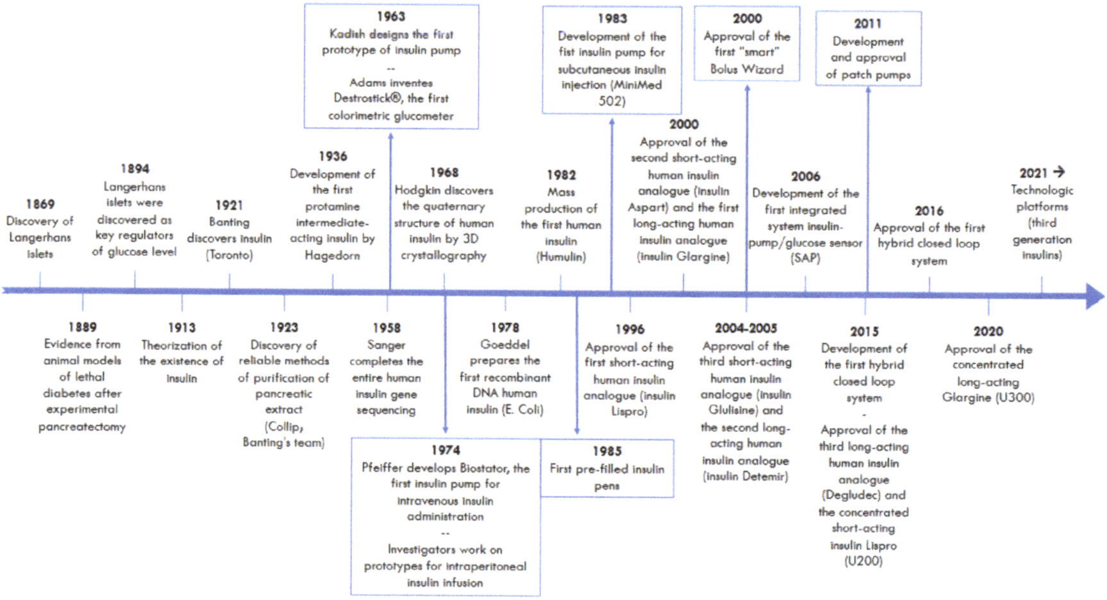

Figure 1. Timeline summarizing the most relevant discoveries and events in the fields of Diabetology, Biotechnology, and Pharmacology that have characterized the last 100 years.

2. Progress in Once-Weekly Insulins

Adequate adherence to pharmacological treatment contributes significantly to achieving and maintaining tailored glucose control, as guidelines recommend, especially in patients with MDI. Novel administration strategies have been studied and proposed, such as once-weekly administered drugs. Once weekly administered drugs represent a significant innovation in the pharmacological management of T2D, as demonstrated mainly by incretin-based injective treatments, such as glucagon-like peptide 1 receptor agonists (GLP-1RAs) and dual GLP-1 and glucose-dependent insulinotropic peptide receptor agonists [14–17]. Possible drawbacks of once-weekly insulins, such as insulin Icodec, are related to their prolonged half-life, leading to less frequent insulin dose adjustments compared to once-daily analogs that, in turn, could generate some concerns in managing glucose variability, especially in insulinopenic diabetes while using the basal-bolus regimen. Therefore, it is mandatory to address the efficacy and safety of insulin Icodec in various insulin regimens, particularly the basal-bolus regimen, in both types of diabetes, which was the aim of our systematic review. Moreover, insulin Icodec direct costs are expected to be higher than those of currently available basal insulin analogs. Large-scale, cost-effective trials are needed to comprehensively estimate the direct and indirect costs of insulin Icodec compared to once-daily insulin analogs.

Ultra-long compared to once-daily insulin analogs should not simply have a longer half-life; instead, they should ensure the lower variability of plasma concentration, a stronger affinity for serum albumin, and significantly lower affinity for insulin receptors, slowing down the receptor-mediated clearance of the insulin analog.

The first ultra-long insulin analog, Icodec (Awiqli®), was approved in March 2024 to treat T2D in Europe [18]. The novel analog should be administered subcutaneously once a week in sites conventionally used to administer other insulin analogs, including the thigh, abdomen, and upper arm [19]. Icodec can be marketed in three different packages, including pens of 1 mL, 1.5 mL, and 3 mL with a standard concentration of 700 IU/mL [20]. The Icodec dose should be calculated and adjusted weekly. The starting dose in insulin-naïve patients should be 70 IU/week, a dose paralleled to 10 IU per day of once-daily insulins. Patients who are switched from other basal insulins to Icodec should be replaced by maintaining a 1:1 ratio with the weekly dose of the basal analog, except for the first administration, which is recommended to increase the dose by 50 to 100% according to baseline-fasting glucose levels. The steady state is achieved after four weeks, and titration should be accomplished weekly (±20 IU) with a recommended fasting/pre-breakfast self-monitored glucose target of 80–130 mg/dL [21].

The pharmacokinetic profile of Icodec is not affected by mild, moderate, or severe hepatic impairment. A slight but statistically significant increase in Icodec exposure was reported along with a declining glomerular filtration rate; nevertheless, the clinical relevance of this phenomenon could be negligible and easily managed with proper titration [22].

Icodec results from molecular bioengineering that introduce several changes in the native structure of other insulin analogs starting from an oral insulin prototype (OI388) [23]. The addition of a C20 fatty diacid-containing side chain (acylation) induces robust and reversible binding to serum albumin, while three amino acid substitutions (chain A, 14E; chain B, 16H, and 25H) provide molecular stability and reduce binding to insulin receptor and clearance [24,25]. Overall, these changes prolong the half-life of Icodec, resulting in 196 h, which is compatible with once-weekly dosing. Moreover, the lower affinity of insulin Icodec, compared to native insulin, for both the insulin and insulin-like growth factor-1 receptors were proven to reduce the mitogenic effect of Icodec in various human cells.

Another once-weekly insulin analog is currently under investigation, namely, the Basal Insulin Fc (BIF, LY3209590, or insulin Efsitora alfa), which is composed of a novel single-chain variant of insulin fused to a human immunoglobulin G2 fragment and crystallizable region of an antibody domain using a peptide linker [26]. Three phase 2 trials have already been completed, and the published results demonstrate that insulin Efsitora alfa is effective and safe in patients with T1D [27] when compared to once-daily insulin Degludec U100 and both T2D insulin-naïve [28] and insulin users [29]. Five phase 3 trials are ongoing to investigate the efficacy and safety of insulin Efsitora alfa as the most relevant part of the once-weekly Insulin Therapy clinical program [30].

3. Efficacy and Safety of Insulin Icodec: The State of the Art

3.1. Phase 2 Trials

A summary of the phase 2 trial results is shown in Table 1. Icodec, compared to Glargine U100, was administered daily and achieved a non-inferiority endpoint that improved glucose control with a similar risk of level 2 and 3 hypoglycemia in insulin-naïve T2D individuals [31].

Titration is essential to achieve optimal glucose control without increasing the risk of hypoglycemia, as demonstrated by another phase 2 trial [32]. The best result in terms of improving glucose control and lowering the risk of hypoglycemia was obtained when Icodec, compared to Glargine U100, was titrated at ±28 IU/week to maintain a fasting/prebreakfast self-monitored glucose level between 80 and 130 mg/dL. The switch to Icodec vs. Glargine U100 in T2D patients who failed to achieve adequate glucose control with other basal insulins was slightly better in terms of the glucose control attained in 15 weeks, especially when a loading dose of Icodec (+100%) was administered at the switching time [33].

Table 1. Overview of phase 2 trials.

	NCT03751657 [27]	NCT03951805 [28]	NCT03922750 [29]
Study design	26-week double-blind, RCT	16-week open-label, randomized, treat-to-target, titration trial with glucose monitoring	16-week open-label, randomized, treat-to-target, switching trial with glucose monitoring
Population	T2D	T2D	T2D
Intervention	Once-weekly insulin Icodec	Once-weekly insulin Icodec Titration A (80–130 mg/dL = adjustment ± 21 IU/week); Titration B (80–130 mg/dL = ±28 IU/week); Titration C (70–108 mg/dL = ±28 IU/week)	Once-weekly insulin Icodec A) with loading dose (a 100% increase from the initial dose) B) without loading dose
Comparator	Once-daily insulin Glargine U100	Once-daily insulin Glargine U100 Titration (80–130 mg/dL = ±4 IU/day)	Once-daily insulin Glargine U100
Baseline characteristics	247 insulin-naïve participants, mean HbA1c 8%, metformin ± DPP-IV inhibitors	205 insulin-naïve participants, mean HbA1c 8.1%, any oral antihyperglycemic agents	154 insulin users (10–50 IU/day): Detemir, Degludec U100, Glargine U100, Glargine U300, mean HbA1c 7.9%
Main findings	Mean change from baseline in HbA1c: −1.33% Icodec vs. −1.15% Glargine U100 (p = 0.08) Hypoglycemia (levels 2 and 3): 0.53 events per patient-year Icodec vs. 0.46 events per patient-year Glargine U100 (RR 1.09; 95%CI, 0.45 to 2.65)	Mean change in TIR (baseline to 15–16 weeks) Icodec A: from 57.0% to 76.6% Icodec B: from 55.2% to 83% Icodec C: from 51.0% to 80.9% Glargine U100: from 55.3% to 75.9% Level 2 hypoglycemia (<54 mg/dL, events per patient-year of exposure) Icodec A: 0.05 Icodec B: 0.15 Icodec C: 0.38 Glargine U100: 0.00 No level 3 hypos were observed.	Mean change in TIR (baseline to 15–16 weeks) Icodec A: from 58.9% to 72.9% Icodec B: from 54.5% to 66.0% Glargine U100: from 58.7% to 65.0% Mean change in HbA1c Icodec A: from 7.9% to 7.1% Icodec B: from 7.9% to 7.4% Glargine U100: from 7.9% to 7.4% Level 1 and 2 hypos were similar (among the 3 groups), and no level 3 hypos were registered

Abbreviations: HbA1c, Glycated hemoglobin; IU, International Unit; T2D, Type 2 Diabetes.

3.2. Phase 3 Trials

3.2.1. Overview of the ONWARDS Clinical Program

The efficacy and safety of insulin Icodec were extensively assessed over six randomized clinical trials (RCTs) of the clinical program ONWARDS (Table 2) [34–39]. Five trials were conducted on T2D patients: 3 in insulin-naïve (ONWARDS 1, 3, and 5) and 2 in insulin-treated (ONWARDS 2 and 4) patients. Only one trial was conducted on T1D (ONWARDS 6). Icodec was compared to once-daily basal insulin types, namely Glargine U100 (ONWARDS 1, 4, and 5), Glargine U300 (ONWARDS 5), and Degludec U100 (ONWARDS 2, 3, and 5), to assess both the efficacy and safety of the novel once-weekly analog.

Table 2. Comprehensive overview of the ONWARDS clinical program.

	ONWARDS 1 [30] (NCT04460885)	ONWARDS 2 [31] (NCT04770532)	ONWARDS 3 [32] (NCT04795531)	ONWARDS 4 [33] (NCT04880850)	ONWARDS 5 [34] (NCT04760626)	ONWARDS 6 [35] (NCT04848480)
Sponsored	Yes	Yes	Yes	Yes	Yes	Yes
Population	Insulin-naïve T2D	Basal insulin-treated T2D	Insulin-naïve T2D	Basal bolus-treated T2D	Insulin-naïve T2D	T1D
Inclusion criteria	Age ≥ 18 yrs, baseline HbA1c 7–11%, baseline BMI ≤ 40 kg/m^2	Age ≥ 18 yrs, baseline HbA1c 7–10%	Age ≥ 18 yrs, baseline HbA1c 7–11%, baseline BMI ≤ 40 kg/m^2	Age ≥ 18 yrs, baseline HbA1c 7–10%	Age ≥ 18 yrs, baseline HbA1c > 7%, for whom insulin treatment is required	HbA1c < 10% At least 1 year of basal-bolus regimen
Study design	Randomized, open-label, treat-to-target phase 3a trial	Randomized, open-label, active-controlled, multicentric, treat-to-target phase 3a trial	Randomized, double-masked, double-dummy, active-controlled, treat-to-target phase 3a trial	Randomized, open-label, multicentric, treat-to-target, non-inferiority trial	Randomized, open-label, multinational trial	Randomized, multicenter, open-label, active-controlled, parallel-group, treat-to-target, phase 3a trial
Study duration, weeks	78 (52 + 26 of extension safety phase) + a 5-week follow-up	26 + a 5-week follow-up	26 + a 5-week follow-up	26 + a 5-week follow-up	52 + a 5-week follow-up	52 (26 + 26 of extension safety phase) + a 5-week follow-up
Pretrial antihyperglycemic drugs	Any non-insulin drugs allowed	Once or twice-daily basal insulins ± non insulin antihyperglycemic agents	Any non-insulin drugs allowed	Any basal-bolus regimen ± non insulin antihyperglycemic agents (>90 days)	Any non-insulin drugs allowed	Basal-bolus regimen (any analogues allowed)
Handling of pretrial antihyperglycemic drugs at the randomization	Pretrial drugs confirmed, except secretagogues	Pretrial drugs confirmed, except secretagogues	Pretrial drugs confirmed at the same dose, including secretagogues (initial dose was reduced by 50%)	Pretrial drugs confirmed, except secretagogues	Pretrial drugs confirmed at the same dose, including secretagogues (initial dose was reduced by 50%)	Pretrial prandial insulins were switched to insulin Aspart
Comorbidities	NA	NA	Arterial hypertension (65%), hepatic steatosis (12.5%), coronary artery disease (10%), renal impairment (8.5%)	NA	Arterial hypertension (70%), hepatic steatosis (9.8%), coronary artery disease (8.5%)	NA

Table 2. *Cont.*

	ONWARDS 1 [30] (NCT04460885)	ONWARDS 2 [31] (NCT04770532)	ONWARDS 3 [32] (NCT04795531)	ONWARDS 4 [33] (NCT04880850)	ONWARDS 5 [34] (NCT04760626)	ONWARDS 6 [35] (NCT04848480)
Intervention	Once-weekly insulin Icodec	Once-weekly insulin Icodec	Once-weekly insulin Icodec + once-daily placebo	Once-weekly insulin Icodec + insulin Aspart	Once-weekly insulin Icodec	Once-weekly insulin Icodec + insulin Aspart
Comparators	Once-daily insulin Glargine U100	Once-daily insulin Degludec U100	Once-daily insulin Degludec U100	Once-daily insulin Glargine U100 + insulin Aspart	Once-daily basal insulins (Glargine U100 or Glargine U300 or Degludec U100)	Once-daily insulin Degludec U100 + insulin Aspart
Sample size: n	Icodec: 492 Glargine: 492	Icodec: 263 Degludec: 263	Icodec: 294 Degludec: 294	Icodec: 292 Glargine: 291	Icodec: 542 OD Basal: 543	Icodec: 290 Degludec: 292
Completed the "in-trial" period: %	Icodec: 96.5% Glargine: 97.4%	Icodec: 97.7% Degludec: 96.2%	Icodec: 95.9% Degludec: 96.2%	Icodec: 94% Glargine: 92%	Icodec: 89.1% OD Basal: 90.8%	Icodec: 90% Glargine: 95%
Primary Outcome	Mean change from baseline to study completion in HbA1c	Mean change from baseline to study completion in HbA1c	Mean change from baseline to study completion in HbA1c	Mean change from baseline to study completion in HbA1c	Mean change from baseline to study completion in HbA1c	Mean change from baseline to study completion (week 26) in HbA1c
Secondary outcomes	Mean change from baseline to study completion in FPG, TIR, weekly insulin dose, body weight	Mean change from baseline to study completion in FPG, TIR, weekly insulin dose, body weight, diabetes satisfaction	Mean change from baseline to study completion in FPG, weekly insulin dose, body weight	Mean change from baseline to study completion in FPG, TIR, weekly insulin dose, body weight	Mean change from baseline to study completion in diabetes satisfaction and compliance, weekly insulin dose and body weight	Mean change from baseline to study completion in FPG, TIR, HbA1c (week 52), body weight, diabetes satisfaction
Safety outcomes	Adverse events, hypoglycemic episodes (levels 1, 2, and 3)	Adverse events, hypoglycemic episodes (levels 1, 2, and 3), daytime and nocturnal hypos	Adverse events, hypoglycemic episodes (levels 1, 2, and 3)	Adverse events, hypoglycemic episodes (levels 1, 2, and 3)	Adverse events, hypoglycemic episodes (levels 1, 2, and 3), daytime and nocturnal hypos	Adverse events, hypoglycemic episodes (levels 1, 2, and 3), daytime and nocturnal hypos
Age, yrs: mean ± sd	Icodec: 59.1 ± 10.1 Glargine: 58.9 ± 9.9	Icodec: 62.3 ± 9.8 Degludec: 62.6 ± 8.4	Icodec: 58 ± 10 Degludec: 59 ± 10	Icodec: 59.7 ± 10.1 Glargine: 59.9 ± 9.9	Icodec: 59.1 ± 10.8 OD Basal: 59.4 ± 10.2	Icodec: 44.1 ± 14.1 Degludec: 44.3 ± 14.1
Diabetes duration, yrs: mean ± sd	Icodec: 11.6 ± 6.7 Glargine: 11.5 ± 6.8	Icodec: 16.5 ± 8.4 Degludec: 16.9 ± 7.9	Icodec: 10.5 Degludec: 10.7	Icodec: 18 ± 9.1 Glargine: 16.3 ± 7.7	Icodec: 11.9 ± 6.9 OD Basal: 12 ± 7.6	Icodec: 20 ± 13.2 Degludec: 19 ± 12.9
Baseline HbA1c, %: mean ± sd	Icodec: 8.5 ± 1 Glargine: 8.4 ± 1	Icodec: 8.17 ± 0.77 Degludec: 8.1 ± 0.77	Icodec: 8.55 ± 1.11 Degludec: 8.48 ± 1.01	Icodec: 8.29 ± 0.86 Glargine: 8.31 ± 0.9	Icodec: 8.96 ± 1.6 OD Basal: 8.88 ± 1.5	Icodec: 7.59 ± 0.96 Degludec: 7.63 ± 0.93
Final HbA1c, %: mean ± sd	Icodec: 6.93 ± 1.33 Glargine: 7.12 ± 1.11	Icodec: 7.2 ± 0.81 Degludec: 7.42 ± 0.97	Icodec: 7 ± 1.09 Degludec: 7.2 ± 0.98	Icodec: 7.14 ± 0.85 Glargine: 7.12 ± 0.85	Icodec: 7.24 ± 2.01 OD Basal: 7.61 ± 2.7	Icodec: 7.15 ± 1.1 Degludec: 7.1 ± 1.1
Baseline FPG, mg/dL: mean ± sd	Icodec: 185.3 ± 49 Glargine: 185.7 ± 51.7	Icodec: 155.2 ± 47 Degludec: 150.7 ± 40.9	Icodec: 187 ± 54 Degludec: 176 ± 46	Icodec: 165.6 ± 54 Glargine: 172.8 ± 63	Icodec: NA OD Basal: NA	Icodec: 179 ± 74 Degludec: 172 ± 72
Final FPG, mg/dL: mean ± sd	Icodec: 125.2 ± 37 Glargine: 125.4 ± 37.3	Icodec: 129.1 ± 29.3 Degludec: 117.7 ± 26	Icodec: 127 ± NA Degludec: 127 ± NA	Icodec: 137 ± 41 Glargine: 132 ± 39	Icodec: NA OD Basal: NA	Icodec: 163.9 ± NA Degludec: 138.3 ± NA
Baseline BMI, kg/m^2: mean ± sd	Icodec: 30 ± 4.8 Glargine: 30.1 ± 5.1	Icodec: 29.5 ± 5.2 Degludec: 29.2 ± 4.9	Icodec: 29.9 ± 5.2 Degludec: 29.2 ± 5.1	Icodec: 30.5 ± 5 Glargine: 30 ± 5	Icodec: 32.6 ± 7 OD Basal: 33 ± 6.9	Icodec: 26.8 ± 5 Degludec: 26.2 ± 4.5
Baseline body weight, kg: mean ± sd	Icodec: 85.2 ± 17.7 Glargine: 84.3 ± 17.6	Icodec: 83.7 ± 18.4 Degludec: 81.5 ± 17.1	Icodec: 85.8 ± 20.1 Degludec: 83.2 ± 18.2	Icodec: 85.5 ± 17.6 Glargine: 83.1 ± 17.3	Icodec: 93.2 ± 22.5 OD Basal: 94.3 ± 21.5	Icodec: 78.6 ± 17.6 Degludec: 77.1 ± 16.8
Final body weight, kg: mean ± sd	Icodec: 87.03 ± 0.21 Glargine: 86.57 ± 0.21	NA	Icodec: 87.3 ± NA Degludec: 86.8 ± NA	Icodec: 88.2 ± NA Glargine: 85.3 ± NA	Icodec: 96 OD Basal: 95.2	Icodec: 79.9 ± NA Degludec: 78.1 ± NA
Starting dose of basal insulin (IU/week)	Icodec: 70 Glargine: 70	1:1 ratio with pretrial basal insulins	Icodec: 70 Degludec: 70	1:1 ratio with pretrial basal insulins	Icodec: 70 Degludec: 70	1:1 ratio with pretrial basal insulins
Weekly insulin dose at the study completion: n (IU)	Icodec: 214 Glargine: 222	Icodec: 268 Degludec: 244	Icodec: 204 Degludec: 186	Icodec: 305 Glargine: 279	Icodec: 227 OD Basal: 185	Icodec: 132 Degludec: 161
Treat-to-target approach	Yes, 80–130 mg/dL	Yes, 80–130 mg/dL	Yes, 80–130 mg/dL	Yes, 80–130 mg/dL	NA	Yes, 80–130 mg/dL
Titration of basal insulin	Icodec: ±20 per week Glargine: ±3 per day	NA	Icodec: ±20 per week Degludec: ±3 per day	Icodec: ±20 per week Glargine: ±3 per day	Icodec: algorithmic-assisted titration Degludec: at the discretion of investigators	Icodec: ±20 per week Degludec: ±3 per day Aspart: dose adjustment (week 0 to 8) or carbohydrate-counting
Frequency of insulin dose adjustment	Once a week	Once a week	Once a week	Once a week	Once a week	Once a week
Additional metrics/tools	Yes, double-blind CGM (weeks 48–52)	Yes, double-blind CGM (weeks 22–26)	None	Yes, double-blind CGM (weeks 22–26)	ICOBOT engine for guiding Icodec titration only	Yes, open CGM (whole study, but not used for insulin titration)
Satisfaction questionnaire	None	Yes, DTSQ	None	None	Yes, DTSQ, TRIM-D	Yes, DTSQ

Abbreviations: CGM, Continuous Glucose Monitoring; DTSQ, Diabetes Treatment Satisfaction Questionnaire; FPG, Fasting Plasma Glucose; HbA1c, Glycated hemoglobin; IU, International Unit; NA, Not Assessed/reported; OD, Once a Day; T1D, Type 1 Diabetes; T2D, Type 2 Diabetes; TIR, Time in Range; TRIM-D, Treatment Related Impact Measure for Diabetes.

Each trial included a 2-week pretrial screening and a 5-week post-trial safety follow-up in which the patients were followed after treatment discontinuation for residual adverse events. The trials ONWARDS 1, 5, and 6 also included a 26-week extension phase during which patients continued the trial treatments in the same way as from the randomization to detect and register efficacy and safety endpoints until the study's completion.

The primary endpoint of all trials was to compare the mean absolute changes in glycated hemoglobin (HbA1c) levels from baseline to study completion, which was set at 26 weeks in ONWARDS and 2, 3, 4, and 6 and 52 weeks in the remaining cohorts. Secondary endpoints included fasting glucose control, time in range (TIR), hypoglycemic risk, other safety outcomes, and patient satisfaction [40].

3.2.2. Procedures

Pretrial Antihyperglycemic Treatment

Any antihyperglycemic drug was allowed before the study entry and during the trials at the same pretrial dose. Sulfonylureas or glinides were discontinued (ONWARDS 1, 2, and 4) or the pretrial dose halved (ONWARDS 3 and 5) because of unacceptable gain in the risk of hypoglycemia when combined with basal insulins.

In ONWARDS 4 and 6, all participants were switched from any pretrial prandial analog to insulin Aspart.

Starting Dose and Titration of Basal Analogs

The starting dose of Icodec and once-daily basal analogs was 70 IU per week (10 IU/day) in insulin-naïve individuals (ONWARDS 1, 3, and 5). In insulin-treated patients (ONWARDS 2, 4, and 6), the starting dose of both Icodec and once-daily basal analogs was the same as the weekly dose of the pretrial basal analog. For the first dose of Icodec, an additional 50% one-time dose was administered. In ONWARDS 6, T1D individuals with a baseline HbA1c > 8% received a 100% once-time additional dose of Icodec in addition to the first administration only.

Basal analogs were titrated weekly using a treat-to-target approach to achieve fasting/prebreakfast glucose levels of 80–130 mg/dL. In ONWARDS 5, the titration of Icodec was assisted by a dose guidance system integrated with a dose recommendation algorithm. Therefore, patients randomized to Icodec received specific training to run the system. Investigators carried out the titration of Degludec at their personal discretion as per standard practice.

Continuous Glucose Monitoring

Continuous glucose monitoring (CGM) was allowed in ONWARDS 1, 2, and 4. It was double-masked over the last four weeks of trials, with only a statistical aim to collect and analyze additional metrics of glucose control, including TIR (70–180 mg/dL), time above range, or TAR (>180 mg/dL), and time spent in clinically relevant hypoglycemia (<54 mg/dL).

In ONWARDS 6, patients with T1D were educated to wear and use an open CGM system to monitor glucose values during the study. However, as per the protocol, any CGM-based insulin adjustment was prohibited.

The GCM system used in all trials was Dexcom G6®.

Safety Endpoints

Safety endpoints were observed and reported over the entire study, including the extension phase and 5-week follow-up. Safety endpoints included any adverse events, such as serious and severe adverse events, events probably and possibly related to insulin use, hypersensitivity, injection-site reactions, hypoglycemia (overall, combined clinically relevant and severe, and nocturnal), and weight gain.

Hypoglycemic events were classified according to a standardized three-level severity scale as follows: level 1 hypoglycemia for glucose levels ranging from 55 to 70 mg/dL, level 2 or clinically significant hypoglycemia for glucose levels $\leq$ 54 mg/dL, and level 3 or severe hypoglycemia to indicate an event characterized by altered mental and/or physical status requiring assistance for the treatment of hypoglycemia, regardless of glucose levels [41].

Satisfaction and Compliance Questionnaires

The Diabetes Treatment Satisfaction Questionnaire and Treatment-Related Impact Measure for Diabetes were used as specific tools to assess secondary endpoints on diabetes satisfaction and compliance in insulin-treated patients in ONWARDS 2, 5, and 6 only.

3.2.3. Methods

Searching, Screening, and Selection of Studies

Two operators (G.L. and A.D.T.) searched databases and registries, including PubMed/MEDLINE, Cochrane Library, and ClinicalTrials.gov, from 1 November 2020 to 9 August 2024, for RCTs assessing the efficacy and safety of insulin Icodec from the ONWARDS clinical program. Keywords and Medical Subject Heading (MeSH) terms included the following: "icodec", "once-weekly basal insulin*", "once-weekly basal analogue*", "basal insulin*", "glargine u100", "glargine u300", and "degludec u100".

Databases were searched independently by each operator to mitigate possible biases. The prespecified clinical question was as follows: "Is insulin Icodec more effective and safer than once-daily basal analogs in improving glycemic parameters of patients with diabetes mellitus who failed to achieve glucose control with non-insulin agents or previous insulin treatment?".

Records were screened and selected by each operator and then compared. The flow diagram illustrating the process of identification, screening, and inclusion of RCTs for this systematic review is shown in the Supplementary Material (Figure S1).

The other three operators (O.E.D., E.G. and V.T.) checked the literature for possible external sources of RCTs.

Inclusion Criteria

Studies were selected based on the following inclusion criteria: patients with uncontrolled T1D or T2D, age $\geq$ 18 years, insulin Icodec vs. active comparators (Degludec U100, Glargine U100, Glargine U300, and Detemir) alone or in combination with prandial analogs, phase 3, multicenter, double-blind or open-label RCTs, and a study duration of 24 weeks or more.

Exclusion Criteria

Non-randomized observational studies and case series were excluded.

Extraction and Synthesis: Comprehensive Details of RCTs

Two operators (G.L. and A.D.T.) extracted data from RCTs. The details of each RCT were extensively reviewed and collected (Table 1). The details include information on the study population, study design and duration, inclusion criteria, baseline antihyperglycemic drugs and the management of pretrial drugs during the trials, frequency of comorbidities, intervention, comparators, sample size, number of patients who completed the "in-trial" period, primary, secondary and safety endpoints, main baseline characteristics, main post-trial characteristics, starting and final weekly doses of insulin analogs, details on basal insulin titration, and additional information.

Extraction and Synthesis: Efficacy Endpoints

Efficacy endpoints were selected according to their clinical relevance, study design, and the heterogeneity of data reporting across all trials. These included (a) the mean absolute change in HbA1c levels from baseline to study completion, summarized as estimated treatment difference (ETD) between the two study groups; (b) the probability of achieving acceptable glucose control (i.e., HbA1c < 7%), summarized as the estimated risk ratio (ERR) or a chance to obtain a specific outcome; (c) the probability of achieving acceptable glucose control without clinically relevant or severe hypoglycemia (i.e., HbA1c < 7% without level 2 or level 3 hypoglycemia, by combining efficacy with a safety endpoint), summarized as ERR or the chance to obtain a specific outcome; (d) the mean absolute difference in TIR after the study completion, summarized as the ERR between the two study groups; and (e) the mean absolute change in fasting plasma glucose (FPG) from baseline to study completion, summarized as ETD between the two study groups.

Technical remark: efficacy endpoints (b) and (c) should be intended as early efficacy endpoints since they are estimated in 12 weeks from randomization in line with clinical practice and current recommendation, suggesting that HbA1c levels should be checked after 2 to 3 months from any therapy adjustment in patients with inadequate glucose control.

Extraction and Synthesis: Safety Endpoints

Safety endpoints were selected according to their clinical relevance, study design, and the heterogeneity of data reporting. These include (a) the mean absolute difference in TAR after the study completion, summarized as ETD between the two study groups; (b) the mean absolute change in body weight from baseline to study completion, summarized as ETD between the two study groups; (c) the probability of presenting with level 2 or level 3 hypoglycemia (combined endpoint), summarized as ERR for the outcome to occur; (d) the probability of presenting with any adverse event, summarized as ERR for the outcome to occur; (e) the probability of presenting with any adverse event probably or possibly related to basal insulin, summarized as ERR for the outcome to occur; (f) the probability of presenting with serious adverse events, summarized as ERR for the outcome to occur; (g) the probability of presenting with serious adverse events probably or possibly related to basal insulin, summarized as ERR for the outcome to occur; and (h) the probability of presenting with injection-site reactions, summarized as ERR for the outcome to occur.

Technical remark: safety analyses were carried out considering the number of patients who experienced a specific event (one or more times) from the total number of participants included in the safety analysis set.

Intention-to-Treat Analysis

All statistics were calculated according to an intention-to-treat analysis. Statistical analyses were conducted on two different clusters of patients according to the prespecified endpoints.

Efficacy endpoints were analyzed using the full-analysis set (randomized participants) and data from the "in-trial" period (from randomization to the last contact, withdrawal, or death).

Safety endpoints were assessed using the safety analysis set (randomized participants who received at least one dose of study drugs) from the "on-treatment" period (from randomization to the trial end).

Participants Who Completed the Trials

The "in-trial" period was completed by more than 90% of randomized participants, except for the Icodec arm in ONWARDS 5 (completion rate 89.1%), with a similar discontinuation rate between the two study groups.

Technical remark: the intention-to-treat analysis aims to reduce the attrition bias due to the relevant dropouts of participants during the follow-up. However, compared to a per-protocol analysis, it was less informative on the real effect of treatments in each stage of the follow-up. A high and symmetric completion rate ensures the readability of intention-to-treat analyses.

Assessment of the Risk of Bias and Publication Bias

The risk of included studies was estimated with the RoB2 assessment tool for individual randomized, parallel-group trials [42]. All trials were extensively evaluated in 5 separate domains, exploring the randomization process, the deviation from the intended interventions, missing data, the measurement of outcomes, and the selection of reported results. The risk of bias was estimated for each outcome (efficacy and safety), and each domain was rated as low, moderate (some concerns), or high (relevant).

Technical remark: primary and secondary endpoints, as well as additional exploratory assessments, were prespecified, except for some evaluations that were carried out post hoc, so when the preliminary or advanced results of RCTs were already available.

With specific regard to the endpoints of interest for our meta-analysis, it should be mentioned that only two variables were listed as not prespecified analyses, namely the variable "probability of experiencing combined clinically significant (level 2) or severe (level 3) hypoglycemia with a given treatment" in ONWARDS 2, and the variable "number of hypoglycemic alerts" in ONWARDS 4 and 6.

Hence, we chose to evaluate the domain bias number five (the selection of the reported results) of ONWARDS 2, 4, and 6 with some concerns (Figure 2).

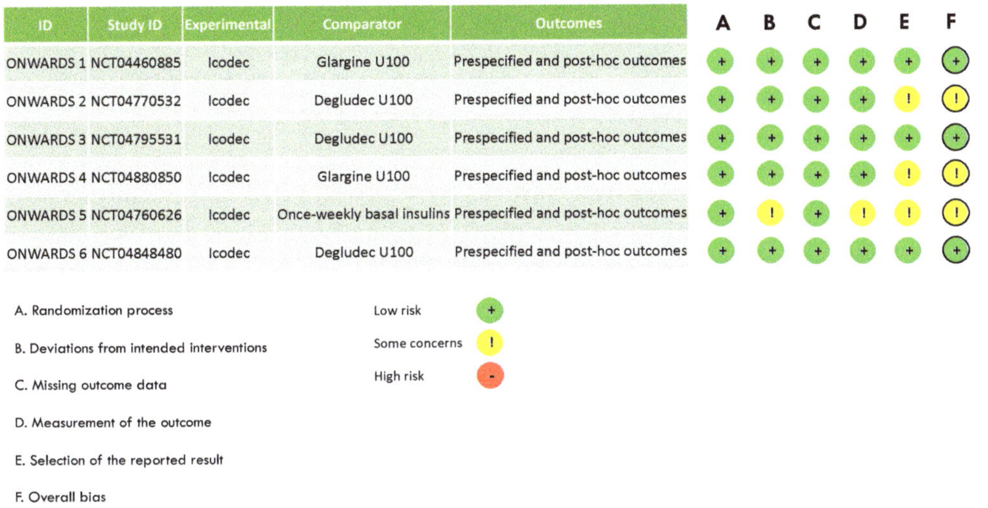

Figure 2. Risk of bias of RCTs included in the systematic review and meta-analysis from the ONWARDS clinical program.

The existence of publication bias for the primary outcome was verified by a funnel plot (Supplementary Material, Figure S2).

Software for Statistics

Forest plots and sensitive analyses were performed by RevMan 5.4.1 with a random-effect model, considering a p-value < 0.05 as statistically significant. Heterogeneity was assessed by I^2. The level of heterogeneity was considered substantial in the case of $I^2 > 60\%$, leading us to explore the possible causes of heterogeneity in the specific result by subgroup analyses [43].

We used the standard error, 95% confidence interval (CI), and interquartile range to estimate the standard deviation when missed.

3.2.4. Results

Synthesis of Data from the ONWARDS Clinical Program

The systematic review and meta-analysis included, for the primary endpoint (the mean absolute change in HbA1c from baseline to study completion), 4347 patients with T1D and T2D inadequately controlled and randomized to receive Icodec (2172) or once-daily basal analogs (2175) for 26 consecutive weeks or more.

The baseline-weighted mean level of HbA1c from the ONWARDS clinical program was 8.4%. Icodec, compared to once-daily insulin analogs, improved glucose control with an ETD of −0.14% [95%CI −0.25; −0.03], $p = 0.01$, and I^2 68% (Figure 3).

Patients randomized to Icodec, compared to those on once-daily basal analogs, had a 16% higher chance to achieve optimal glucose control (i.e., HbA1c < 7%) over 12 weeks from randomization but this difference was not statistically significant with an ERR of 1.16 [95%CI 0.95; 1.42], and I^2 84% (Figure 4).

Study or Subgroup	Icodec Mean	Icodec SD	Icodec Total	Once-daily basal insulin Mean	Once-daily basal insulin SD	Once-daily basal insulin Total	Weight	Mean Difference IV, Random, 95% CI
ONWARDS 5	-1.68	2.3529	542	-1.3	2.3529	543	9.8%	-0.38 [-0.66, -0.10]
ONWARDS 2	-0.93	0.8776	263	-0.71	0.8776	263	17.6%	-0.22 [-0.37, -0.07]
ONWARDS 3	-1.6	0.6186	294	-1.4	0.6186	294	21.5%	-0.20 [-0.30, -0.10]
ONWARDS 1	-1.55	1.3309	492	-1.35	1.3309	492	16.4%	-0.20 [-0.37, -0.03]
ONWARDS 4	-1.16	0.8001	291	-1.18	0.8001	291	19.2%	0.02 [-0.11, 0.15]
ONWARDS 6	-0.47	1.1078	290	-0.51	1.1078	292	15.5%	0.04 [-0.14, 0.22]
Total (95% CI)			2172			2175	100.0%	-0.14 [-0.25, -0.03]

Heterogeneity: Tau² = 0.01; Chi² = 15.46, df = 5 (P = 0.009); I² = 68%
Test for overall effect: Z = 2.50 (P = 0.01)

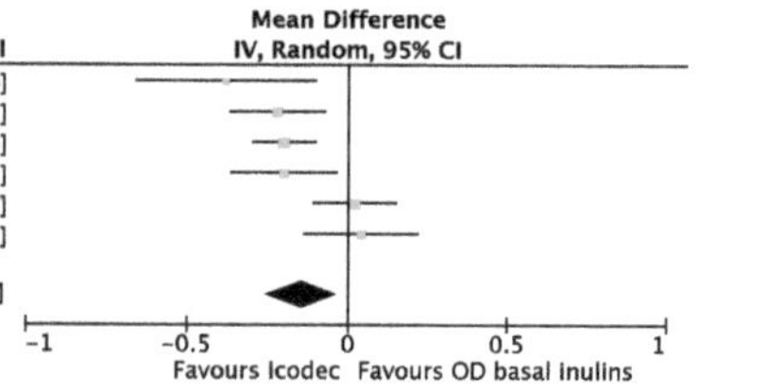

Abbreviations: ETD, Estimated Treatment Difference; OD, Once-Daily.

Figure 3. Forest plot of meta-analysis for mean change in Glycated Hemoglobin (ETD, %) from baseline to study completion (intention-to-treat analysis).

Study or Subgroup	Icodec Events	Icodec Total	Once-daily basal insulin Events	Once-daily basal insulin Total	Weight	Risk Ratio M-H, Random, 95% CI
ONWARDS 6	117	290	133	292	19.9%	0.89 [0.73, 1.07]
ONWARDS 4	119	291	131	291	19.9%	0.91 [0.75, 1.10]
ONWARDS 1	283	492	223	492	22.2%	1.27 [1.12, 1.44]
ONWARDS 3	167	294	122	294	20.6%	1.37 [1.16, 1.62]
ONWARDS 2	105	263	68	263	17.4%	1.54 [1.20, 1.99]
Total (95% CI)		1630		1632	100.0%	1.16 [0.95, 1.42]
Total events	791		677			

Heterogeneity: Tau² = 0.04; Chi² = 25.05, df = 4 (P < 0.0001); I² = 84%
Test for overall effect: Z = 1.49 (P = 0.14)

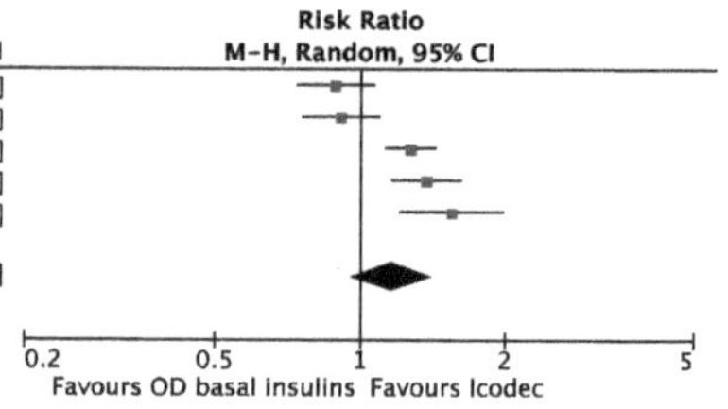

Abbreviations: ERR, Estimated Risk Ratio; OD, Once-Daily.

Figure 4. Forest plot of meta-analysis for probability (ERR) to achieve optimal glucose control (i.e., HbA1c < 7%) from baseline to 12 weeks (intention-to-treat analysis).

Patients randomized to Icodec, compared to those randomized to once-daily basal analogs, had a statistically significant 17% greater chance to achieve optimal glucose control without clinically relevant or severe hypoglycemia (i.e., HbA1c < 7%, without level 2 or 3 hypos) over 12 weeks from randomization (ERR of 1.17 [95%CI 1.01; 1.36], $p = 0.03$, and I^2 66%) (Figure 5).

Study or Subgroup	Icodec Events	Icodec Total	Once-daily basal insulin Events	Once-daily basal insulin Total	Weight	Risk Ratio M-H, Random, 95% CI
ONWARDS 6	28	290	49	292	8.0%	0.58 [0.37, 0.89]
ONWARDS 4	76	291	73	291	13.9%	1.04 [0.79, 1.37]
ONWARDS 1	259	492	210	492	22.5%	1.23 [1.08, 1.41]
ONWARDS 5	222	542	174	543	20.9%	1.28 [1.09, 1.50]
ONWARDS 3	153	294	117	294	19.6%	1.31 [1.09, 1.56]
ONWARDS 2	97	263	71	263	15.1%	1.37 [1.06, 1.76]
Total (95% CI)		2172		2175	100.0%	1.17 [1.01, 1.36]
Total events	835		694			

Heterogeneity: Tau² = 0.02; Chi² = 14.57, df = 5 (P = 0.01); I² = 66%
Test for overall effect: Z = 2.13 (P = 0.03)

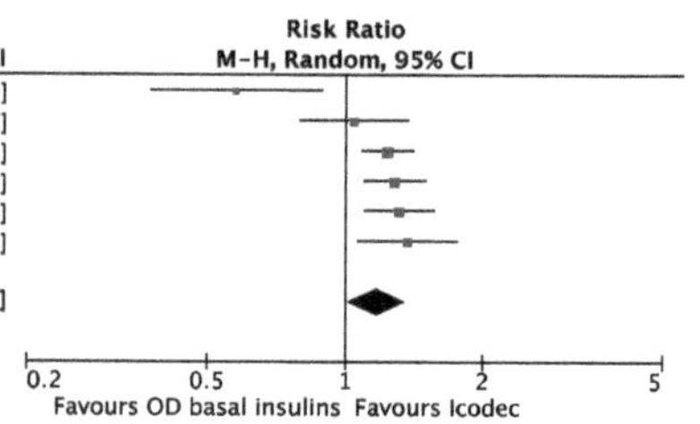

Abbreviations: ERR, Estimated Risk Ratio; OD, Once-Daily.

Figure 5. Forest plot of meta-analysis for probability (ERR) to achieve optimal glucose control (i.e., HbA1c < 7%) without clinically relevant (level 2) or severe (level 3) hypoglycemic events from baseline to 12 weeks (intention-to-treat analysis).

The baseline-weighted mean FPG from the ONWARDS clinical program was 174.7 mg/dL. ETD between Icodec and once-daily basal insulin doses was 2.44 mg/dL in favor of once-daily basal insulins, but this result was not statistically significant [95%CI −2.95; 7.82], I^2 70% (Supplementary Material, Figure S3).

Data from CGMs indicated that TIR was slightly higher with Icodec than once-daily basal insulins with an ETD of 1.64% (around 23 min/day), which was not statistically significant with 95%IC [−1.65; 4.93] and I^2 79%. At the same time, the ETD in TAR between patients on Icodec compared to those on once-daily basal insulins was −2.34% [95%CI

−5.51; 0.83], and I^2 76%, parallel to a non-statistically significant lower exposure to potentially dangerous hyperglycemia (≥180 mg/dL) at around 35 min/day (Supplementary Material, Figures S4 and S5).

The baseline-weighted mean body weight from the ONWARDS clinical program was 85.8 kg. Treatment with basal insulin analogs increased body weight; however, Icodec, compared to once-daily insulins, induced a slight but statistically significant weight gain of 0.62 kg [95%CI 0.25; 0.99], $p = 0.001$, and I^2 25% (Figure 6).

	Icodec			Once-daily basal insulin				Mean Difference
Study or Subgroup	Mean	SD	Total	Mean	SD	Total	Weight	IV, Random, 95% CI
ONWARDS 6	1.29	3.9388	290	1.01	3.9388	292	22.2%	0.28 [−0.36, 0.92]
ONWARDS 1	2.29	4.6414	492	1.83	4.6414	492	25.2%	0.46 [−0.12, 1.04]
ONWARDS 3	2.8	4.2683	294	2.3	4.2683	294	20.0%	0.50 [−0.19, 1.19]
ONWARDS 4	2.7	5.1176	291	2.2	6.8235	291	11.7%	0.50 [−0.48, 1.48]
ONWARDS 5	2.28	10.079	542	1.45	10.079	542	8.3%	0.83 [−0.37, 2.03]
ONWARDS 2	1.4	5.4997	263	−0.3	5.4997	263	12.5%	1.70 [0.76, 2.64]
Total (95% CI)			**2172**			**2174**	**100.0%**	**0.62 [0.25, 0.99]**

Heterogeneity: Tau² = 0.05; Chi² = 6.70, df = 5 (P = 0.24); I² = 25%
Test for overall effect: Z = 3.28 (P = 0.001)

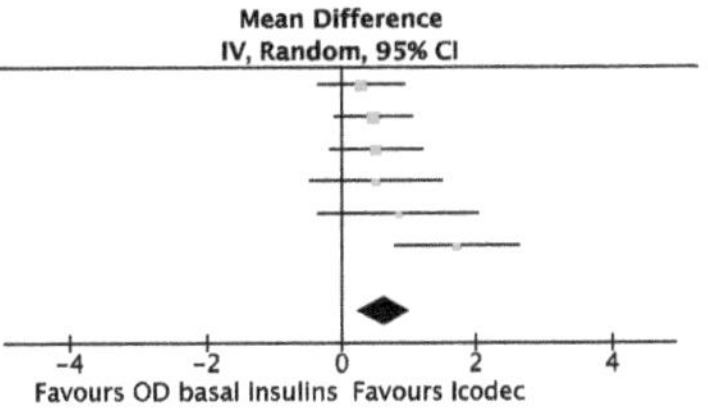

Abbreviations: ETD, Estimated Treatment Difference; OD, Once-Daily.

Figure 6. Forest plot of meta-analysis for mean change in body weight (ETD, kg) from baseline to study completion (intention-to-treat analysis).

The combined endpoint summarizing the risk of clinically relevant or severe hypoglycemic events (combined level 2 or level 3 hypoglycemia) revealed that a greater but not statistically significant number of patients randomized to Icodec than once-daily basal analogs had hypoglycemic events, with an ERR of 1.16 [95%CI 0.95; 1.41], I^2 75% (Figure 7).

	Icodec		Once-daily basal insulin			Risk Ratio
Study or Subgroup	Events	Total	Events	Total	Weight	M-H, Random, 95% CI
ONWARDS 1	48	492	52	492	14.1%	0.92 [0.64, 1.34]
ONWARDS 4	150	291	162	291	24.3%	0.93 [0.80, 1.08]
ONWARDS 6	282	290	223	292	27.5%	1.27 [1.19, 1.36]
ONWARDS 2	37	262	29	263	11.3%	1.28 [0.81, 2.02]
ONWARDS 5	64	542	45	538	14.5%	1.41 [0.98, 2.03]
ONWARDS 3	26	293	18	294	8.3%	1.45 [0.81, 2.59]
Total (95% CI)		**2170**		**2170**	**100.0%**	**1.16 [0.95, 1.41]**
Total events	607		529			

Heterogeneity: Tau² = 0.04; Chi² = 20.18, df = 5 (P = 0.001); I² = 75%
Test for overall effect: Z = 1.44 (P = 0.15)

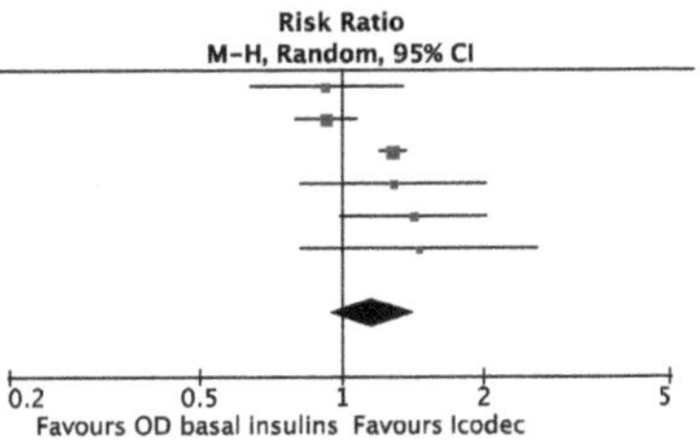

Abbreviations: ERR, Estimated Risk Ratio; OD, Once-Daily.

Figure 7. Forest plot of meta-analysis for probability (ERR, %) of experiencing clinically relevant (level 2) or severe (level 3) hypoglycemic events from baseline study completion (intention-to-treat analysis).

Adverse events, mostly mild-to-moderate, were reported in a more relevant number of participants randomized to Icodec than in once-daily basal analogs with an ERR of 1.04 [95%CI 1.00; 1.08], $p = 0.07$ and I^2 0%, indicating an almost statistically significant 4% increase in the overall risk of adverse events. However, only a minority of events was finally adjudicated as possibly or probably related to basal insulin use, with a non-statistically significant difference in specific endpoint, with an ERR of 1.22 [95%CI 0.99; 1.49], $p = 0.07$, and I^2 20% (Supplementary Material, Figures S6 and S7).

Serious adverse events were registered in a lower absolute number of patients randomized to Icodec than those given once-daily basal insulin doses with an ERR of 0.94 [95%CI 0.78; 1.13] and I^2 0%, which was not statistically relevant. Serious adverse events possibly or probably related to basal insulin use were reported in an equal number of patients randomized to Icodec rather than those given once-daily basal insulin doses with a non-significant ERR of 1.08 [95%CI 0.66; 1.76] and I^2 13% (Supplementary Material, Figures S8 and S9).

The number of patients who presented with injection-site reactions was similar between the two arms, with an ERR of 1.08 [95%CI 0.62; 1.90] and I^2 21% (Supplementary Material, Figure S10).

Exploring the Heterogeneity of the Results

The meta-analysis revealed substantial heterogeneity in the results from the RCTs of the ONWARDS clinical, especially among the efficacy endpoints, TAR, and the risk of combined level 2 or 3 hypoglycemia. The leading causes of heterogeneity were explored across several factors, including baseline demographics, glucose control, insulin-naïve vs. insulin-treated patients, the type of once-daily basal insulin used as a comparator to Icodec, the concomitant use of sulfonylureas or glinides during the trials, the basal-bolus vs. basal only regimen, and the risk of bias (low vs. moderate risk).

Subgroup analyses revealed that heterogenicity disappeared when grouping the results of trials according to the type of intervention. More precisely, the efficacy and safety of Icodec were examined by considering how it worked in the context of a basal only rather than in a basal-bolus regimen. When used in the context of the basal-only regimen, Icodec obtained better results in terms of glucose control (ETD in HbA1c of −0.22%), probability to achieve glucose control (+33%) and glucose control without clinically relevant or severe hypoglycemia (+28%), with more time spent in target (+4.55%, around 65 min/day) and less time spent in hyperglycemia (−5.14%, 74 min/day) (Table 3).

Table 3. Subgroup analyses exploring the heterogeneity of results in efficacy and safety from the ONWARDS clinical program.

Main Outcomes with Significant Heterogenicity (I^2 >60%)	Icodec in the Context of Basal Regimen (Subgroup 1-ONWARDS 1, 2, 3, and 5)	Icodec in the Context of Basal-Bolus Regimen (Subgroup 2-ONWARDS 4 and 6)
ETD [95%CI], I^2 in HbA1c	**−0.22% [−0.29; −0.14], I^2 0% Favors Icodec**	0.03% [−0.08; 0.13], I^2 0%
ERR [95%CI], I^2 in probability to achieve HbA1c < 7% *	**1.33 [1.21; 1.47], I^2 2% Favors Icodec**	0.90 [0.79; 1.02], I^2 0%
ERR [95%CI], I^2 in probability to achieve HbA1c < 7% without experiencing clinically relevant or severe hypoglycemia	**1.28 [1.17; 1.39], I^2 0% Favors Icodec**	0.79 [0.44; 1.42], I^2 81%
ETD [95%CI], I^2 in TIR **	**4.55% [2.01; 7.08], I^2 0% Favors Icodec**	−0.88% [−2.97; 1.20], I^2 28%
ETD [95%CI], I^2 in FPG ***	0.1 mg/dL [−3.01; 3.20], I^2 0%	8.05 mg/dL [−12.99; 29], I^2 91%
ETD [95%CI], I^2 in TAR **	**−5.14% [−7.27; −3.01], I^2 0% Favors Icodec**	0.07% [−2; 2.15], I^2 0%
ERR [95%CI], I^2 in the probability of experiencing combined level 2 or 3 hypoglycemic events ****	1.12 [0.98; 1.15], I^2 0%	1.09 [0.76; 1.57], I^2 95%

* Subgroup 1-ONWARDS 1, 2, and 3; Subgroup 2-ONWARDS 4 and 6. ** GCM data were available only from ONWARDS 1, 2, 4, and 6. Subgroup 1—ONWARDS 1 and 2; Subgroup 2—ONWARDS 4 and 6. *** FPG not assessed or reported in ONWARDS 5. Subgroup 1-ONWARDS 1, 2, and 3; Subgroup 2-ONWARDS 4 and 6. Substantial variability is attributable to the results of the ONWARDS 6 only. **** Substantial variability attributable to the results of the ONWARDS 6 only. Statistically significant differences are in bold. Abbreviations: Estimated Risk Ratio, ERR; Estimate Treatment Difference, ETD.

The combined risk of experiencing level 2 or 3 hypoglycemia was statistically significant in ONWARDS 6 but not in ONWARDS 4. Patients were treated with basal-bolus regimens in both trials, but only patients with T1D had a statistically significant increase in the risk of combined level 2 or 3 hypoglycemia. Moreover, the risk of clinically relevant or severe hypoglycemic events was significantly higher when background glinides and sulfonylureas were included as an add-on to basal analogs (ONWARDS 3 and 5) with an ERR of 1.42 [95%CI 1.05; 1.93], and I^2 0%.

4. Discussion

The results of this systematic review and meta-analysis provide an update on Insulin Icodec in both T1D and T2D beyond previously published results [44–47]. So far, insulin Icodec has been demonstrated to be slightly better than daily administered basal analogs in terms of glucose control and the chance to achieve targeted glucose levels without a relevant gain in the risk of hypoglycemia in T2D. Specific comparisons between Icodec and either Glargine U100 or Degludec U100 showed that Icodec was slightly superior to Degludec U100 and equal to Glargine U100 in improving glucose control. At the same time, Icodec, compared to Degludec U100, increased the risk of any hypoglycemic events with moderate-to-substantial heterogenicity of the results [48].

Icodec was found to perform equally in insulin-naïve and insulin-treated T2D individuals, indicating that baseline antihyperglycemic treatment does not affect the clinical response to Icodec when stated de novo or switched from another basal analog [49].

Our data indicate that Icodec is effective in reducing HbA1c levels starting from 26 and up to 78 weeks of treatment. Compared to once-daily basal insulins, namely Glargine U100, Glargine U300, and Degludec U100, Icodec provide a statistically significant absolute mean change in HbA1c of −0.14%. Moreover, we found that Icodec, compared to once-daily basal insulins, increases the probability of achieving adequate glucose control (i.e., HbA1c < 7%) safely without level 2 or 3 hypoglycemic events by 17%. The therapeutic targets can be obtained after 12 weeks of treatment, which means just in time or soon before the second check of HbA1c levels after therapy adjustment.

Overall, the above-mentioned glycemic benefits did not translate into relevant changes in TIR registered by a CGM system during the last four weeks of the trials. No difference in FPG was also reported, probably because of the rigorous treat-to-target approach that investigators used in all trials. No data on FPG were assessed or reported in ONWARDS 5, which is a trial in which different methods of titration were applied to the two study groups. Patients randomized to insulin Icodec were guided by an app-based algorithmic tool to titrate basal insulin weekly, while patients randomized to once-daily basal insulins received instruction directly from investigators as per standard practice. It is unclear and complicated to predict how missing data could have influenced the cumulative weight of the FPG endpoint in our meta-analysis.

Most patients experienced slight weight gain during the trials, estimated at 2 kg as a mean. Icodec was responsible for an additional weight gain of 0.62 kg over once-daily basal analogs. This effect could be attributable to a slightly higher weekly dose of Icodec than basal analogs in all trials.

The number of patients experiencing hypoglycemic events was similar for Icodec and once-daily basal insulin doses in T2D [50] but not T1D (ONWARDS 6), where Icodec was associated with a statistically significant higher risk of clinically relevant or severe hypoglycemic events. This result cannot be explained entirely by the concomitant administration of a prandial analog in the context of a basal-bolus regimen since the risk of level 2 or 3 hypos was not increased in T2D (ONWARDS 4). The main explanation is the specific effect of Icodec on glucose variability in T1D and requires more investigation [51]. The combined risk of clinically relevant or severe hypoglycemic events was also higher among patients on Icodec than once-daily basal analogs in trials where sulfonylureas and glinides were not discontinued (ONWARDS 3 and 5). Although the pretrial dose of secretagogues was halved during both trials, the combination of sulfonylureas and glinides with Icodec resulted in a 42% increase in the risk of potentially dangerous hypoglycemic events. Therefore, this specific association should be avoided in clinical practice.

Safety endpoints were similar between Icodec and once-daily basal analogs. The overall risk of any adverse events was not statistically significant, and it was mitigated by the systematic revision of any signs and symptoms potentially related to insulin use (possibly or probably).

Injection-site reactions, as well as serious adverse events, were infrequent and statistically similar between the two groups.

Last, insulin Icodec works better when used in a basal regimen only rather than in the context of a basal-bolus regimen, resulting in a greater ETD in HbA1c (−0.22%), with a higher chance of achieving HbA1c < 7% (+33%) and HbA1c < 7% without clinically relevant or severe hypoglycemia (+28%), and a higher TIR (around 65 min/day) and lower

TAR (−74 min/day) compared to once-daily basal analogs. These results were statistically relevant and occurred independently of pretrial treatments (both insulin and non-insulin agents) but could be attributable to a poorer baseline glucose control and lower duration of diabetes (ONWARDS 1, 2, 3, and 5).

5. Study Limitations

The leading limitation of the ONWARDS program trials is the sample size, which is adequate for the primary outcome (changes in HbA1c) only but does not allow subgroup analyses that are desirable for this kind of trials.

Second, most relevant safety outcomes, such as the estimation of hypoglycemic risk, were not included in the prespecified analyses and were calculated post hoc, thus potentially reducing the level of evidence of this relevant outcome.

Third, data from real-time glucose monitoring were scarce. CGM data were available only in four trials, but only in one (ONWARDS 6, in T1D) were data registered and analyzed during the entire study period. Consequently, information on glucose variability, daytime, and nocturnal hypoglycemic risk were limited and required to be better analyzed with additional trials.

6. Conclusions

Insulin Icodec, the first approved once-weekly insulin analog, provides evidence of substantial non-inferiority compared to once-daily basal analogs in diabetes management in both insulin-naïve and insulin-treated patients who failed to achieve adequate glucose control. Icodec works slightly better than once-daily basal analogs in T2D individuals, especially when used in the context of basal-only rather than a basal-bolus regimen.

Weight gain is highly predictable after insulin initiation, and Icodec confirms this well-known trend. Providing patients with effective non-pharmacological and pharmacological intervention is reasonable to avoid weight gain or promote weight loss when necessary.

Specific trials are expected to address the impact of Icodec on glycemic variability in individuals with T1D. Moreover, other trials are needed to comprehensively evaluate the best clinical scenario in which insulin Icodec can be cost-effective compared to once-daily insulin analogs.

Supplementary Materials: The following supporting information can be downloaded at: https://www.mdpi.com/article/10.3390/biomedicines12081852/s1, Figure S1. PRISMA 2020 flow diagram for the systematic review; Figure S2. Funnel plot for the estimation of publication bias; Figure S3. Forest plot of meta-analysis for mean change in fasting plasma glucose levels (ETD, mg/dL) from baseline to study completion (intention-to-treat analysis); Figure S4. Forest plot of meta-analysis for mean change in time in range (ETD, %) throughout the last 4 weeks of trials (intention-to-treat analysis); Figure S5. Forest plot of meta-analysis for mean change in time above range (ETD, %) throughout the last 4 weeks of trials (intention-to-treat analysis); Figure S6. Forest plot of meta-analysis for probability of experiencing any adverse event (ERR, %) from baseline to study completion; Figure S7. Forest plot of meta-analysis for probability of experiencing any adverse event (ERR, %) probably or possibly related to insulin use from baseline to study completion; Figure S8. Forest plot of meta-analysis for probability of experiencing serious adverse event (ERR, %) from baseline to study completion; Figure S9. Forest plot of meta-analysis for probability of experiencing serious adverse event (ERR, %) probably or possibly related to insulin use from baseline to study completion; Figure S10. Forest plot of meta-analysis for probability of experiencing injection-site reaction (ERR, %) from baseline to study completion.

Author Contributions: G.L. and A.D.T.: conceptualization, database search, data collection, drafting original paper, review, correction, and visualization. O.E.D., V.T. and E.G.: conceptualization, validation, review, and correction. V.D.G., V.A.G. and G.P.: validation, review, and visualization. All authors have read and agreed to the published version of the manuscript.

Funding: This research received no external funding.

Data Availability Statement: Data supporting the findings of this systematic review and meta-analysis are available from the first, last, or corresponding author on reasonable request.

Conflicts of Interest: The authors declare that the research was conducted in the absence of commercial or financial relationships that could be interpreted as potential conflicts of interest.

Abbreviations

CGM	Continuous glucose monitoring
CI	Confidence interval
ERR	Estimated risk ratio
ETD	Estimated treatment difference
FPG	Fasting plasma glucose
GLP-1RA	Glucagon-like peptide 1 receptor agonists
HbA1c	Glycated hemoglobin
MDI	Multiple daily injections
RCT	Randomized clinical trial
T1D	Type 1 diabetes
T2D	Type 2 diabetes
TAR	Time above range
TIR	Time in range

References

1. Jörgens, V.; Porta, M. Unveiling Diabetes—Historical Milestones in Diabetology. In *Frontiers in Diabetes*; Karger: Basel, Switzerland, 2020; 25p. [CrossRef]
2. Banting, F.G.; Best, C.H.; Collip, J.B.; Campbell, W.R.; Fletcher, A.A. Pancreatic Extracts in the Treatment of Diabetes Mellitus. *Can. Med. Assoc. J.* **1922**, *12*, 141–146. [PubMed]
3. Bliss, M. The history of insulin. *Diabetes Care* **1993**, *16*, 4–7. [CrossRef] [PubMed]
4. Stretton, A.O. The first sequence—Fred Sanger and insulin. *Genetics* **2002**, *162*, 527–532. [CrossRef] [PubMed]
5. Quianzon, C.C.; Cheikh, I. History of insulin. *J. Community Hosp. Intern. Med. Perspect.* **2012**, *2*, 18701. [CrossRef] [PubMed]
6. Goeddel, D.V.; Kleid, D.G.; Bolivar, F.; Heyneker, H.L.; Yansura, D.G.; Crea, R.; Hirose, T.; Kraszewski, A.; Itakura, K.; Riggs, A.D. Expression in *Escherichia coli* of chemically synthesized genes for human insulin. *Proc. Natl. Acad. Sci. USA* **1979**, *76*, 106–110. [CrossRef] [PubMed]
7. Iyer, G.; Dyawanapelly, S.; Jain, R.; Dandekar, P. An overview of oral insulin delivery strategies (OIDS). *Int. J. Biol. Macromol.* **2022**, *208*, 565–585. [CrossRef] [PubMed]
8. Primavera, R.; Kevadiya, B.D.; Swaminathan, G.; Wilson, R.J.; De Pascale, A.; Decuzzi, P.; Thakor, A.S. Emerging Nano- and Micro-Technologies Used in the Treatment of Type-1 Diabetes. *Nanomaterials* **2020**, *10*, 789. [CrossRef] [PubMed]
9. Jarosinski, M.A.; Dhayalan, B.; Rege, N.; Chatterjee, D.; Weiss, M.A. 'Smart' insulin-delivery technologies and intrinsic glucose-responsive insulin analogues. *Diabetologia* **2021**, *64*, 1016–1029. [CrossRef] [PubMed]
10. Sun, H.; Saeedi, P.; Karuranga, S.; Pinkepank, M.; Ogurtsova, K.; Duncan, B.B.; Stein, C.; Basit, A.; Chan, J.C.N.; Mbanya, J.C.; et al. IDF Diabetes Atlas: Global, regional and country-level diabetes prevalence estimates for 2021 and projections for 2045. *Diabetes Res. Clin. Pract.* **2022**, *183*, 109119, Erratum in *Diabetes Res. Clin. Pract.* **2023**, *204*, 110945. [CrossRef] [PubMed]
11. Park, J.; Kim, G.; Kim, B.S.; Han, K.D.; Kwon, S.Y.; Park, S.H.; Lee, Y.B.; Jin, S.M.; Kim, J.H. Insulin Fact Sheet in Type 1 and 2 Diabetes Mellitus and Trends of Antidiabetic Medication Use in Insulin Users with Type 2 Diabetes Mellitus: 2002 to 2019. *Diabetes Metab. J.* **2023**, *47*, 211–219. [CrossRef]
12. Pitak, P.; Tasai, S.; Kumpat, N.; Na Songkla, P.; Fuangchan, A.; Krass, I.; Dhippayom, T. The prevalence of glycemic control in patients with type 2 diabetes treated with insulin: A systematic review and meta-analysis. *Public Health* **2023**, *225*, 218–228. [CrossRef] [PubMed]
13. Blonde, L.; Aschner, P.; Bailey, C.; Ji, L.; Leiter, L.A.; Matthaei, S.; Global Partnership for Effective Diabetes Management. Gaps and barriers in the control of blood glucose in people with type 2 diabetes. *Diabetes Vasc. Dis. Res.* **2017**, *14*, 172–183. [CrossRef] [PubMed]
14. Rubino, D.M.; Greenway, F.L.; Khalid, U.; O'Neil, P.M.; Rosenstock, J.; Sørrig, R.; Wadden, T.A.; Wizert, A.; Garvey, W.T.; STEP 8 Investigators. Effect of Weekly Subcutaneous Semaglutide vs. Daily Liraglutide on Body Weight in Adults with Overweight or Obesity without Diabetes: The STEP 8 Randomized Clinical Trial. *JAMA* **2022**, *327*, 138–150. [CrossRef] [PubMed]
15. Dungan, K.M.; Povedano, S.T.; Forst, T.; González, J.G.; Atisso, C.; Sealls, W.; Fahrbach, J.L. Once-weekly dulaglutide vs. once-daily liraglutide in metformin-treated patients with type 2 diabetes (AWARD-6): A randomised, open-label, phase 3, non-inferiority trial. *Lancet* **2014**, *384*, 1349–1357, Erratum in *Lancet* **2014**, *384*, 1348. [CrossRef] [PubMed]
16. Philis-Tsimikas, A.; Wysham, C.H.; Hardy, E.; Han, J.; Iqbal, N. Efficacy and tolerability of exenatide once weekly over 7 years in patients with type 2 diabetes: An open-label extension of the DURATION-1 study. *J. Diabetes Complicat.* **2019**, *33*, 223–230. [CrossRef] [PubMed]

17. Lisco, G.; Disoteo, O.E.; De Geronimo, V.; De Tullio, A.; Giagulli, V.A.; Guastamacchia, E.; De Pergola, G.; Jirillo, E.; Triggiani, V. Is Tirzepatide the New Game Changer in Type 2 Diabetes? *Endocrines* **2024**, *5*, 72–86. [CrossRef]
18. Blair, H.A. Insulin Icodec: First Approval. *BioDrugs* **2024**, *38*, 1–8. [CrossRef] [PubMed]
19. Plum-Mörschel, L.; Andersen, L.R.; Hansen, S.; Hövelmann, U.; Krawietz, P.; Kristensen, N.R.; Lehrskov, L.L.; Haahr, H. Pharmacokinetic and Pharmacodynamic Characteristics of Insulin Icodec After Subcutaneous Administration in the Thigh, Abdomen or Upper Arm in Individuals with Type 2 Diabetes Mellitus. *Clin. Drug Investig.* **2023**, *43*, 119–127. [CrossRef] [PubMed]
20. Available online: https://www.novonordisk.ca/content/dam/nncorp/ca/en/products/awiqli-en-consumer-information-12-march-2024.pdf (accessed on 7 July 2024).
21. Kalra, S.; Bhattacharya, S.; Kapoor, N. Counseling for Insulin Icodec: A Proposed Practitioner's Guide. *Diabetes Ther.* **2024**, *15*, 1491–1499. [CrossRef] [PubMed]
22. Haahr, H.; Cieslarová, B.; Hingst, J.R.; Jiang, S.; Kristensen, N.R.; Kupčová, V.; Nørgreen, L.; Wagner, F.H.; Ignatenko, S. The Effect of Various Degrees of Renal or Hepatic Impairment on the Pharmacokinetic Properties of Once-weekly Insulin Icodec. *Clin. Pharmacokinet.* **2024**, *63*, 819–830. [CrossRef] [PubMed]
23. Hubálek, F.; Refsgaard, H.H.F.; Gram-Nielsen, S.; Madsen, P.; Nishimura, E.; Münzel, M.; Brand, C.L.; Stidsen, C.E.; Claussen, C.H.; Wulff, E.M.; et al. Molecular engineering of safe and efficacious oral basal insulin. *Nat. Commun.* **2020**, *11*, 3746, Erratum in *Nat. Commun.* **2020**, *11*, 4232. [CrossRef] [PubMed]
24. Kjeldsen, T.B.; Hubálek, F.; Hjørringgaard, C.U.; Tagmose, T.M.; Nishimura, E.; Stidsen, C.E.; Porsgaard, T.; Fledelius, C.; Refsgaard, H.H.F.; Gram-Nielsen, S.; et al. Molecular Engineering of Insulin Icodec, the First Acylated Insulin Analog for Once-weekly Administration in Humans. *J. Med. Chem.* **2021**, *64*, 8942–8950. [CrossRef] [PubMed]
25. Nishimura, E.; Pridal, L.; Glendorf, T.; Hansen, B.F.; Hubálek, F.; Kjeldsen, T.; Kristensen, N.R.; Lützen, A.; Lyby, K.; Madsen, P.; et al. Molecular and pharmacological characterization of insulin icodec: A new basal insulin analog designed for Once-weekly dosing. *BMJ Open Diabetes Res. Care* **2021**, *9*, e002301. [CrossRef] [PubMed]
26. Moyers, J.S.; Hansen, R.J.; Day, J.W.; Dickinson, C.D.; Zhang, C.; Ruan, X.; Ding, L.; Brown, R.M.; Baker, H.E.; Beals, J.M. Preclinical Characterization of LY3209590, a Novel Weekly Basal Insulin Fc-Fusion Protein. *J. Pharmacol. Exp. Ther.* **2022**, *382*, 346–355. [CrossRef] [PubMed]
27. Kazda, C.M.; Bue-Valleskey, J.M.; Chien, J.; Zhang, Q.; Chigutsa, E.; Landschulz, W.; Wullenweber, P.; Haupt, A.; Dahl, D. Novel Once-weekly Basal Insulin Fc Achieved Similar Glycemic Control with a Safety Profile Comparable to Insulin Degludec in Patients With Type 1 Diabetes. *Diabetes Care* **2023**, *46*, 1052–1059. [CrossRef]
28. Bue-Valleskey, J.M.; Kazda, C.M.; Ma, C.; Chien, J.; Zhang, Q.; Chigutsa, E.; Landschulz, W.; Haupt, A.; Frias, J.P. Once-weekly Basal Insulin Fc Demonstrated Similar Glycemic Control to Once-Daily Insulin Degludec in Insulin-Naive Patients with Type 2 Diabetes: A Phase 2 Randomized Control Trial. *Diabetes Care* **2023**, *46*, 1060–1067. [CrossRef] [PubMed]
29. Frias, J.; Chien, J.; Zhang, Q.; Chigutsa, E.; Landschulz, W.; Syring, K.; Wullenweber, P.; Haupt, A.; Kazda, C. Safety and efficacy of Once-weekly basal insulin Fc in people with type 2 diabetes previously treated with basal insulin: A multicentre, open-label, randomised, phase 2 study. *Lancet Diabetes Endocrinol.* **2023**, *11*, 158–168. [CrossRef] [PubMed]
30. Bergenstal, R.M.; Philis-Tsimikas, A.; Wysham, C.; Carr, M.C.; Bue-Valleskey, J.M.; Botros, F.T.; Blevins, T.; Rosenstock, J. Once-weekly insulin efsitora alfa: Design and rationale for the QWINT phase 3 clinical development programme. *Diabetes Obes. Metab.* **2024**, *26*, 3020–3030. [CrossRef] [PubMed]
31. Rosenstock, J.; Bajaj, H.S.; Janež, A.; Silver, R.; Begtrup, K.; Hansen, M.V.; Jia, T.; Goldenberg, R.; NN1436-4383 Investigators. Once-weekly Insulin for Type 2 Diabetes without Previous Insulin Treatment. *N. Engl. J. Med.* **2020**, *383*, 2107–2116. [CrossRef]
32. Lingvay, I.; Buse, J.B.; Franek, E.; Hansen, M.V.; Koefoed, M.M.; Mathieu, C.; Pettus, J.; Stachlewska, K.; Rosenstock, J. A Randomized, Open-Label Comparison of Once-weekly Insulin Icodec Titration Strategies vs. Once-Daily Insulin Glargine U100. *Diabetes Care* **2021**, *44*, 1595–1603. [CrossRef] [PubMed]
33. Bajaj, H.S.; Bergenstal, R.M.; Christoffersen, A.; Davies, M.J.; Gowda, A.; Isendahl, J.; Lingvay, I.; Senior, P.A.; Silver, R.J.; Trevisan, R.; et al. Switching to Once-weekly Insulin Icodec vs. Once-Daily Insulin Glargine U100 in Type 2 Diabetes Inadequately Controlled on Daily Basal Insulin: A Phase 2 Randomized Controlled Trial. *Diabetes Care* **2021**, *44*, 1586–1594. [CrossRef] [PubMed]
34. Rosenstock, J.; Bain, S.C.; Gowda, A.; Jódar, E.; Liang, B.; Lingvay, I.; Nishida, T.; Trevisan, R.; Mosenzon, O.; ONWARDS 1 Trial Investigators. Weekly Icodec vs. Daily Glargine U100 in Type 2 Diabetes without Previous Insulin. *N. Engl. J. Med.* **2023**, *389*, 297–308. [CrossRef] [PubMed]
35. Philis-Tsimikas, A.; Asong, M.; Franek, E.; Jia, T.; Rosenstock, J.; Stachlewska, K.; Watada, H.; Kellerer, M. Switching to Once-weekly insulin icodec vs. once-daily insulin degludec in individuals with basal insulin-treated type 2 diabetes (ONWARDS 2): A phase 3a, randomised, open label, multicentre, treat-to-target trial. *Lancet Diabetes Endocrinol.* **2023**, *11*, 414–425, Erratum in *Lancet Diabetes Endocrinol.* **2023**, *11*, e9. [CrossRef] [PubMed]
36. Lingvay, I.; Asong, M.; Desouza, C.; Gourdy, P.; Kar, S.; Vianna, A.; Vilsbøll, T.; Vinther, S.; Mu, Y. Once-weekly Insulin Icodec vs Once-Daily Insulin Degludec in Adults with Insulin-Naive Type 2 Diabetes: The ONWARDS 3 Randomized Clinical Trial. *JAMA* **2023**, *330*, 228–237. [CrossRef] [PubMed]

37. Mathieu, C.; Ásbjörnsdóttir, B.; Bajaj, H.S.; Lane, W.; Matos, A.L.S.A.; Murthy, S.; Stachlewska, K.; Rosenstock, J. Switching to Once-weekly insulin icodec vs. once-daily insulin glargine U100 in individuals with basal-bolus insulin-treated type 2 diabetes (ONWARDS 4): A phase 3a, randomised, open-label, multicentre, treat-to-target, non-inferiority trial. *Lancet* **2023**, *401*, 1929–1940. [CrossRef] [PubMed]
38. Bajaj, H.S.; Aberle, J.; Davies, M.; Donatsky, A.M.; Frederiksen, M.; Yavuz, D.G.; Gowda, A.; Lingvay, I.; Bode, B. Once-weekly Insulin Icodec with Dosing Guide App vs. Once-Daily Basal Insulin Analogues in Insulin-Naive Type 2 Diabetes (ONWARDS 5): A Randomized Trial. *Ann. Intern. Med.* **2023**, *176*, 1476–1485; Erratum in *Ann. Intern. Med.* **2023**, *176*, 1688. [CrossRef] [PubMed]
39. Russell-Jones, D.; Babazono, T.; Cailleteau, R.; Engberg, S.; Irace, C.; Kjaersgaard, M.I.S.; Mathieu, C.; Rosenstock, J.; Woo, V.; Klonoff, D.C. Once-weekly insulin icodec vs. once-daily insulin degludec as part of a basal-bolus regimen in individuals with type 1 diabetes (ONWARDS 6): A phase 3a, randomised, open-label, treat-to-target trial. *Lancet* **2023**, *402*, 1636–1647. [CrossRef] [PubMed]
40. Philis-Tsimikas, A.; Bajaj, H.S.; Begtrup, K.; Cailleteau, R.; Gowda, A.; Lingvay, I.; Mathieu, C.; Russell-Jones, D.; Rosenstock, J. Rationale and design of the phase 3a development programme (ONWARDS 1-6 trials) investigating Once-weekly insulin icodec in diabetes. *Diabetes Obes. Metab.* **2023**, *25*, 331–341. [CrossRef] [PubMed]
41. Agiostratidou, G.; Anhalt, H.; Ball, D.; Blonde, L.; Gourgari, E.; Harriman, K.N.; Kowalski, A.J.; Madden, P.; McAuliffe-Fogarty, A.H.; McElwee-Malloy, M.; et al. Standardizing Clinically Meaningful Outcome Measures beyond HbA1c for Type 1 Diabetes: A Consensus Report of the American Association of Clinical Endocrinologists, the American Association of Diabetes Educators, the American Diabetes Association, the Endocrine Society, JDRF International, The Leona M. and Harry B. Helmsley Charitable Trust, the Pediatric Endocrine Society, and the T1D Exchange. *Diabetes Care* **2017**, *40*, 1622–1630. [CrossRef] [PubMed]
42. Sterne, J.A.C.; Savović, J.; Page, M.J.; Elbers, R.G.; Blencowe, N.S.; Boutron, I.; Cates, C.J.; Cheng, H.Y.; Corbett, M.S.; Eldridge, S.M.; et al. RoB 2: A revised tool for assessing risk of bias in randomised trials. *BMJ* **2019**, *366*, l4898. [CrossRef] [PubMed]
43. Higgins, J.P.; Thompson, S.G. Quantifying heterogeneity in a meta-analysis. *Stat. Med.* **2002**, *21*, 1539–1558. [CrossRef] [PubMed]
44. Karakasis, P.; Patoulias, D.; Pamporis, K.; Popovic, D.S.; Stachteas, P.; Bougioukas, K.I.; Fragakis, N.; Rizzo, M. Efficacy and safety of Once-weekly vs. once-daily basal insulin analogues in the treatment of type 2 diabetes mellitus: A systematic review and meta-analysis. *Diabetes Obes. Metab.* **2023**, *25*, 3648–3661. [CrossRef] [PubMed]
45. Ribeiro ESilva, R.; de Miranda Gauza, M.; Guisso, M.E.S.; da Silva, J.O.N.; Kohara, S.K. Once-weekly Insulin Icodec vs. Once-Daily Insulin Glargine U100 for type 2 diabetes: A systematic review and meta-analysis of phase 2 randomized controlled trials. *Arch. Endocrinol. Metab.* **2023**, *67*, e000614. [CrossRef]
46. Dutta, D.; Nagendra, L.; Bhat, S.; Mohindra, R.; Surana, V.; Misra, A. Optimal use of once weekly icodec insulin in type-2 diabetes: An updated meta-analysis of phase-2 and phase-3 randomized controlled trials. *Diabetes Metab. Syndr.* **2023**, *17*, 102877. [CrossRef] [PubMed]
47. Wang, X.; Xiao, W.; Liang, Z.; Li, S.; Tang, Q. Efficacy and safety of Once-weekly basal insulin vs. once-daily basal insulin in patients with type 2 diabetes: A systematic review and meta-analysis. *Medicine* **2023**, *102*, e36308. [CrossRef] [PubMed]
48. Shetty, S.; Suvarna, R. Efficacy and safety of Once-weekly insulin icodec in type 2 diabetes: A meta-analysis of ONWARDS phase 3 randomized controlled trials. *Diabetes Obes. Metab.* **2024**, *26*, 1069–1081. [CrossRef] [PubMed]
49. Ahmed, M.; Shafiq, A.; Javaid, H.; Jain, H.; Nashwan, A.J.; Tul-Ain, Q.; Basit, J. Clinical Outcomes with Once-weekly Insulin Icodec vs. Once-Daily Insulin Glargine U100 in Insulin-Naïve and Previously Insulin-Treated Individuals with Type 2 Diabetes: A Meta-Analysis of Randomised Controlled Trials. *Endocrinol. Diabetes Metab.* **2024**, *7*, e00480. [CrossRef] [PubMed]
50. Bajaj, H.S.; Ásbjörnsdóttir, B.; Bari, T.J.; Begtrup, K.; Vilsbøll, T.; Rosenstock, J. Once-weekly insulin icodec compared with daily basal insulin analogues in type 2 diabetes: Participant-level meta-analysis of the ONWARDS 1-5 trials. *Diabetes Obes. Metab.* **2024**, *26*, 3810–3820. [CrossRef] [PubMed]
51. Hövelmann, U.; Engberg, S.; Heise, T.; Kristensen, N.R.; Nørgreen, L.; Zijlstra, E.; Ribel-Madsen, R. Pharmacokinetic and pharmacodynamic properties of Once-weekly insulin icodec in individuals with type 1 diabetes. *Diabetes Obes. Metab.* **2024**, *26*, 1941–1949. [CrossRef] [PubMed]

MDPI AG
Grosspeteranlage 5
4052 Basel
Switzerland
Tel.: +41 61 683 77 34

Biomedicines Editorial Office
E-mail: biomedicines@mdpi.com
www.mdpi.com/journal/biomedicines

www.ingramcontent.com/pod-product-compliance
Lightning Source LLC
Chambersburg PA
CBHW061451210926
51850CB00008B/1681
* 9 7 8 3 7 2 5 8 7 3 0 8 1 *